UVEITIS MANAGEMENT

A Clinical Handbook

Other Titles by Susan Lightman

Immunology of Eye Diseases
Steroid Hormones and the T-Cell Cytokine Profile
Uveitis
Diabetes and the Eye
HIV and the Eye
Fundamentals of Clinical Ophthalmology (Series Editor)

UVEITIS MANAGEMENT
A Clinical Handbook

Editors

Oren Tomkins-Netzer
Carmel Medical Centre, Israel &
Technion-Israel Institute of Technology, Israel

Rachael Niederer
University of Auckland, New Zealand &
Auckland District Health Board, New Zealand

Susan Lightman
University College London, UK &
Moorfields Eye Hospital, UK

World Scientific

NEW JERSEY • LONDON • SINGAPORE • BEIJING • SHANGHAI • HONG KONG • TAIPEI • CHENNAI • TOKYO

Published by

World Scientific Publishing Co. Pte. Ltd.
5 Toh Tuck Link, Singapore 596224
USA office: 27 Warren Street, Suite 401-402, Hackensack, NJ 07601
UK office: 57 Shelton Street, Covent Garden, London WC2H 9HE

Library of Congress Cataloging-in-Publication Data
Names: Tomkins-Netzer, Oren, editor. | Niederer, Rachael, editor. | Lightman, Susan, editor.
Title: Uveitis management : a clinical handbook / editors, Oren Tomkins-Netzer, Rachael Niederer, Susan Lightman.
Description: New Jersey : World Scientific, [2023] | Includes bibliographical references and index.
Identifiers: LCCN 2022013672 | ISBN 9789811251467 (hardcover) | ISBN 9789811251474 (ebook) | ISBN 9789811251481 (ebook other)
Subjects: MESH: Uveitis--diagnosis | Uveitis--therapy
Classification: LCC RE351 | NLM WW 240 | DDC 617.7/2--dc23/eng/20220819
LC record available at https://lccn.loc.gov/2022013672

British Library Cataloguing-in-Publication Data
A catalogue record for this book is available from the British Library.

For any available supplementary material, please visit
https://www.worldscientific.com/worldscibooks/10.1142/12701#t=suppl

Desk Editor: Shaun Tan Yi Jie

Typeset by Stallion Press
Email: enquiries@stallionpress.com

https://doi.org/10.1142/9789811251474_fmatter

Preface

Welcome to this book, which is a very practical guide to the assessment and management of patients with uveitis. Good clinical examination is key from the start, so that the extent and type of the ocular problem is defined quickly. For each patient, thinking in terms of etiology of infection, inflammation or masquerade provides a framework for careful thinking and then further investigation and management. The layout is logical in its approach with excellent clinical illustrations from the practices of the authors, and the book can be read from front to back or in a clinical situation. Chapter 12 provides a rapid résumé of what to think about and do!

For trainees there is a useful list of key learning points at the end of each chapter. Appendix A gives you a list of the commonly used drugs and doses and Appendix B a list of frequently asked questions.

We hope this will provide you with the confidence to manage these patients who can be very frightening and can lose vision very quickly without proper management.

Wishing you all the very best from all of us.

Sue Lightman
Rachael Niederer
Oren Tomkins-Netzer

About the Editors

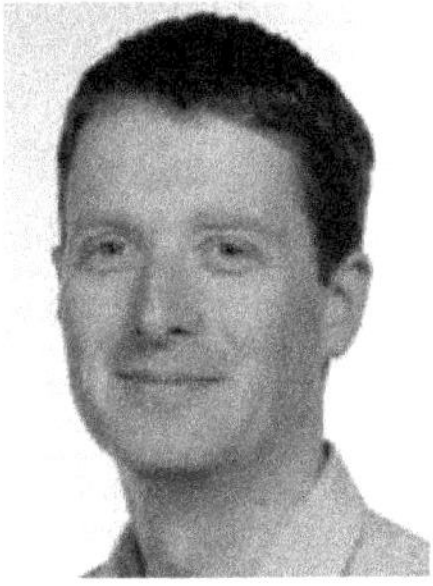

Professor Oren Tomkins-Netzer is Director of Ophthamology at Carmel Medical Centre, Israel and Associate Professor at Technion-Israel Institute of Technology, Israel where he specializes in Uveitis, and teaches courses in Ophthalmology and Practical Uveitis. He was previously Clinical Associate Professor at University College London, UK. He has published over 100 papers and book chapters, and is on several editorial boards.

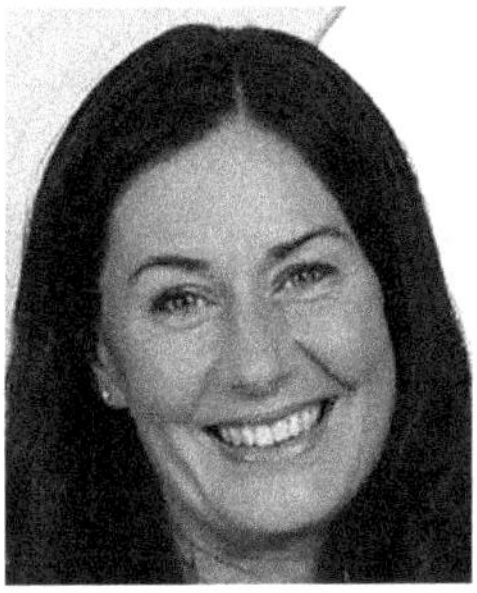

Dr. Rachael Niederer is Senior Lecturer at the Department of Ophthalmology in the University of Auckland, New Zealand, as well as Senior Medical Ophthalmologist specializing in Uveitis at Auckland District Health Board, where she runs the training programme for ophthalmology residents (and is recipient of the Distinguished Clinical Tutor Award). She has won many illustrious honors, such as the Sir William McKenzie Prize in Ophthalmology for Early Excellence in Eye Research, the Vice Chancellor's Award for Best Doctoral Thesis, and the Howsam Gold Medal for Excellence for highest mark in the RANZCO fellowship examination. She has a research interest in uveitis with over 70 publications.

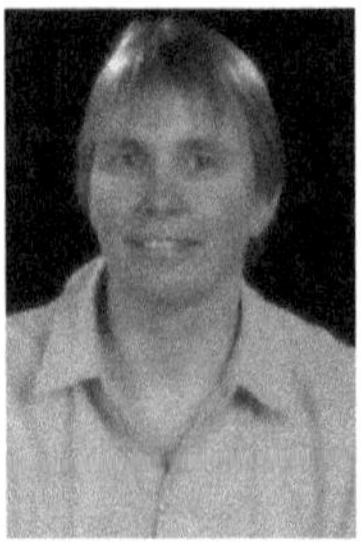

Professor Susan Lightman was Professor of Clinical Ophthalmology at University College London, UK and Consultant Ophthalmologist at Moorfields Eye Hospital from 1987–2018. She is a Fellow of the Royal College of Physicians (FRCP), Fellow of the Royal College of Ophthalmologists (FRCOphth), Fellow of the Academy of Medical Sciences (FMedSci), Fellow of the Association for Research in Vision and Ophthalmology (FARVO), Fellow of the Academy of Medical Educators (FAcadMEd), and Fellow of the Higher Education Academy (FHEA). She has published over 400 papers and written/edited 6 books.

Professor Lightman is regarded as an international authority on the subject of ocular inflammatory and diseases, having run one of the world's busiest clinics in general uveitis, pediatric uveitis, and ocular inflammation and infection for over 30 years at Moorfields, London. Additionally, she oversaw an active clinical research program in the diagnosis and management of ocular inflammatory diseases, supervising over 40 candidates for research degrees and over 200 students who attended the very popular MSc courses and Summer Schools she ran for many years. She now concentrates on teaching nationally and internationally in the field of ocular inflammation. She has received many international awards, including the American Academy Achievement Award, the Bjerrum Medal from the Danish Ophthalmological Society, as well as the Lifetime Achievement Award from the Hellenic Society for the Study of Ocular Inflammation and Infection.

About the Contributors

Chapter 1 — Classification of Uveitis

Shaul Sar,* Hana Shyriaieva,* Oren Tomkins-Netzer*,†
*Uveitis Service, Ophthalmology Department, Lady Davis Carmel Medical Center, Haifa, Israel
†Ruth and Bruch Rappaport Faculty of Medicine, Technion — Israel Institute of Technology, Haifa, Israel

Chapter 2 — Clinical Assessment in Uveitis

Priya Samalia
Royal Victorian Eye and Ear, Melbourne, Australia

Chapter 3 — Imaging in Uveitis

François Pépin,* Lilian Koh†
*CHU de Québec — Université Laval, Quebec, Canada
†Department of Ophthalmology, Woodlands Health, National Healthcare Group Eye Institute, Singapore

Chapter 4 — Systemic Investigations in Uveitis

Lazha Sharief
Ophthalmology Department, King's College Hospital NHS Foundation Trust, London, UK

Chapter 5 — Non-Infectious Uveitis

Yael Sharon,*,† Michal Kramer*,†
*Department of Ophthalmology, Rabin Medical Center, Petah-Tikva, Israel
†Sackler Faculty of Medicine, Tel Aviv University, Tel Aviv, Israel

Chapter 6 — Infectious Uveitis

Sophia L Zagora
Sydney Eye Hospital, Sydney, Australia
Clinical Senior Lecturer, University of Sydney, Sydney, Australia
Westmead Children's Hospital, New South Wales, Australia

Chapter 7 — Masquerade Syndromes

Yi-Hsing Chen,[*,†,‡] Yih-Shiou Hwang[†,‡]
*UCL Institute of Ophthalmology, University College London, London, UK
†Department of Ophthalmology, Chang Gung Memorial Hospital, Taoyuan, Taiwan
‡College of Medicine, Chang Gung University, Taoyuan, Taiwan

Chapter 8 — Complications of Uveitis

Jay Meyer,[*,†] Sonya Bennett,* Daniel Gosling,* Haya Al-Ani,* Sarah Welch,* Rachael Niederer[*,†]
*Department of Ophthalmology, Auckland District Health Board, Auckland, New Zealand
†University of Auckland, Auckland, New Zealand

Chapter 9 — Medical Management of Uveitis

Asaf Bar,[*,†] Tal Koval,[*,†] Eli Neimark,[*,†] Ron Eremenko[*,†]
*Ophthalmology Department, E. Wolfson Medical Center, Holon, Israel
†Sackler Faculty of Medicine, Tel Aviv, Israel

Chapter 10 — Surgical Management of Complications of Uveitis

Sonya Bennett,* Sarah Welch,* Jay Meyer,[*,†] Daniel Gosling,* Rachael Niederer[*,†]
*Department of Ophthalmology, Auckland District Health Board, Auckland, New Zealand
†Department of Ophthalmology, University of Auckland, Auckland, New Zealand

Chapter 11 — Cataract Surgery in Uveitis

Priya D Samalia,* Joanne L Sims[†]

*The Royal Victorian Eye and Ear Hospital, Melbourne, Australia
[†]Greenlane Clinical Centre, Auckland District Health Board, Auckland, New Zealand

Chapter 12 — Practical Approach to Managing the Uveitis Patient

Rachael Niederer,[*,†] Sue Lightman,[‡,§] Oren Tomkins-Netzer[¶,||]
*Department of Ophthalmology, Auckland District Health Board, Auckland, New Zealand
[†]University of Auckland, Auckland, New Zealand
[‡]UCL Institute of Ophthalmology, University College London, London, UK
[§]University of the Highlands and Islands, Inverness, UK
[¶]Uveitis Service, Ophthalmology Department, Lady Davis Carmel Medical Center, Haifa, Israel
[||]Ruth and Bruch Rappaport Faculty of Medicine, Technion — Israel Institute of Technology, Haifa, Israel

Teaching Points

Elewys Hearne
Severn Deanery, UK

Contents

Abbreviations

AAU	Acute anterior uveitis
ACE	Angiotensin-converting enzyme
ACIOL	Anterior chamber intraocular lens
ANA	Antinuclear antibody
APMPPE	Acute posterior multifocal placoid pigment epitheliopathy
ASPPC	Acute syphilitic posterior placoid chorioretinitis
ARN	Acute retinal necrosis
ART	Antiretroviral therapy
AU	Anterior uveitis
AZOOR	Acute zonal occult outer retinopathy
BCG	Bacillus Calmette-Guérin
BCR	Birdshot chorioretinitis
BCVA	Best corrected visual acuity
BD	Behçet disease
BHL	Bihilar lymphadenopathy
BRB	Blood retinal barrier
CBC	Complete blood count
CI	Confidence interval
CME	Cystoid macular edema
CMV	Cytomegalovirus
CN	Cranial nerve
CNS	Central nervous system
CNV	Choroidal neovascularization
CNVM	Choroidal neovascular membrane
CRP	C-reactive protein
CSCR	Central serous chorioretinopathy
CST	Central subfoveal thickness
CT	Computed tomography

CXR	Chest X-ray
DNA	Deoxyribonucleic acid
dsDNA	Double-stranded DNA
DUSN	Diffuse unilateral subacute neuroretinitis
DVT	Deep vein thrombosis
EBV	Epstein-Barr virus
ECHO	Echocardiography
EDI-OCT	Extended depth imaging ocular coherence tomography
EDTA	Ethylenediaminetetraacetic acid
ELISA	Enzyme-linked immunosorbent assay
ERG	Electroretinogram
ERM	Epiretinal membrane
ESR	Erythrocyte sedimentation rate
EVS	Endophthalmitis vitrectomy study
FAF	Fundus autofluorescence
FAST	First-line antimetabolites as steroid-sparing treatment
FFA	Fundus fluorescein angiography
FML	Fluoromethalone
FTA-ABS	Fluorescent treponemal antibody absorption
GON	Glaucomatous optic neuropathy
HAART	Highly active antiretroviral therapy
HAV-Ab	Hepatitis A virus antibody
HBcAb	Hepatitis B core antibody
HBsAb	Hepatitis B surface antibody
HBsAg	Hepatitis B surface antigen
HBV	Hepatitis B virus
HCV	Hepatitis C virus
HCV-Ab	Hepatitis C virus antibody
HIV	Human immune deficiency virus
HLA	Human leukocyte antigen
HPV	Human papilloma virus
HR	Hazard ratio
HSV	Herpes simplex virus
HTLV	Human T-lymphotrophic virus
HZO	Herpes zoster ophthalmicus
ICG	Indocyanine green
ICGA	Indocyanine green angiography

ICI	Immune checkpoint inhibitor
IDI	Intravitreal dexamethasone implant
IFA	Indirect fluorescent antibody assay
Ig	Immunoglobulin
IGRA	Interferon-gamma release assay
IL	Interleukin
IMT	Immunomodulatory therapy
IOFB	Intraocular foreign body
IOL	Intraocular lens
IOP	Intraocular pressure
IRVAN	Idiopathic retinal vasculitis-aneurysms-neuroretinitis syndrome
ITA	Intravitreal triamcinolone acetate
IU	Intermediate uveitis
IVDU	Intravenous drug user
J-H	Jarisch-Herxheimer
JIA	Juvenile idiopathic arthritis
kg	Kilogram
KP	Keratic precipitate
LFT	Liver function tests
MEK	Mitogen-activated protein kinase
MEWDS	Multiple evanescent white dot syndrome
MFC	Multifocal choroiditis
MFC-PU	Multifocal choroiditis with panuveitis
mg	Milligram
μg	Microgram
MIGS	Microincision glaucoma surgery
MMC	Mitomycin-C
MMF	Mycophenolate mofetil
MMR	Measles, mumps and rubella
MRI	Magnetic resonance imaging
MS	Multiple sclerosis
MUST	Multicenter Uveitis Steroid Treatment
Nd:YAG	Neodynium-doped yttrium aluminium garnet
NIU	Non-infectious uveitis
NPV	Negative predictive value
OCP	Ocular cicatricial pemphigoid

OCT	Ocular coherence tomography
OCT-A	Ocular coherence tomography angiography
OHT	Ocular hypertension
PanU	Panuveitis
PAS	Peripheral anterior synechiae
PCR	Polymerase chain reaction
PE	Pulmonary embolism
PI	Peripheral iridotomy
PIC	Punctate inner choroidopathy
POHS	Presumed ocular histoplasmosis syndrome
POINT	Periocular vs Intravitreal corticosteroids for uveitic macular edema
PORN	Progressive outer retinal necrosis
PostU	Posterior uveitis
PPD	Purified protein derivative
PPV	Positive predictive value
PTA	Periocular triamcinolone acetate
PTK	Photorefractive keratectomy
PVR	Proliferative vitreoretinopathy
PVRL	Primary vitreoretinal lymphoma
RD	Retinal detachment
RF	Rheumatoid factor
RFT	Renal function tests
RNFL	Retinal nerve fiber layer
RP	Retinitis pigmentosa
RPE	Retinal pigment epithelium
RPR	Rapid plasma reagin
RRD	Rhegmatogenous retinal detachment
SLE	Systemic lupus erythematosus
SUN	Standardization of uveitis nomenclature
TB	Tuberculosis
TINU	Tubulointerstitial nephritis and uveitis
TNF	Tumor necrosis factor
TPHA	Treponema pallidum hemagglutination test
TPMT	Thiopurine methyltransferase
TPPA	Treponema pallidum particle agglutination
UMS	Uveitis masquerade syndrome

U.S.	United States
UWF	Ultra-wide field
VDRL	Venereal Disease Research Laboratory
VEGF	Vascular endothelial growth factor
VKH	Vogt-Koyanagi-Harada syndrome
VZV	Varicella zoster virus
YAG	Yttrium aluminum garnet

https://doi.org/10.1142/9789811251474_0001

Chapter 1

Classification of Uveitis

Shaul Sar, Hana Shyriaieva,* Oren Tomkins-Netzer*,†*

Uveitis is defined as inflammation of the iris, ciliary body, vitreous, retina, or choroid. It has an incidence of 10.5–52/100,000 person-years with a prevalence of 38–284/100,000 persons.[1] A study of medical insurance claims for 4 million individuals in the USA reported a prevalence of 133/100,000 persons with a predominance of non-infectious uveitis (90.7%) and anterior uveitis (80%). It accounts for 10% to 15% of all causes of blindness among people of working age in the developed world.[2] Other ocular pathologic features such as diabetic retinopathy and age-related macular degeneration are more prevalent with older age, but most cases of uveitis occur in young active people and therefore any vision loss has a longer effect. This can lead to a loss of productive work years and affects patient independence. Uveitis can have a significant impact on social and medical services, because these patients cannot be managed by general practitioners and require frequent hospital attendance.[3]

Causes of uveitis are classified into infectious causes (herpes simplex anterior uveitis, syphilitic retinitis, Bartonella-associated neuroretinitis, toxoplasmic retinitis, etc.), inflammatory diseases (sarcoidosis-associated uveitis, HLA-B27-associated anterior uveitis, Behçet's disease uveitis, etc.) and masquerade syndromes (CNS lymphoma, leukemia, metastatic disease, intraocular foreign body, retinal detachment). While the prevalence of some causes of uveitis varies according to genetic and geographic factors (Behçet's disease, sarcoidosis, tuberculosis, Lyme disease), the clinical diagnosis is based on relevant medical history in combination with signs and symptoms.

*Uveitis Service, Ophthalmology Department, Lady Davis Carmel Medical Center, Haifa, Israel
†Ruth and Bruch Rappaport Faculty of Medicine, Technion — Israel Institute of Technology, Haifa, Israel

Table 1.1. Anatomic classification of uveitis.

Type	Primary site of inflammation	Includes
Anterior uveitis	Anterior chamber	Iritis, iridocyclitis, anterior cyclitis
Intermediate uveitis	Vitreous	Pars planitis, posterior cyclitis, hyalitis
Posterior uveitis	Retina or choroid	Focal/multifocal/diffuse choroiditis, chorioretinitis, retinochoroiditis, retinitis, neuroretinitis
Panuveitis	Anterior chamber, vitreous, and retina or choroid	

Adapted from Jabs DA, Nussenblatt RB, Rosenbaum JT. Standardization of uveitis nomenclature for reporting clinical data. Results of the first international workshop. Am J Ophthalmol 2005;140(3): 509–16.[4]

In an attempt to create a standardized nomenclature for diagnosing and describing uveitis, the Standardization of Uveitis Nomenclature (SUN) Working Group developed in 2005 an anatomical classification system, descriptors, standardized grading system and terminology.[4]

Uveitis is classified based on anatomical location and divided into anterior, intermediate, posterior and panuveitis (Table 1.1).

The clinical course of anterior uveitis can be acute, in which the disease persists for less than 3 months (as seen in cases of HLA-B27-associated anterior uveitis, herpes simplex anterior uveitis), or chronic, in which the disease persists for 3 months or longer (Behçet's disease, sarcoidosis-associated uveitis). Chronic anterior uveitis is more likely to cause ocular complications such as cataract, glaucoma, band keratopathy, and posterior synechiae (Table 1.2).[5]

To determine disease severity the SUN developed criteria to describe inflammation activity according to anterior chamber cells, flare counts and vitreous haze. The grade of anterior cells is determined as the number of cells seen through a 1 × 1 mm slit lamp beam through the anterior chamber. The grade of flare is based on the appearance of a 1 × 1 mm beam through the anterior chamber. Vitreous haze grading is based on retinal visualization using an indirect ophthalmoscope (Table 1.3).[4,6]

The SUN report published standardized definitions for disease outcome including inactive disease, improvement and worsening of the inflammation. An inactive disease is typically defined as absence of anterior chamber cells and flare, no active inflammatory chorioretinal and/or

Table 1.2. Descriptors of uveitis.

Category	Descriptor	Comment
Onset	Sudden	
	Insidious	
Duration	Limited	≤ 3 months duration
	Persistent	>3 months duration
Course	Acute	Episode characterized by sudden onset and limited duration
	Recurrent	Repeated episodes separated by periods of inactivity without treatment ≥3 months in duration
	Chronic	Persistent uveitis with relapse in <3 months after discontinuing treatment

Adapted from Jabs DA, Nussenblatt RB, Rosenbaum JT. Standardization of uveitis nomenclature for reporting clinical data. Results of the first international workshop. Am J Ophthalmol 2005;140(3): 509–16.[4]

Table 1.3. Grading scheme for anterior chamber cells, flare and vitreous haze.

Anterior Chamber Cells	
Grade	*Cells in Field*
0	<1
0.5+	1–5
1+	6–15
2+	16–25
3+	26–50
4+	>50
Anterior Chamber Flare	
Grade	*Description*
0	None
1+	Faint
2+	Iris and lens details are clear
3+	Iris and lens details are hazy
4+	Fibrin or plastic aqueous
Vitreous Haze	
Grade	*Description*
0	Clear retinal image
0.5+	Traces
1+	Clear optic disc and vessels, hazy nerve fiber layer

(*Continued*)

Table 1.3. (*Continued*)

2+	Hazy optic disc and vessels
3+	Optic disc is visible
4+	Optic disc is not visible

Adapted from Jabs DA, Nussenblatt RB, Rosenbaum JT. Standardization of uveitis nomenclature for reporting clinical data. Results of the first international workshop. Am J Ophthalmol 2005;140(3):509–16.[4]

Table 1.4. Activity of uveitis terminology.

Term	Definition
Inactive	No cells/flare/active inflammatory chorioretinal and/or retinal vascular lesions
Worsening	Two-step increase in level of inflammation (e.g., anterior chamber cells, vitreous haze) or increase from grade 3+ to 4+
Improving	Two-step decrease in level of inflammation (e.g., anterior chamber cells, vitreous haze) or decrease to grade 0
Remission	Inactive disease for ≥3 months after discontinuing all treatment for eye disease

Adapted from Jabs DA, Nussenblatt RB, Rosenbaum JT. Standardization of uveitis nomenclature for reporting clinical data. Results of the first international workshop. Am J Ophthalmol 2005;140(3):509–16.[4]

retinal vascular lesions. Disease remission was defined as inactive disease for more than 3 months after discontinuing all treatment for eye disease (Table 1.4).

Following the establishment of standardized disease assessment criteria, the SUN issued separate consensus reports on the definition of 25 specific uveitides (Table 1.5). For each disease hundreds of cases were collected globally and expert committees reached consensus agreements on disease definition and diagnosis. Almost 6,000 cases of the most common uveitides were collected retrospectively between 2010 and 2016. The chosen diseases included both infectious and non-infectious conditions. The aim was to develop structural criteria for the diagnosis of each disease, based on clinical findings and ancillary tests.[7–32]

Examples for disease criteria include birdshot chorioretinitis (based on 207 cases) and toxoplasmic retinitis (174 cases). For birdshot chorioretinitis, diagnosis is based on typical clinical findings (multifocal cream-colored or yellow-orange, oval or round choroidal lesions) and a

Table 1.5. Uveitides for which SUN consensus criteria were developed.

Anatomic class	Infectious	Systemic disease-associated	Eye-limited
Anterior	Cytomegalovirus anterior uveitis, Herpes simplex virus anterior uveitis, syphilitic anterior uveitis	Juvenile idiopathic arthritis-associated anterior uveitis, spondyloarthritis/HLA-B27-associated anterior uveitis, sarcoidosis-associated anterior uveitis	Fuchs' uveitis syndrome
Intermediate	Syphilitic intermediate uveitis	Multiple sclerosis-associated intermediate uveitis, sarcoidosis-associated intermediate uveitis	Pars planitis, intermediate uveitis non-pars planitis type
Posterior	Acute retinal necrosis, cytomegalovirus retinitis, syphilitic posterior uveitis, toxoplasmosis retinitis, tuberculous posterior uveitis	Sarcoidosis-associated panuveitis	Acute posterior multifocal placoid pigment epitheliopathy, birdshot chorioretinitis, multiple evanescent white dot syndrome, multifocal choroiditis with panuveitis, punctate inner choroiditis, serpiginous choroiditis
Panuveitis	Syphilitic panuveitis, tuberculous panuveitis	Behçet's disease uveitis, sarcoidosis-associated panuveitis, Vogt-Koyanagi-Harada disease	Sympathetic ophthalmia

Adapted from Van Gelder RN, Sen HN, Tufail A, Lee AY. Here Comes the SUN (Part 2): Standardization of uveitis nomenclature for disease classification criteria. Am J Ophthalmol 2021;228:A2–A6.[33]

positive HLA-A29 test, or alternatively when absent to mild anterior and vitreous activity is found (Table 1.6, Figure 1.1).[30] For toxoplasmosis retinitis, distinct clinical features (presence of hyperpigmented and/or atrophic chorioretinal scar adjacent to retinitis lesions) are paramount for diagnosis and can be replaced by a positive serology or PCR test in the presence of focal or paucifocal necrotizing retinitis (Table 1.7, Figures 1.2 and 1.3).[11]

Table 1.6. Classification criteria for birdshot chorioretinitis.

Criteria: 1, 2 and 3 OR 4

1. Characteristic bilateral multifocal choroiditis on ophthalmoscopy (multifocal cream-colored or yellow-orange, oval or round choroidal lesions)
   AND
2. Absent to mild anterior chamber inflammation:
   a) No keratic precipitates **AND**
   b) No synechiae **AND**
   c) Absent to mild anterior chamber cells
   AND
3. Absent to moderate vitritis
   OR
4. Multifocal choroiditis with
   a) Positive HLA-A29 test **AND** (b or c)
   b) Characteristic "birdshot" spots on ophthalmoscopy **OR**
   c) Characteristic indocyanine green angiogram (multifocal hypocyanescent spots) without characteristic "birdshot" spots on ophthalmoscopy

Exclusions:

1. Positive serologic test for syphilis using a treponema test
2. Evidence of sarcoidosis (either bilateral hilar adenopathy on chest imaging or tissue biopsy demonstrating noncaseating granuloma)*
3. Evidence of intraocular lymphoma on diagnostic vitrectomy or tissue biopsy

**Possible sarcoidosis should be evaluated with chest imaging at a minimum.*

Adapted from Standardization of Uveitis Nomenclature Working G. Classification criteria for birdshot chorioretinitis. Am J Ophthalmol 2021;228:65–71.[30]

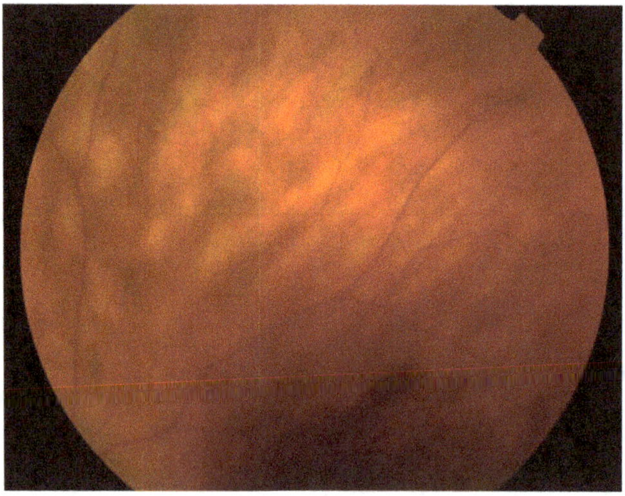

Figure 1.1. Birdshot chorioretinitis.

Table 1.7. Classification criteria for toxoplasmosis retinitis.

Criteria: Focal or paucifocal necrotizing retinitis* AND (1 or 2)

1. Evidence of infection with *Toxoplasma Gondii*
   a) Positive PCR for *Toxoplasma Gondii* from either the aqueous or vitreous specimen
      OR
   b) Positive serum IgM antibodies against *Toxoplasma Gondii*
   OR
2. Characteristic clinical ocular features
   a) Hyperpigmented and/or atrophic chorioretinal scar **AND** (b or c)
   b) Round or oval retinitis lesions **OR**
   c) Recurrent acute (episodic) course

Exclusions:

1. Both negative IgG AND IgM antibodies against *Toxoplasma Gondii* (unless there is positive PCR for *Toxoplasma Gondii* from aqueous or vitreous specimen)
2. Positive serology for syphilis using a treponemal test
3. Intraocular specimen PCR — positive for herpes simplex virus, varicella zoster or cytomegalovirus (unless there is immune compromise, morphologic evidence for >1 infection, the picture of toxoplasmic retinitis and the intraocular fluid specimen also has a positive PCR for *T. Gondii*)

**Active retinitis lesions in immunocompetent patients. Immunocompromised patients may have a multifocal or diffuse necrotizing retinitis. Number of scars may be >5.*

Adapted from Standardization of Uveitis Nomenclature Working G. Classification criteria for toxoplasmic retinitis. Am J Ophthalmol 2021;228:134–41.[11]

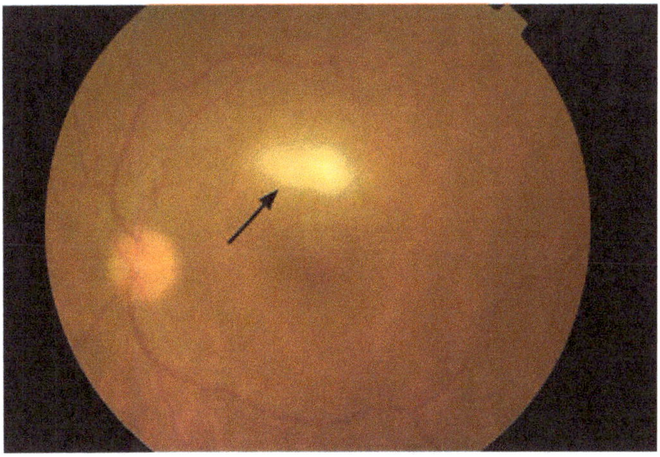

Figure 1.2. Acute toxoplasmosis retinitis (arrow).

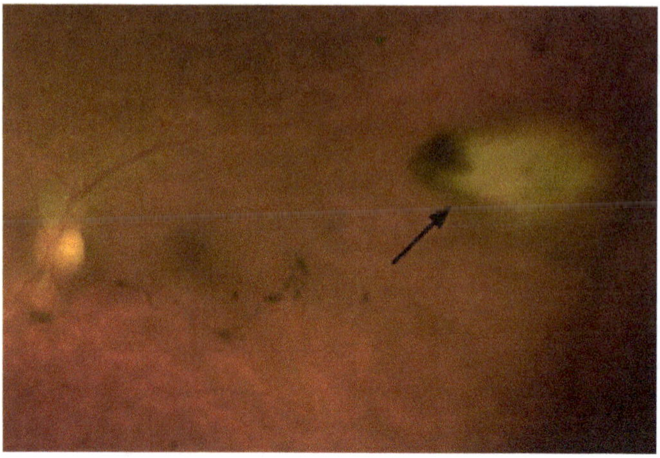

Figure 1.3. Toxoplasmosis retinitis reactivation along the border of an old scar (arrow).

The SUN classification developed consistent criteria that provides standardized nomenclature and grading for disease diagnosis, describing disease activity and assessing treatment response. It creates a structure for uniform reporting and terminology, expanding future clinical research.[7]

Teaching Points

- Uveitis is classified into
  - Infectious causes
  - Inflammatory diseases
  - Masquerade syndromes
- Standardization of Uveitis Nomenclature (SUN) Working Group have developed:
  - A uveitis anatomical classification system
  - Descriptors of uveitis (onset/duration/course)
  - Standardized grading system for anterior chamber cells, flare and vitreous haze (0–4+)
  - Terminology for the activity of uveitis (inactive/worsening/improving/remission)
  - 25 specific uveitides diagnostic criteria, using a combination of clinical findings and ancillary tests

References

1. Prete M, Dammacco R, Fatone MC, Racanelli V. Autoimmune uveitis: clinical, pathogenetic, and therapeutic features. *Clin Exp Med* 2016;16(2):125–36.
2. Thorne JE, Suhler E, Skup M, *et al.* Prevalence of noninfectious uveitis in the United States: a claims-based analysis. *JAMA Ophthalmol* 2016;134(11): 1237–45.
3. Tomkins-Netzer O, Talat L, Bar A, *et al.* Long-term clinical outcome and causes of vision loss in patients with uveitis. *Ophthalmology* 2014;121(12):2387–92.
4. Jabs DA, Nussenblatt RB, Rosenbaum JT. Standardization of uveitis nomenclature for reporting clinical data. Results of the first international workshop. *Am J Ophthalmol* 2005;140(3):509–16.
5. Sobrin L, Pistilli M, Dreger K, *et al.* Factors predictive of remission of chronic anterior uveitis. *Ophthalmology* 2020;127(6):826–34.
6. Nussenblatt RB, Palestine AG, Chan CC, Roberge F. Standardization of vitreal inflammatory activity in intermediate and posterior uveitis. *Ophthalmology* 1985;92(4):467–71.
7. Standardization of Uveitis Nomenclature Working G. Development of classification criteria for the uveitides. *Am J Ophthalmol* 2021;228:96–105.
8. Standardization of Uveitis Nomenclature Working G. Classification criteria for tubulointerstitial nephritis with uveitis syndrome. *Am J Ophthalmol* 2021;228:255–61.
9. Standardization of Uveitis Nomenclature Working G. Classification criteria for multiple evanescent white dot syndrome. *Am J Ophthalmol* 2021;228: 198–204.
10. Standardization of Uveitis Nomenclature Working G. Classification criteria for multiple sclerosis-associated intermediate uveitis. *Am J Ophthalmol* 2021;228:72–9.
11. Standardization of Uveitis Nomenclature Working G. Classification criteria for toxoplasmic retinitis. *Am J Ophthalmol* 2021;228:134–41.
12. Standardization of Uveitis Nomenclature Working G. Classification criteria for acute posterior multifocal placoid pigment epitheliopathy. *Am J Ophthalmol* 2021;228:174–81.
13. Standardization of Uveitis Nomenclature Working G. Classification criteria for juvenile idiopathic arthritis-associated chronic anterior uveitis. *Am J Ophthalmol* 2021;228:192–7.
14. Standardization of Uveitis Nomenclature Working G. Classification criteria for syphilitic uveitis. *Am J Ophthalmol* 2021;228:182–91.
15. Standardization of Uveitis Nomenclature Working G. Classification criteria for cytomegalovirus anterior uveitis. *Am J Ophthalmol* 2021;228:89–95.

16. Standardization of Uveitis Nomenclature Working G. Classification criteria for Vogt-Koyanagi-Harada disease. *Am J Ophthalmol* 2021;228:205–11.
17. Standardization of Uveitis Nomenclature Working G. Classification criteria for multifocal choroiditis with panuveitis. *Am J Ophthalmol* 2021;228:152–8.
18. Standardization of Uveitis Nomenclature Working G. Classification criteria for cytomegalovirus retinitis. *Am J Ophthalmol* 2021;228:245–54.
19. Standardization of Uveitis Nomenclature Working G. Classification criteria for tubercular uveitis. *Am J Ophthalmol* 2021;228:142–51.
20. Standardization of Uveitis Nomenclature Working G. Classification criteria for serpiginous choroiditis. *Am J Ophthalmol* 2021;228:126–33.
21. Standardization of Uveitis Nomenclature Working G. Classification criteria for acute retinal necrosis syndrome. *Am J Ophthalmol* 2021;228:237–44.
22. Standardization of Uveitis Nomenclature Working G. Classification criteria for punctate inner choroiditis. *Am J Ophthalmol* 2021;228:275–80.
23. Standardization of Uveitis Nomenclature Working G. Classification criteria for varicella zoster virus anterior uveitis. *Am J Ophthalmol* 2021;228:165–73.
24. Standardization of Uveitis Nomenclature Working G. Classification criteria for herpes simplex virus anterior uveitis. *Am J Ophthalmol* 2021;228:231–6.
25. Standardization of Uveitis Nomenclature Working G. Classification criteria for Behçet disease uveitis. *Am J Ophthalmol* 2021;228:80–8.
26. Standardization of Uveitis Nomenclature Working G. Classification criteria for Fuchs uveitis syndrome. *Am J Ophthalmol* 2021;228:262–7.
27. Standardization of Uveitis Nomenclature Working G. Classification criteria for pars planitis. *Am J Ophthalmol* 2021;228:268–74.
28. Standardization of Uveitis Nomenclature Working G. Classification criteria for sympathetic ophthalmia. *Am J Ophthalmol* 2021;228:212–9.
29. Standardization of Uveitis Nomenclature Working G. Classification criteria for spondyloarthritis/HLA-B27-associated anterior uveitis. *Am J Ophthalmol* 2021;228:117–25.
30. Standardization of Uveitis Nomenclature Working G. Classification criteria for birdshot chorioretinitis. *Am J Ophthalmol* 2021;228:65–71.
31. Standardization of Uveitis Nomenclature Working G. Classification criteria for sarcoidosis-associated uveitis. *Am J Ophthalmol* 2021;228:220–30.
32. Standardization of Uveitis Nomenclature Working G. Classification criteria for intermediate uveitis, non-pars planitis type. *Am J Ophthalmol* 2021;228:159–64.
33. Van Gelder RN, Sen HN, Tufail A, Lee AY. Here Comes the SUN (Part 2): Standardization of uveitis nomenclature for disease classification criteria. *Am J Ophthalmol* 2021;228:A2–A6.

https://doi.org/10.1142/9789811251474_0002

Chapter 2 Clinical Assessment in Uveitis

*Priya Samalia**

2.1 Introduction

A wide range of infectious and non-infectious conditions present as uveitis. Additionally, uveitis can be the first manifestation of systemic disease. Genetic, geographic and environmental factors all impact on the underlying uveitic etiology. It is therefore important to assess these subjects systematically in order to reach an underlying diagnosis. For this a thorough history and review of systems is required, followed by careful clinical examination. Subsequent investigations should be tailored to the history, examination findings and clinical suspicion rather than an exhaustive list of tests.

2.2 History Taking

2.2.1 *Demographics*

2.2.1.1 *Age*

Some conditions are more prevalent in certain age groups. Infectious uveitis is more common in extremes of age (especially <16 and >60 years) and autoimmune uveitis has a predilection for middle age.[1]

Examples of common conditions with age predilection include:

- Children/adolescence (<16 years): juvenile idiopathic arthritis (JIA), tubulointerstitial nephritis with uveitis syndrome (TINU), toxocariasis[1]

* Royal Victorian Eye and Ear, Melbourne, Australia

- Young adults to middle age (20–50): autoimmune disorders[1]
- Older age (>60 years): primary vitreoretinal lymphoma, birdshot chorioretinitis[3]

2.2.1.2 *Gender*

Certain entities are more likely to affect a specific gender.[4] For example:

- Males: ankylosing spondylitis, reactive arthritis, Behçet's disease
- Females: rheumatoid arthritis, JIA, scleroderma, antiphospholipid syndrome

2.2.1.3 *Ethnicity*

An understanding of the individual's ethnic background is necessary as some conditions are more likely to occur in certain ethnicities.[4]

- Caucasian: Birdshot chorioretinitis, HLA-B27-associated uveitis
- Asian: Behçet's disease, Vogt-Koyanagi-Harada (VKH) disease
- Pigmented ethnicities: sarcoidosis, VKH

2.2.1.4 *Geographic Location*

The prevalence of uveitic entities vary depending on geographic location due to influences of ecological factors and the predominant pathogens in a particular location.

Most common causes of infectious uveitis are toxoplasmosis, herpetic uveitis and tuberculosis. In developing countries other causes must be considered including onchocerciasis, leprosy, leptospirosis and other parasitic diseases.[1]

- Tuberculosis (TB)-related uveitis: India
- Lyme disease: Europe, Northern America
- Toxoplasmosis: Brazil
- Onchocerciasis: South America, Africa

Common non-infectious causes[1]:

- Behçet's disease: Turkey, Saudi Arabia, Israel, China, Iran, Japan
- VKH: Japan

2.2.2 *Social History*

Work and recreational activities can also give insights into the underlying diagnosis as these activities can predispose or increase the risk of certain conditions.[4]

Examples of conditions more likely depending on social history:

- Gardeners: Whipple's disease
- Plumbers, sewer workers: leptospirosis
- Raw meat diet: toxoplasmosis
- Contact with puppies: toxocariasis
- Contact with cats: toxoplasmosis
- Intravenous drug use: endogenous endophthalmitis, human immunodeficiency virus (HIV)
- Unsafe sexual practices: syphilis, HIV

2.2.3 *Medication History*

Some prescription medication can cause uveitis. It is therefore important to take a thorough drug history.[5]

Examples of drugs causing uveitis include:

- Bisphosphonates: anterior uveitis, scleritis, orbital inflammatory disease
- Cancer immune therapies such as immune check point inhibitors: uveitis, retinal vasculitis, VKH-like inflammation
- TNF-α inhibitors: paradoxically can induce sarcoid-like granulomatous inflammation, etanercept may cause flare of HLA-B27-associated uveitis
- Vaccination may be associated with uveitis

2.2.4 *Past Ocular History*

- History of trauma/intraocular surgery: sympathetic ophthalmia
- Myopia: punctate inner choroiditis

- Pseudophakia: uveitis-glaucoma-hyphema syndrome
- Iris implants: uveitis-glaucoma-hyphema syndrome
- Ocular surgery: surgically induced scleritis, endophthalmitis

2.2.5 *Pre-existing Systemic Conditions*

In some instances, individuals have a known systemic diagnosis prior to the onset of uveitis. Additionally, systemic conditions can predispose individuals to develop certain types of uveitis. Particular attention should be paid to immunosuppression, as this may increase the likelihood of developing infectious uveitis. Immune suppression may also mask some of the typical signs of infectious uveitis and give an atypical presentation.

Other pre-existing systemic conditions may predispose to non-infectious uveitis, in particular ankylosing spondylitis, inflammatory bowel disease (ulcerative colitis, Crohn's disease), psoriatic arthritis, collagen vascular diseases, Behçet's disease, sarcoidosis and multiple sclerosis.

2.3 Ocular Symptoms

2.3.1 *Symptoms*

Presenting ocular symptoms can help determine the anatomic location.

- Anterior uveitis: pain, redness, photophobia
- Intermediate uveitis: floaters, reduced vision
- Posterior uveitis: floaters, photopsia, metamorphopsia, visual field scotomas, reduced vision
- Scleritis: pain on eye movements, facial pain, pain waking from sleep

Children may be asymptomatic and only present due to complications such as cataract and band keratopathy. This may happen more commonly in unilateral disease as well as in JIA-associated uveitis. Children with JIA should be screened periodically for uveitis in an attempt to diagnose uveitis early, prior to uveitis-related complications (Table 2.1).[7]

2.3.2 *Onset*

The rate of onset of uveitis may help to determine the underlying cause.

Table 2.1. **Screening frequency for juvenile idiopathic arthritis (JIA).**

Type of uveitis	Screening frequency
Oligoarticular/pauciarticular (RF negative)/psoriatic/undifferentiated **ANA+ve**	≤6 years old at onset screen 3-monthly for 2 years then 6-monthly for 5 years >6 years old at onset screen 6-monthly for 2 years then annually for 3 years
Oligoarticular/pauciarticular (RF negative)/psoriatic/undifferentiated **ANA-ve**	≤6 years old at onset screen 6-monthly for 2 years then annually for 3 years >6 years old at onset screen annually for 5 years or until 11 years old
Polyarthritis RF positive/systemic	Annually for 5 years or until 11 years old
Enthesitis-related arthritis	Either as above, or initial screen and discharge with precautions to parents
Onset after 12 years	Screen 6-monthly × 2
Any patient stopping IMT or biologic IMT	Screen 3-monthly for one year

RF = rheumatoid factor, ANA = antinuclear antibody, IMT = immunomodulatory therapy

- Sudden onset: sympathetic ophthalmia, VKH, Behçet's disease
- Insidious: intermediate uveitis, birdshot chorioretinitis, primary vitreoretinal lymphoma

2.3.3 *Laterality*

Certain conditions can present with simultaneous bilateral uveitis for example:

- TINU
- JIA
- VKH
- Birdshot chorioretinitis
- Acute posterior multifocal placoid pigment epitheliopathy (APMPPE)

2.3.4 *Systemic Symptoms*

Systems review is important in uveitis to detect previously undiagnosed systemic illness. See Table 2.2 for possible symptoms as a clue to the underlying etiology.

Table 2.2. **Major body systems in the review of symptoms.**

Body system	Example of symptom & potential uveitic cause
Constitutional Symptoms	• **Fever:** endogenous endophthalmitis, sarcoidosis, Kawasaki, Lyme • **Weight loss:** sarcoidosis, lymphoma
Ear, Nose, Mouth, Throat	• **Mouth ulcers:** Behçet's disease, syphilis, systemic lupus erythematosus (SLE) • **Hutchinson's teeth:** congenital syphilis • **Strawberry gingivitis:** granulomatosis with polyangiitis (GPA) • **Hearing loss:** VKH, sarcoidosis, Cogan's syndrome, syphilis, relapsing polychondritis, Susac syndrome • **Saddle nose deformity:** congenital syphilis, GPA, relapsing polychondritis, leprosy, lymphoma, trauma • **Nose bleeds:** GPA • **Chronic sinusitis:** GPA • **Perichondritis/swelling or painful ears:** relapsing polychondritis • **Voice change:** relapsing polychondritis
Cardiovascular	• **Palpitations:** sarcoidosis, Takayasu, SLE • **Chest pain:** SLE, sarcoidosis
Respiratory	• **Dyspnea, cough, wheeze:** sarcoidosis, TB • **Hemoptysis:** TB
Gastrointestinal	• **Diarrhea:** inflammatory bowel disease, Whipple's disease
Genitourinary	• **Dysuria:** reactive arthritis, syphilis • **Genital ulcers:** reactive arthritis, syphilis, Behçet's disease • **Hematuria:** polyarteritis nodosa, GPA • **Epididymitis:** Behçet's disease • History of **recurrent miscarriage:** SLE, antiphospholipid syndrome
Musculoskeletal	• **Arthralgia:** HLA-B27, JIA, rheumatoid arthritis, Behçet's disease, psoriatic arthritis, relapsing polychondritis, Lyme disease • **Plantar fasciitis:** HLA-B27 • **Sclerodactyly:** scleroderma • **Raynaud's phenomenon:** rheumatoid arthritis, dermatomyositis, polymyositis
Integumentary	• **Poliosis:** VKH, sympathetic ophthalmia • **Alopecia:** sarcoidosis, SLE, syphilis, VKH • **Skin rash:** vasculitides, sarcoidosis, syphilis, HLA-B27 • **Skin photosensitivity:** SLE • **Nails:** psoriatic arthritis, reactive arthritis • **Tattoo reaction:** sarcoidosis, tattoo-induced uveitis
Hematologic	• **Deep vein thrombosis:** antiphospholipid syndrome • **Petechia, purpura:** Kawasaki disease

Table 2.2. (*Continued*)

Body system	Example of symptom & potential uveitic cause
Neurological	• **Headache:** APMPPE, sarcoidosis, Behçet's disease, Lyme, VKH • **Vestibular:** Cogan's syndrome, VKH • **Meningeal irritation:** VKH • **Paresthesia:** multiple sclerosis • **Seizures:** SLE, sarcoidosis, antiphospholipid syndrome
Psychiatric	• **Personality change:** neurosarcoid, Behçet's with neurologic involvement, SLE, polyarteritis nodosa
Endocrine	• **Polyuria, polydipsia:** diabetes with diabetes-associated uveitis
Hematologic/ Lymphatic	• **Lymphadenopathy:** lymphoma, Bartonelliosis, sarcoidosis, TB

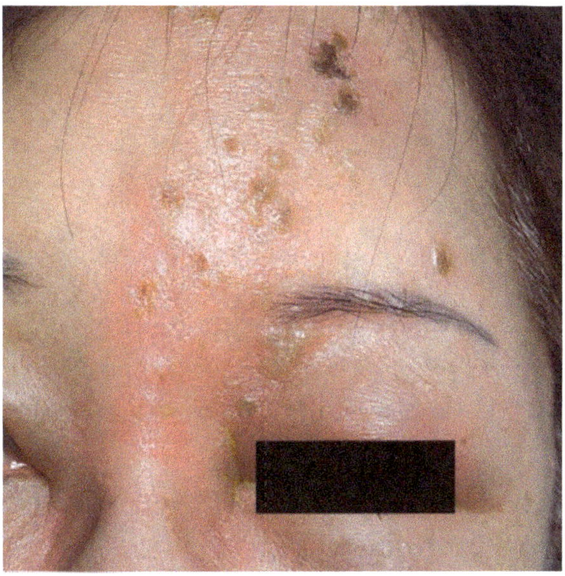

Figure 2.1. Skin lesions in herpes zoster ophthalmicus.

2.4 Ocular Examination

2.4.1 *Orbit and Adnexa*

- Vesicles: herpes zoster virus (Figure 2.1), herpes simplex virus (Figure 2.2)

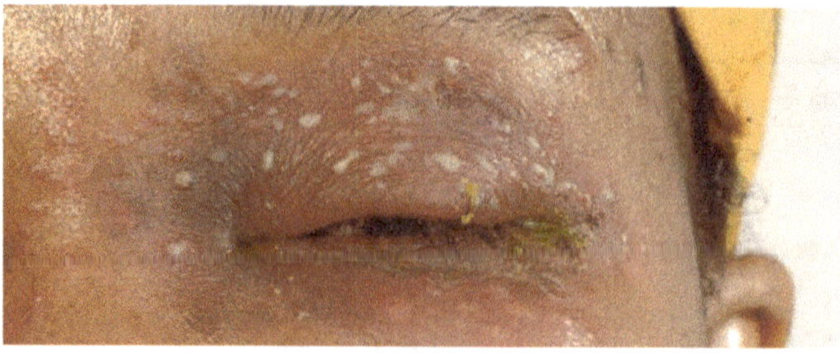

Figure 2.2. Skin lesions in herpes simplex.

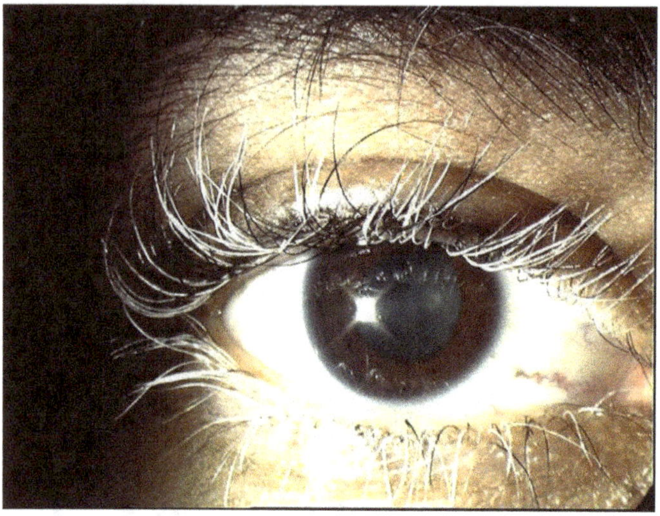

Figure 2.3. Poliosis of the upper eyelid lashes in a patient with VKH.

- Poliosis: VKH, sympathetic ophthalmia (Figure 2.3)
- Nodules: sarcoidosis, leprosy
- Madarosis: leprosy
- Proptosis: posterior scleritis, orbital inflammatory disease, GPA
- Lacrimal gland enlargement: orbital inflammatory disease, sarcoidosis (Figure 2.4)
- Nasolacrimal duct obstruction: GPA

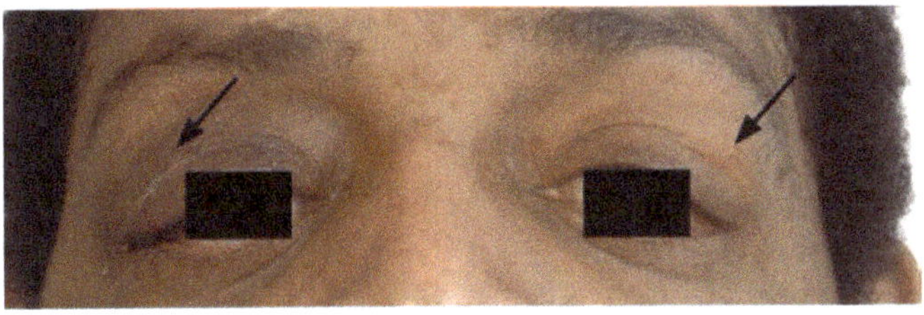

Figure 2.4. Bilateral lacrimal gland enlargement due to sarcoidosis (arrows).

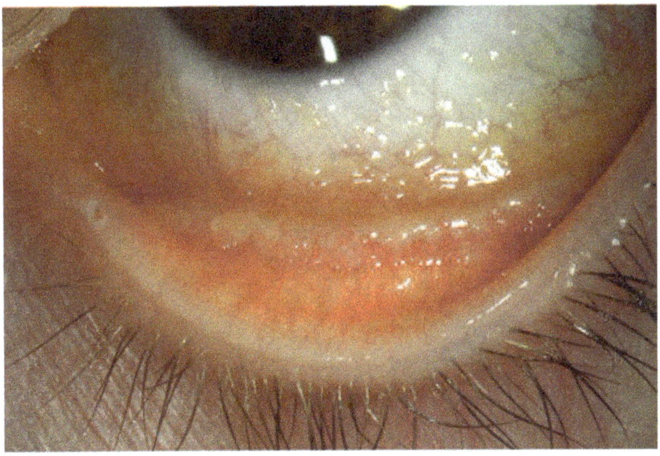

Figure 2.5. Conjunctival granulomas in sarcoidosis.

2.4.2 Conjunctiva

Gross examination in ambient illumination should be performed initially, prior to slit lamp examination, to detect subtle color changes such as the violaceous hue of scleritis.

- Conjunctival injection
- Conjunctival granuloma: sarcoidosis (Figure 2.5)
- Phlyctenulosis: generally a delayed hypersensitivity reaction. Less commonly occurs with TB and worm infestation, particularly in developing countries.

2.4.3 Cornea

2.4.3.1 Dendrites

Herpetic disease may present with epithelial dendrites. In herpes simplex these appear as branching dendritic lesions which may be stained with fluorescein (Figure 2.6). In herpes zoster ophthalmicus there may be pseudodendrites which tend to be smaller in size, lack terminal bulbs and have a relative lack of central staining (Figure 2.7).

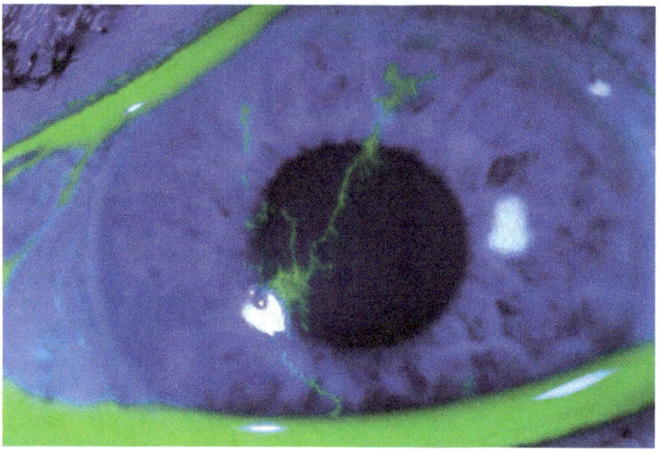

Figure 2.6. Dendritic ulcer in a patient with herpes simplex keratouveitis.

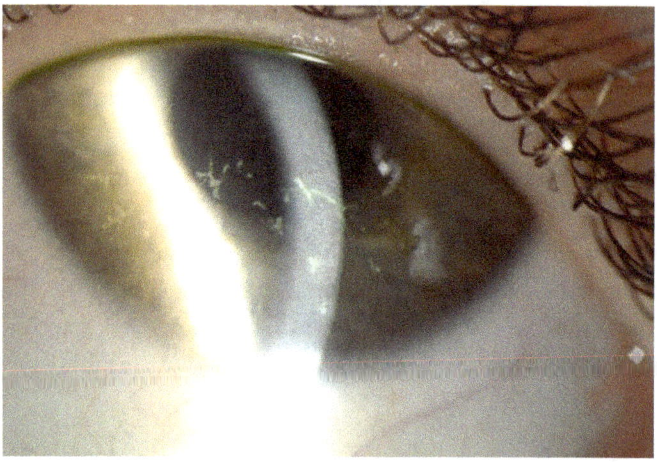

Figure 2.7. Pseudodendrites in a patient with herpes zoster ophthalmicus.

2.4.3.2 Keratic Precipitates

Keratic precipitates (KPs) are deposits on the corneal endothelium composed of aggregates of inflammatory cells including polymorphonuclear cells, lymphocytes and epithelioid cells. KPs can be large (granulomatous, Figure 2.8) or small (non-granulomatous, Figure 2.9). While the shape and

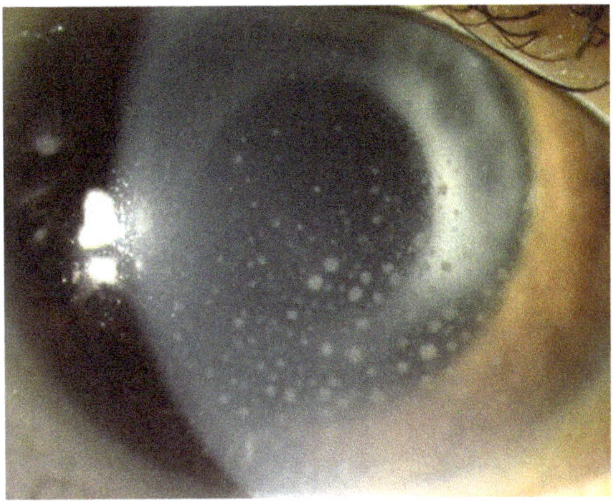

Figure 2.8. Large granulomatous keratic precipitates distributed along Arlt's triangle due to sarcoidosis.

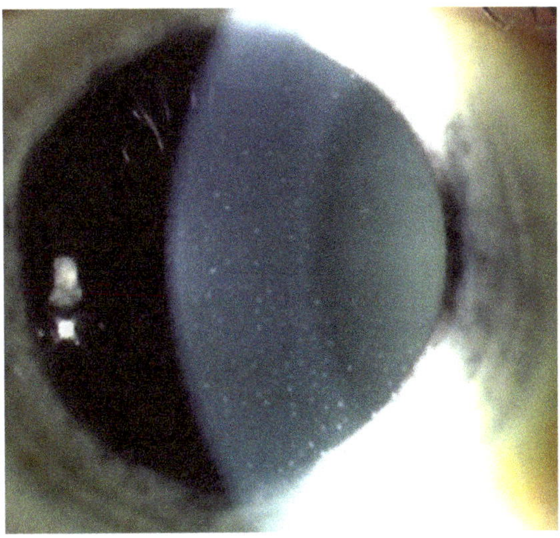

Figure 2.9. Non-granulomatous, stellate keratic precipitates diffusely distributed in a patient with Fuchs' uveitis syndrome.

distribution of the KPs can help in the diagnosis of certain diseases (e.g., diffuse stellae KPs in Fuchs' uveitis syndrome), their appearance in many diseases can be variable.

Generally KPs align along Arlt's triangle due to gravitational effects and aqueous fluid convection currents in the anterior chamber. Arlt's triangle is a triangle from the central to inferior cornea with the apex centrally and the base inferiorly.

Grey-white stellate KPs distributed generally over the entire corneal endothelium is seen in viral uveitis and FUS.

2.4.3.3 *Band Keratopathy*

This is the deposition of calcium within the sub-epithelium, Bowman's layer and anterior stroma (Figure 2.10). It generally indicates a degree of chronicity and is also more common in childhood uveitis, particularly JIA.

2.4.3.4 *Interstitial Keratitis*

Interstitial keratitis is characterized by inflammation primarily in the corneal stroma (Table 2.3).

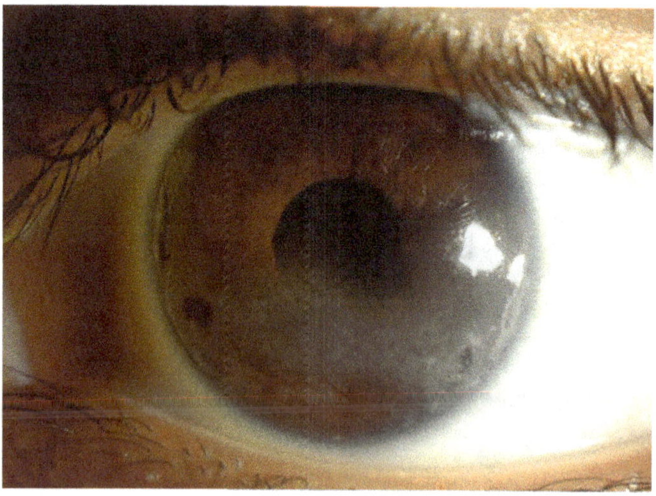

Figure 2.10. Band keratopathy in chronic uveitis.

Table 2.3. Differential diagnosis for major causes of interstitial keratitis.

Infective	Non-infective
Congenital or acquired syphilis	Cogan's syndrome
Tuberculosis	Sarcoidosis
Leprosy	GPA
Herpes simplex virus	Rheumatoid arthritis
Onchocerciasis	Relapsing polychondritis
Lyme disease	

GPA = granulomatosis with polyangiitis

Table 2.4. SUN Working Group grading for anterior chamber cells.[8]

Grade	Cell number
0	<1
0.5+	1–5
1+	6–15
2+	16–25
3+	25–50
4+	>50

2.4.3.5 *Corneal Sensation*

Certain uveitic conditions can affect corneal nerves resulting in an anesthetic cornea. Major uveitic causes of corneal hypoesthesia:

- Herpes simplex virus
- Herpes zoster virus
- Leprosy

2.4.4 *Anterior Segment*

2.4.4.1 *White Blood Cells*

The degree of anterior segment inflammation is classified by the SUN criteria by determining the number of white blood cells seen per high power field (1×1 mm slit beam) on slit lamp examination (Table 2.4).

Table 2.5. Differential diagnosis for the common uveitic causes of hypopyon.

Infective	Non-infective	Masquerade
Exogenous endophthalmitis	HLA-B27	Leukemia
Endogenous endophthalmitis	Behçet's disease	Lymphoma
Toxocariasis	Lens-associated	Retinoblastoma
Leprosy	TASS	Melanoma
		Metastasis
		Drug induced, e.g., rifabutin

TASS = toxic anterior segment syndrome

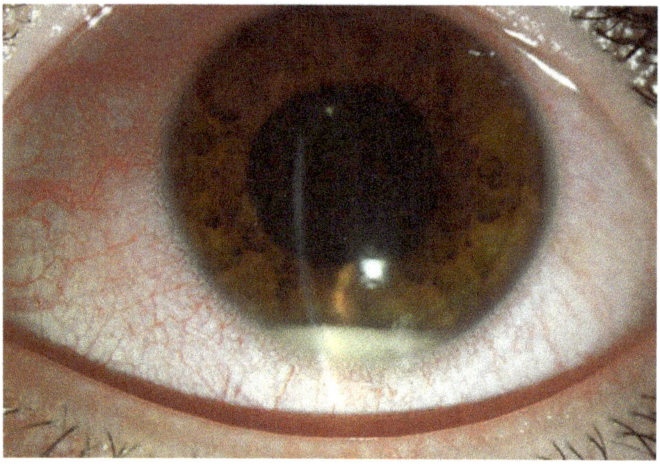

Figure 2.11. Hypopyon in HLA-B27-associated uveitis.

Intensive anterior chamber inflammation can lead to hypopyon formation (Table 2.5, Figure 2.11).

2.4.4.2 *Protein*

Ocular inflammation can disrupt the blood-aqueous barrier leading to increased protein content. Increased protein content leads to scattering of light causing the fluid to appear turbid, termed aqueous flare (Table 2.6, Figure 2.12).

Table 2.6. SUN Working Group grading for anterior chamber flare.[8]

Grade	Flare Description
0	None
1+	Faint
2+	Moderate (iris and lens details clear)
3+	Marked (iris and lens details hazy)
4+	Intense (fibrin or plastic aqueous, Figure 2.12)

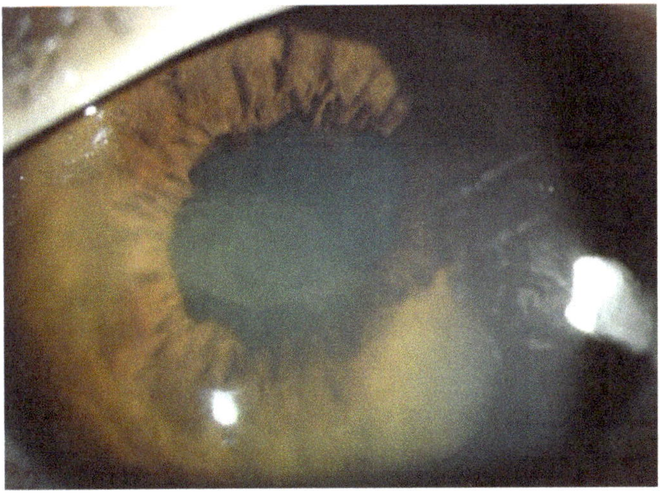

Figure 2.12. Fibrin in the anterior chamber.

2.4.4.3 *Red Blood Cells*

Hyphema can occur with viral uveitis, FUS and uveitis-glaucoma-hyphema syndrome.

2.4.5 Gonioscopy

Gonioscopic examination can reveal characteristic findings of certain conditions. Periodic gonioscopic examination is also important in the

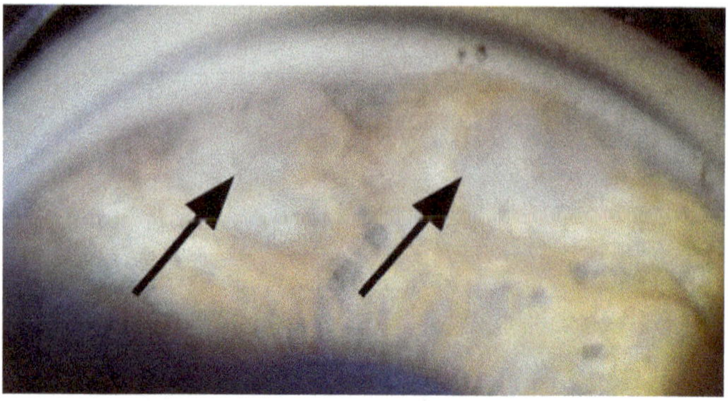

Figure 2.13. Gonioscopy of tent-shaped peripheral anterior synechia (arrows) in a patient with sarcoidosis.

ongoing management to observe for peripheral anterior synechiae (PAS) that can increase the risk of uveitic glaucoma.[9]

- Tent-shaped PAS: sarcoidosis (Figure 2.13)
- Iridocorneal nodules: sarcoidosis
- Radial vessels: FUS

2.4.6 *Iris*

2.4.6.1 *Heterochromia*

Differences in iris color are easiest examined before dilation in ambient daylight. Hypochromic heterochromia is where the abnormal iris is lighter in color and hyperchromic heterochromia is the reverse (see Chapter 5, Figure 5.7).

- Hypochromic heterochromia: FUS, Posner-Schlossman syndrome, herpes zoster uveitis, herpes simplex uveitis, leprosy, juvenile xanthogranuloma
- Hyperchromic heterochromia: FUS in blue eyes as stromal atrophy allows the posterior pigmented layer of the iris to show through

2.4.6.2 *Posterior Synechia*

The iris can become adherent to the anterior lens capsule forming posterior synechia (Figure 2.14). Posterior synechia are common with acute

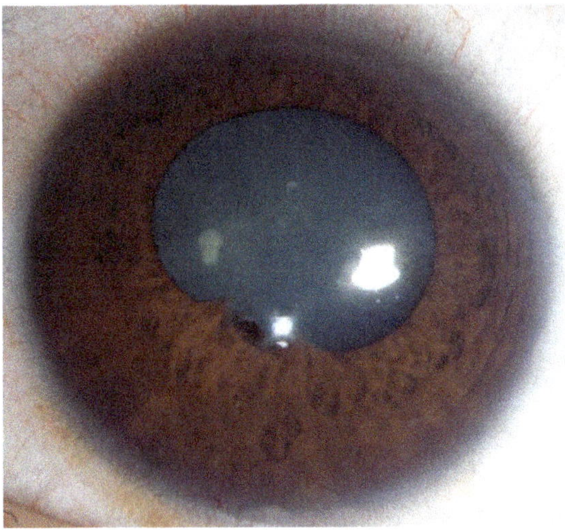

Figure 2.14. Posterior synechiae.

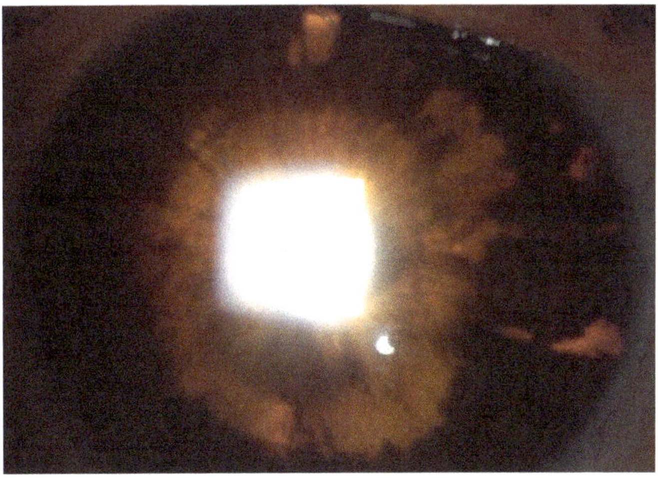

Figure 2.15. Iris transillumination defects on retroillumination slit lamp exam.

anterior uveitis but there are a few conditions where they are generally absent such as FUS and birdshot chorioretinitis.

2.4.6.3 *Transillumination Defects*

Retroillumination on slit lamp exam can reveal iris transillumination defects (Figure 2.15).

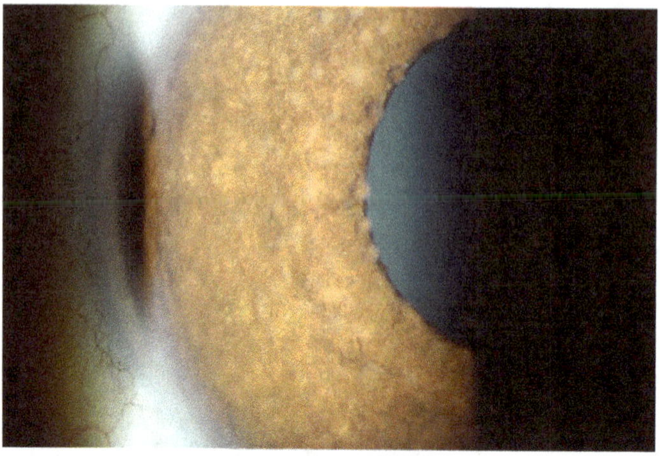

Figure 2.16. Koeppe nodules secondary to sarcoidosis.

- Sectoral iris atrophy: herpetic uveitis
- Iris transillumination defect usually along intraocular lens haptic: uveitis-glaucoma-hyphema syndrome

2.4.6.4 *Nodules*

- Koeppe nodules: along the pupillary border, occur in both granulomatous and non-granulomatous uveitis (Figure 2.16)
- Bussaca nodules: Located in the mid-periphery of the iris, seen in granulomatous inflammation (Figure 2.17)
- Iris crystals (Russell bodies): immunoglobulin-containing structures derived from plasma cells seen in chronic uveitic entities such as FUS
- Iris pearls: leprosy[10]

2.4.6.5 *Pupillary Membranes*

Can occur with severe uveitis (Figure 2.18). Controlling inflammation and mydriatic therapy can sometimes break these; however, in unresponsive cases surgical intervention may be required.

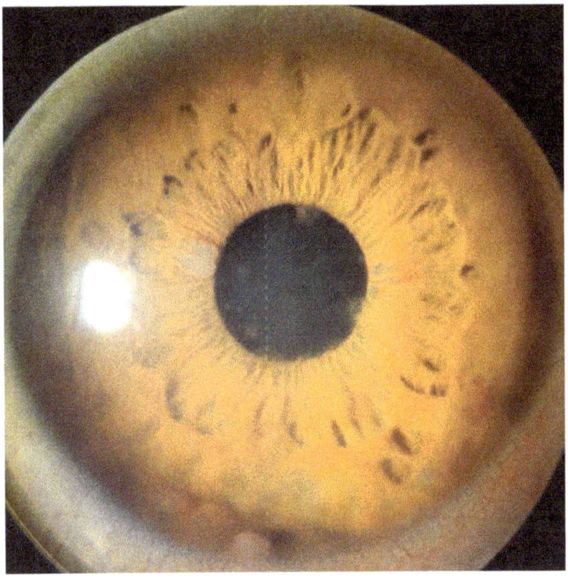

Figure 2.17. Koeppe nodules and Bussaca nodules secondary to sarcoidosis.

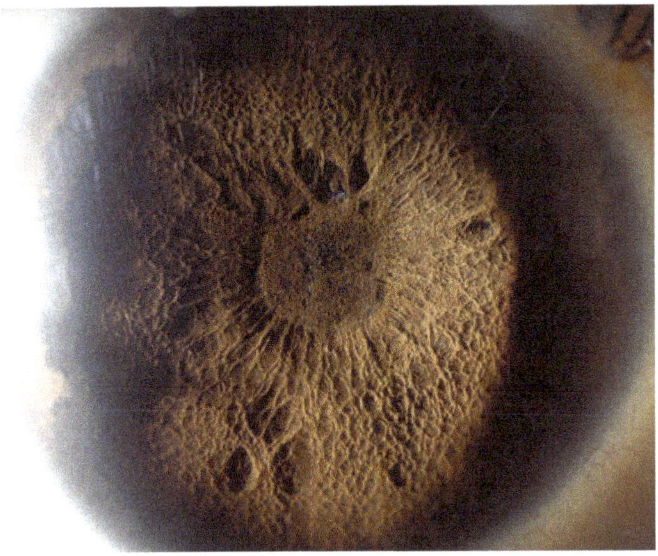

Figure 2.18. Extensive pupillary membrane resulting in acoria.

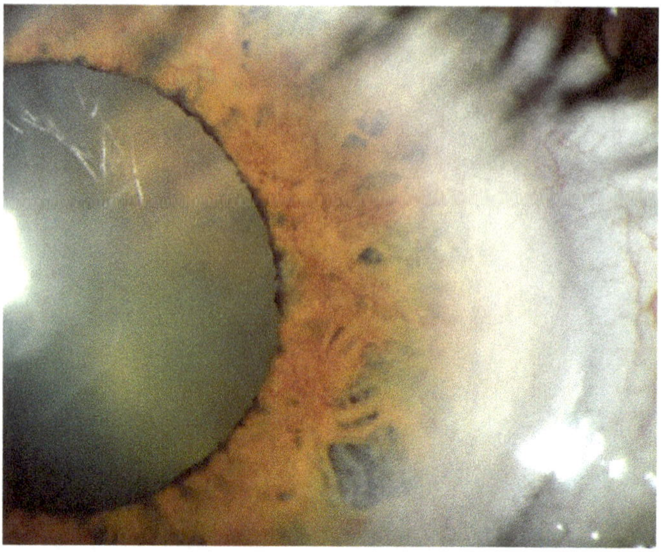

Figure 2.19. Rubeosis iridies.

2.4.6.6 *Rubeosis Iridies*

Prominent dilated iris vessels can be seen in severe inflammation and also as a late complication of uveitis (Figure 2.19).

- Iris Roseola: yellow nodules associated with dilated iris vessels, described as a "classic sign" of syphilis

2.4.7 Lens

Cataract can develop with chronic uveitis. The most common type of cataract is posterior subcapsular cataract (Figure 2.20). Glaukomflecken, anterior lens opacities can occur with hypertensive uveitis.

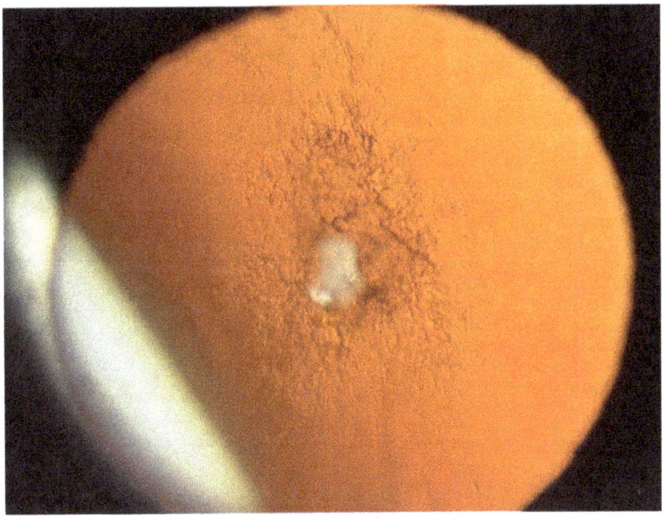

Figure 2.20. Posterior subcapsular cataract due to uveitis secondary to sarcoidosis.

Table 2.7. U.S. National Eye Institute grading scheme for vitreous cell.[11]

Grade	Cell Number	Description
0	0–1	Clear
Trace	2–20	Few opacities
1+	21–50	Scattered opacities
2+	51–100	Moderate opacities
3+	101–250	Many opacities
4+	>251	Dense opacities

2.4.8 *Vitreous*

2.4.8.1 *Vitreous Cell*

The U.S. National Eye Institute has a grading system in an attempt to standardize vitreous cell description. This is based on the number of vitreous cells seen in the posterior chamber (Table 2.7).

Vitreous inflammatory cells can accumulate in clumps to cause snowballs (Table 2.8, Figure 2.21) and snowbanks (Figure 2.22). Strings of snowballs, termed "string of pearls", appear in conditions such as vitreoretinal lymphoma, tubercular uveitis or candida endophthalmitis (Figure 2.23).

Table 2.8. Major causes of vitreous snowballs.

Infective	Non-infective	Masquerade
Candidiasis	Intermediate uveitis	Lymphoma
Whipple's disease	Sarcoidosis	Amyloid
Syphilis	Multiple sclerosis	Seeding of endophytic retinoblastoma
Lyme disease		

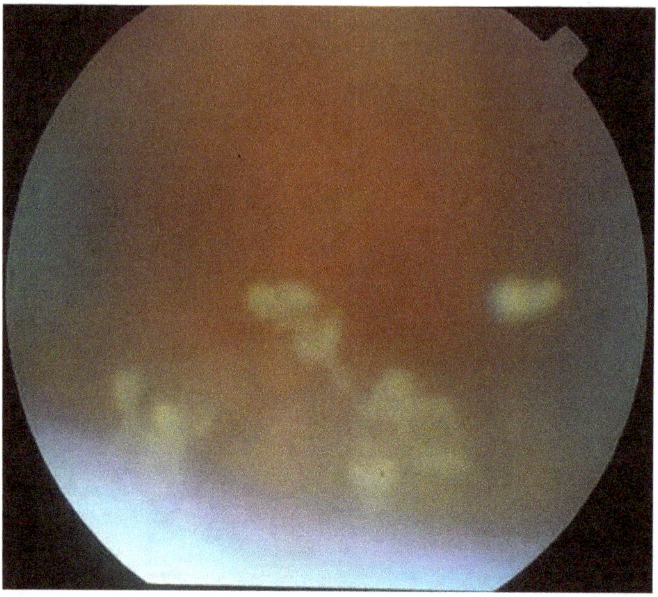

Figure 2.21. Snowballs in intermediate uveitis.

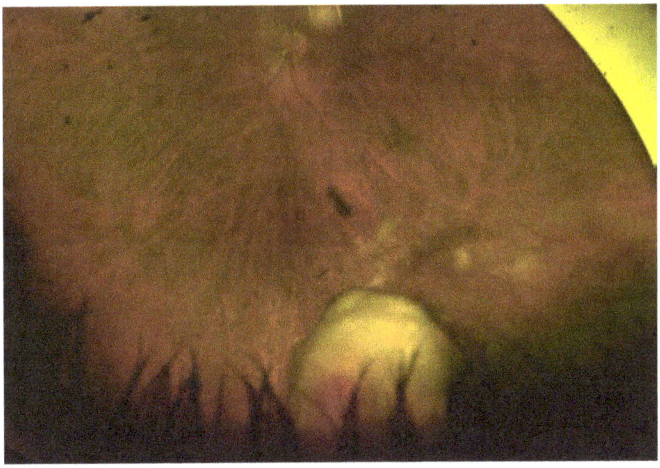

Figure 2.22. Snowbank in a patient with idiopathic intermediate uveitis. Note the neovascularization over the snowbank.

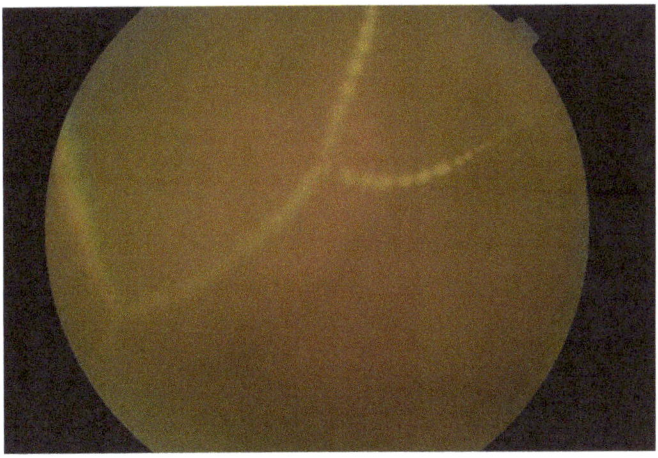

Figure 2.23. String of pearls in patient with tuberculosis uveitis.

Table 2.9. U.S. National Eye Institute grading for vitreous haze grading.[12]

Grade	Description
0	Clear
0.5+	Trace
1+	Few opacities, mild blurring
2+	Significant blurring but still visible
3+	Optic nerve visible, no vessels seen
4+	Dense opacity obscures the optic nerve head

2.4.8.2 *Vitreous Haze*

Vitreous haze is the obscuration of fundal details due to proteinaceous material within the vitreous, analogous to aqueous flare. It is assessed by fundal examination using an indirect lens (Table 2.9).

2.4.9 *Retina*

A careful dilated retinal exam is an important part of the assessment.

2.4.9.1 *Retinitis*

Active retinal inflammation appears as fluffy yellow-white areas with poorly defined edges which can be focal or multifocal (Table 2.10).

Table 2.10. Differential diagnosis for major causes of retinitis.

	Focal Retinitis	Multifocal Retinitis
Infective	Toxoplasmosis (Figure 2.24) Onchocerciasis Cysticercosis	Syphilis Acute retinal necrosis (Figure 2.25) Cytomegalovirus Candidiasis Progressive outer retinal necrosis DUSN Bartonellosis
Non-infective	Behçet's disease	Behçet's disease Sarcoidosis
Masquerade	Masquerade	Masquerade

DUSN = diffuse unilateral subacute neuroretinitis

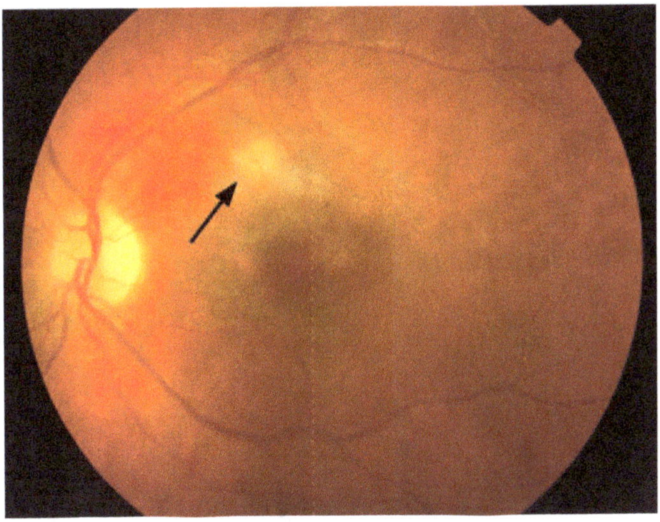

Figure 2.24. **Focal retinitis due to primary acquired toxoplasmosis (arrow).**

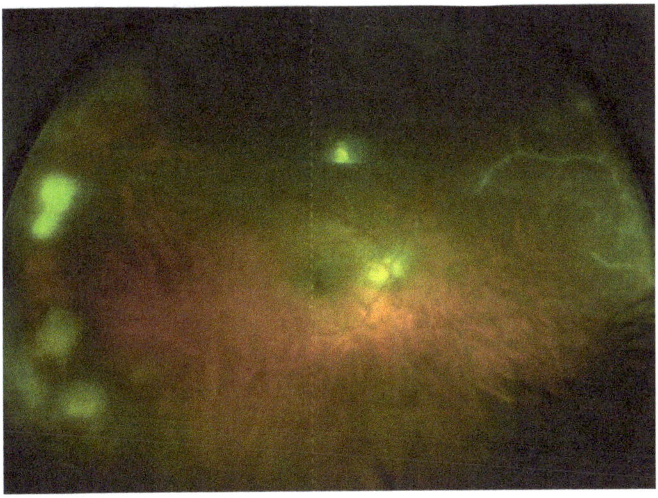

Figure 2.25. **Multifocal retinitis with vitritis causing a hazy fundal view due to acute retinal necrosis.**

2.4.9.2 *Exudative Macular Detachment*

Exudative macular detachment can occur in certain uveitic entities. Common causes include:

- VKH
- Sympathetic ophthalmia (Figure 2.26)
- Posterior scleritis
- Necrotizing retinitis
- Uveal effusion syndrome

2.4.9.3 *Retinal Vasculature*

Retinal vasculitis can affect predominantly arteries, veins or both (Table 2.11).

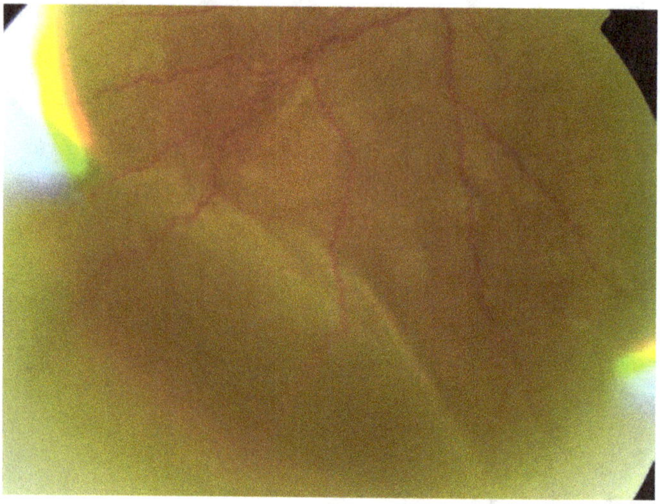

Figure 2.26. Exudative retinal detachment in sympathetic ophthalmitis.

Table 2.11. Differential diagnosis for common causes of retinal vasculitis.

	Predominantly Arteritis	**Predominantly Phlebitis**	**Arteritis + Phlebitis**
Non-infectious	SLE Polyarteritis nodosa Dermatomyositis Churg-Strauss Susac syndrome GPA Kawasaki disease IRVAN	Sarcoidosis (Figure 2.27) MS Pars planitis Behçet's disease Birdshot chorioretinitis VKH	Crohn's disease/UC Behçet's disease (Figure 2.28) Frosted branch angiitis

Table 2.11. (*Continued*)

	Predominantly Arteritis	Predominantly Phlebitis	Arteritis + Phlebitis
Infectious	ARN/PORN Toxoplasmosis Syphilis	HIV-associated retinal vasculitis Tuberculosis Toxoplasmosis Syphilis CMV Cat-scratch disease (Bartonellosis) Whipple's	ARN/PORN Toxoplasmosis Syphilis Tuberculosis CMV
Masquerade	Masquerade	Masquerade	Masquerade

SLE = systemic lupus erythematosus, GPA = granulomatosis with polyangiitis, ARN = acute retinal necrosis, PORN = progressive outer retinal necrosis, MS = multiple sclerosis, VKH = Vogt-Koyanagi-Harada, CMV = cytomegalovirus, UC = ulcerative colitis, IRVAN = idiopathic retinal vasculitis aneurysms and neuroretinitis

Adapted from Rosenbaum JT, Sibley CH, Lin P. Retinal vasculitis. Curr Opin Rheumatol 2016;28(3):228–35.[13]

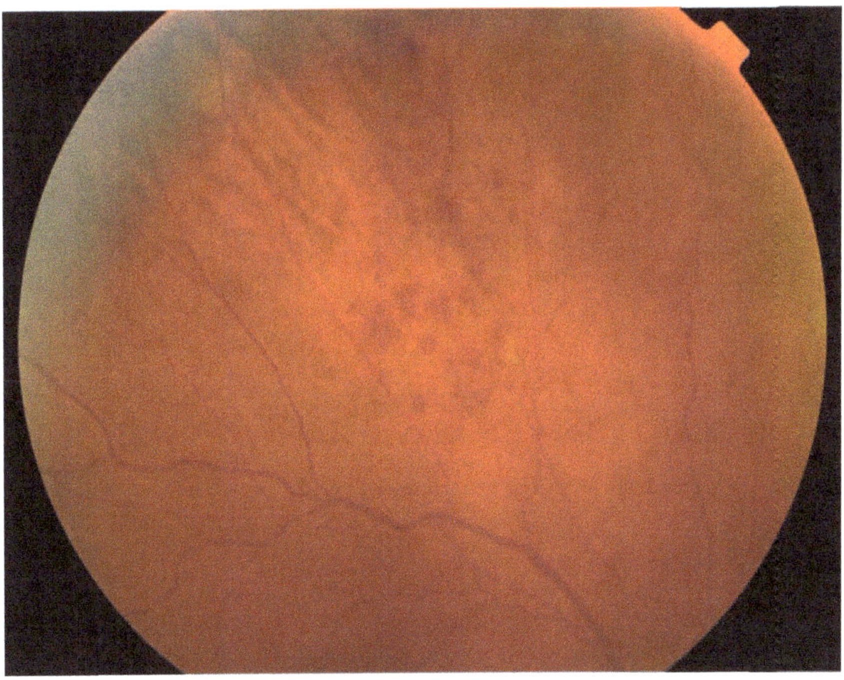

Figure 2.27. Occlusive phlebitis in sarcoidosis.

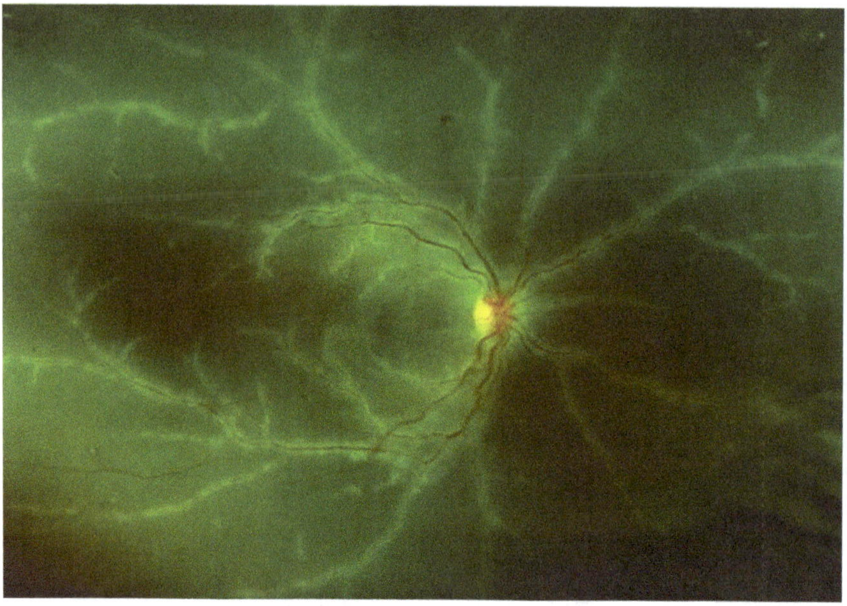

Figure 2.28. Extensive retinal vasculitis involving both arteries and veins in Behçet's disease.

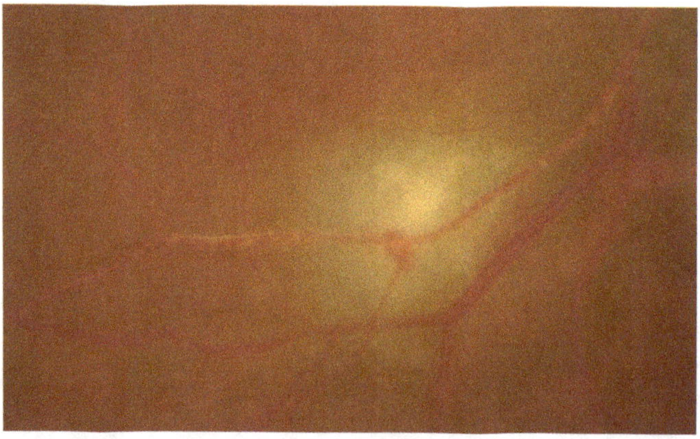

Figure 2.29. Kyrieleis phenomenon in ocular toxoplasmosis.

2.4.9.4 *Kyrieleis Phenomenon*

This is retinal peri-arterial plaques like beads on a string. This sign is characteristic of ocular toxoplasmosis (Figure 2.29), but can also occur in ARN.

2.4.9.5 *Posterior Segment Uveitic Complications Observed on Fundal Exam*

- Cystoid macular edema
- Macular lamellar hole
- Choroidal neovascular membrane
- Retinal pigment epithelial clumping
- Retinal neovascularization
- Sunset glow fundus: seen in convalescent VKH and chronic sympathetic ophthalmia
- Vitreous hemorrhage
- Retinal dragging secondary to traction: toxocariasis
- Rhegmatogenous retinal detachment

2.4.10 *Choroid*

Choroidal inflammation can be focal or multifocal choroiditis (Table 2.12).

Table 2.12. Differential diagnosis for major causes of choroiditis.

	Focal choroiditis	Multifocal choroiditis
Infective	Tuberculosis (Figure 2.30) Toxocariasis Nocardia Candidiasis Chikungunya virus	Histoplasmosis (Figure 2.32) Pneumocystis choroiditis Tuberculosis (Figure 2.33) Cryptococcus West Nile virus
Non-infective	Sarcoidosis (Figure 2.31)	Sarcoidosis Idiopathic multifocal choroiditis Birdshot chorioretinitis (Figure 2.34) APMPPE (Figure 2.35) Punctate inner choroiditis Idiopathic serpiginous (Figure 2.36)
Masquerade	Lymphoma Choroidal metastases	Lymphoma Choroidal metastases

APMPPE = acute posterior multifocal placoid pigment epitheliopathy

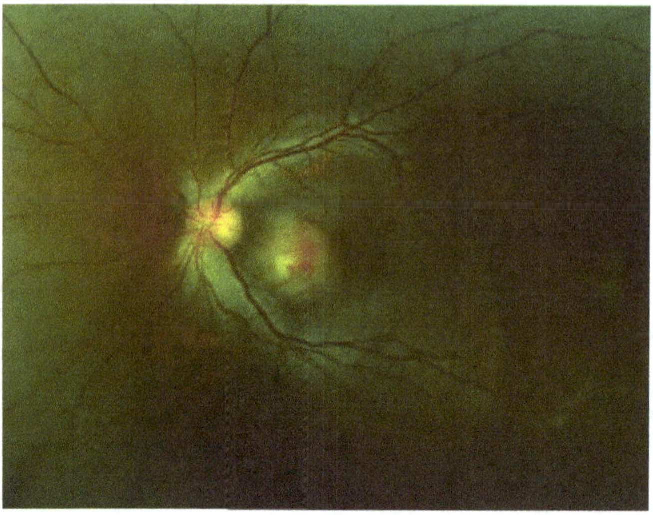

Figure 2.30. Focal choroidal granuloma with associated subretinal fluid secondary to tuberculosis.

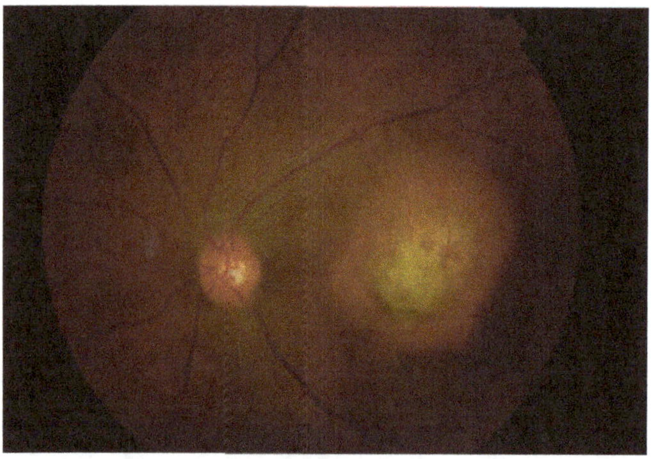

Figure 2.31. Solitary choroidal granuloma in sarcoidosis uveitis.

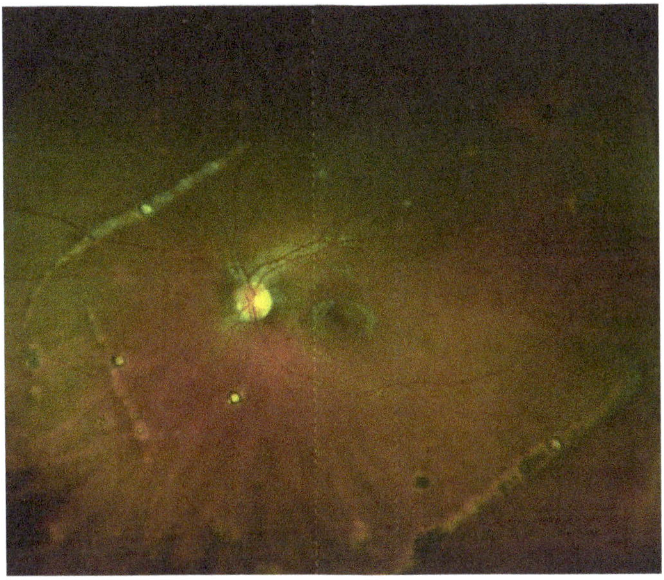

Figure 2.32. Multifocal choroidal lesions ("punched out" lesions) and choroidal tracks ("snail tracks") in a patient with presumed ocular histoplasmosis.

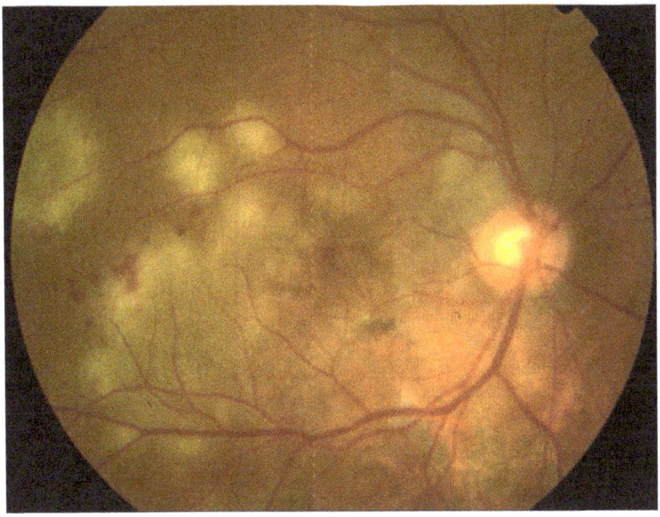

Figure 2.33. Multifocal choroiditis from tuberculosis-associated serpiginous-like choroidopathy.

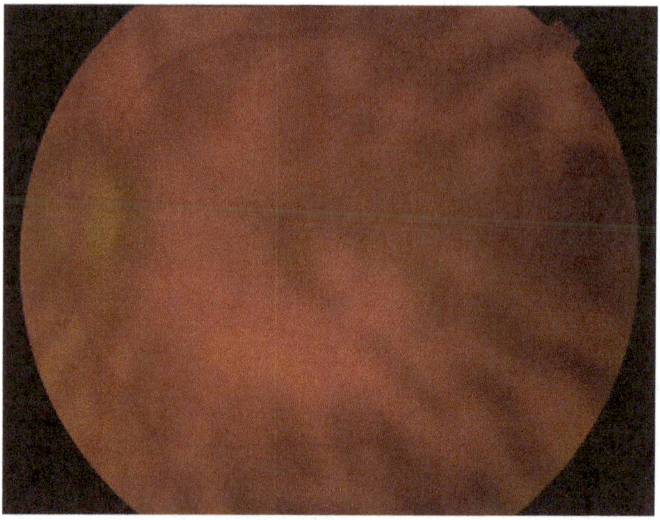

Figure 2.34. Multifocal choroiditis in birdshot chorioretinitis. Note the oval yellow lesions radiating from the optic nerve.

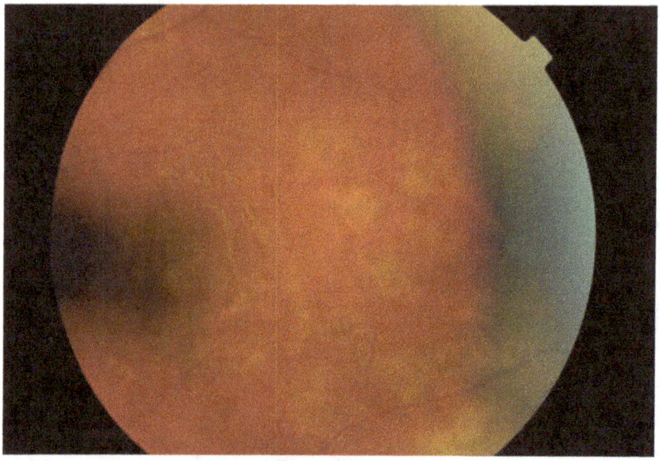

Figure 2.35. Multifocal choroiditis in a patient with APMPPE. Note the plaque-like shape of the lesions.

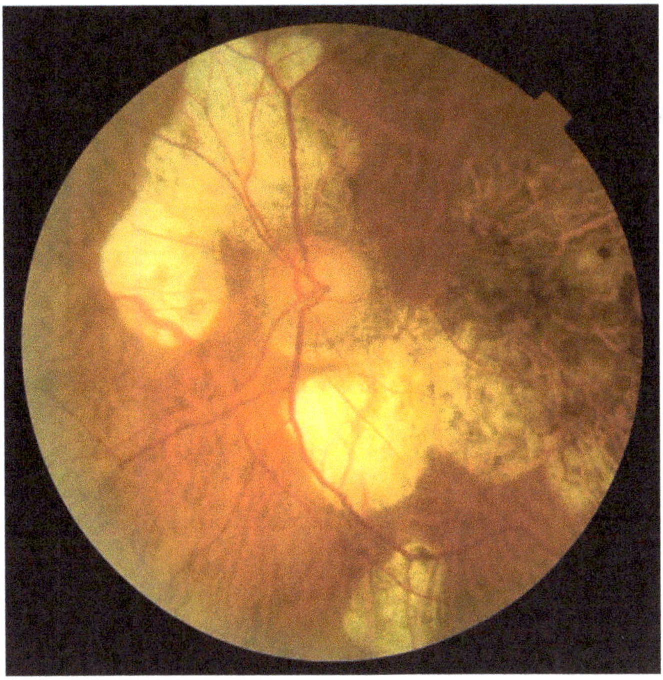

Figure 2.36. Serpiginous choroiditis.

2.4.11 *Neuro-Ophthalmic Exam*

2.4.11.1 *Pupil Assessment*

- Miosis: due to posterior synechiae
- Mydriasis: Posner-Schlossman syndrome[14]
- Light-Near dissociation: neurosyphilis, herpes zoster virus
- Relative afferent pupillary defect: indicates optic neuritis component

2.4.11.2 *Optic Nerve*

It is important to test optic nerve function in the setting of inflammatory papillitis.

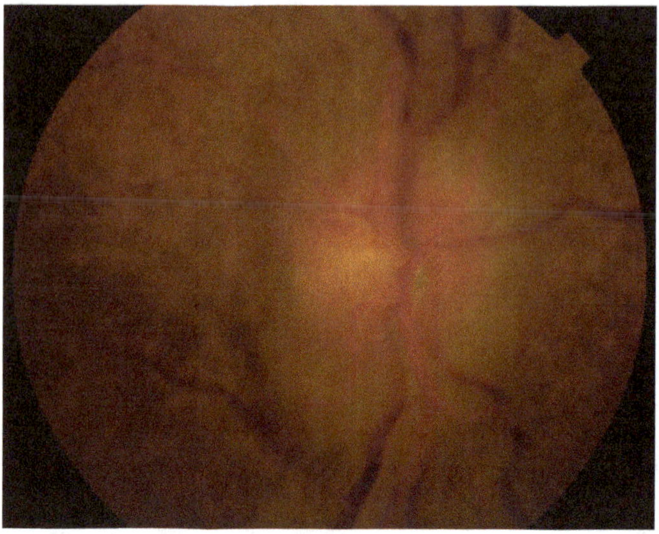

Figure 2.37. Extensive optic nerve head swelling due to sarcoidosis.

Inflammatory papillitis associated with optic nerve dysfunction indicates an optic neuritis component. Differential diagnosis for major causes:

- Multiple sclerosis
- Sarcoidosis (Figure 2.37)
- Syphilis

2.4.11.3 *Other Cranial Nerve Involvement*

- Bell's palsys: sarcoidosis (Heerfordt syndrome: anterior uveitis, parotid gland enlargement, facial palsy, fever)
- Facial nerve palsy: leprosy
- Cranial nerve IV, V, VI: orbital inflammatory syndrome

2.4.12 ***Intraocular Pressure***

2.4.12.1 *Ocular Hypertension*

Elevated intraocular pressure (IOP) at presentation, so called hypertensive uveitis, is defined as an IOP of 24 mmHg or greater.[8] Though ocular

Table 2.13. Differential diagnosis for common causes of hypertensive uveitis.

Infective	Non-infective
Herpetic (HSV, VZV, CMV)	Posner-Schlossman syndrome
Toxoplasmosis	Fuchs' uveitis syndrome
Rarely endophthalmitis	

HSV = herpes simplex virus, VZV = varicella zoster virus, CMV = cytomegalovirus

Table 2.14. SUN Working Group anatomic classification for uveitis.[8]

Type	Primary site of inflammation
Anterior uveitis	Anterior chamber
Intermediate uveitis	Vitreous
Posterior uveitis	Retina and choroid
Panuveitis	All compartments of the eye

hypertension can be found in many cases of acute uveitis, it is a suggesting sign of specific etiologies (Table 2.13). During the course of uveitis, raised IOP can occur due to uveitic glaucoma or in response to steroid treatment.[9]

2.4.12.2 *Hypotony*

Hypotony is an IOP of less than 6 mmHg. It is more common in childhood and longstanding uveitis.[15]

Acute hypotony is due to ciliary body hyposecretion and increased uveoscleral outflow and is typically reversible. Chronic hypotony, however, is irreversible and progression to phthisis bulbi can occur. Chronic hypotony is due to ciliary body atrophy or the development of cyclitic membranes pulling the ciliary body causing ciliary body detachment or tractional cyclodialysis, leading to increased outflow.[15]

2.4.13 *Anatomic Location of Uveitis*

The type of uveitis is based on the site with the most prominent inflammation (Table 2.14). The site of uveitis is suggestive of certain etiologies (Tables 2.15 and 2.16).

Table 2.15. Differential diagnosis for major causes of panuveitis and posterior uveitis.

Infective	Non-infective	Masquerade
Tuberculosis	Sympathetic ophthalmia	Endophthalmitis
Syphilis	VKH	Lymphoma
Leprosy	Sarcoidosis	Trauma
Herpetic	Behçet's disease	
Lyme disease	JIA	
Toxoplasmosis		
Endophthalmitis		
Candidiasis		

JIA = juvenile idiopathic arthritis

Table 2.16. Differential diagnosis for major causes of intermediate uveitis.

Infective	Non-infective	Masquerade
Syphilis	Idiopathic (pars planitis)	Lymphoma
Lyme disease	Sarcoidosis	Waldenström macroglobulinemia
Whipple's disease	Multiple sclerosis	
	Inflammatory bowel disease	

2.5 Special Notes on Infectious Uveitis and Syphilis

Anti-inflammatory treatment with corticosteroid or other immunosuppressive agents are used to treat non-infectious uveitis. Unopposed steroid/immunosuppressive agents in the setting of infectious uveitis can worsen outcomes. It is therefore important to rule out an infective cause.

Risk factors for infectious uveitis:

- Immunocompromised: HIV, AIDS, iatrogenic immunosuppression
- Trauma
- External infectious source

Clinical cues and features of infective cause:

- Unilateral uveitis
- Moderate to large KP

- Raised IOP
- Retinitis
- Immunocompromised patient
- Constellation of signs:
  - Iris transillumination and hypertensive uveitis: herpes virus
  - Macular star: Bartonellosis

Syphilis is a great masquerader and should be considered in any individual with ocular inflammation.[16]

Teaching Points

- A systematic approach is required to gain the correct uveitis diagnosis. A comprehensive history including a full review of systems, drug history, and a detailed examination should point you towards specific investigations.
- Children with JIA may be asymptomatic with their uveitis, and only present with complications such as cataract and band keratopathy. Therefore, regular screening is imperative (see Table 2.1).
- The size and distribution of KPs can support specific diagnoses, but bear in mind, they can be variable. Large KPs indicate a granulomatous condition, whilst small KPs are indicative of a non-granulomatous condition. KPs mostly align along Arlt's triangle, but if they are grey-white stellate KPs spread over the entire endothelium then think of viral uveitis and FUS.
- On gonioscopy examination, tented peripheral anterior synechiae and iridocorneal nodules can be seen in sarcoidosis, and radial vessels in FUS.
- Common causes of exudative macular detachment include: VKH, sympathetic ophthalmia, posterior scleritis, necrotizing retinitis and uveal effusion syndrome.
- In retinal vasculitis, whether there is predominantly an arteritis or a phlebitis, or an equal amount of both, can help direct your differential diagnosis (see Table 2.11). In choroiditis, whether it is focal or multifocal will direct your differential diagnosis (see Table 2.12).
- Retinal peri-arterial plaques, like beads on a string, are known as Kyrieleis phenomenon. This is characteristic of ocular toxoplasmosis but can also be seen in ARN.

References

1. Rathinam SR, Namperumalsamy P. Global variation and pattern changes in epidemiology of uveitis. *Indian J Ophthalmol* 2007;55:173–83.
2. Cunningham Jr ET, Smith JR, Tugal-Tutkun I, Rothova A, Zierhut M. Uveitis in children and adolescents. *Ocul Immunol Inflamm* 2016;24(4):365–71.
3. Samalia P, Hawley L, Niederer RL, Sims J. A review of de novo uveitis in older adults presenting to a large tertiary centre. *Br J Ophthalmol* 2021;in press. doi: 10.1136/bjophthalmol-2020-318657.
4. Rathinam SR, Babu M. Algorithmic approach in the diagnosis of uveitis. *Indian J Ophthalmol* 2013;61:255–62.
5. Samalia P, Sims J, Niederer RL. Drug-induced ocular inflammation. *NZ Med J* 2020;133(1527):83–94.
6. Samalia P, Welch S, Polkinghorne P, Niederer RL. Endogenous endophthalmitis: a 21-year review of cases at a tertiary eye care centre. *Ocul Immunol Inflamm* 2020;7:1–6.
7. Smith JR, Matthews JM, Conrad D, Hall AJ, Niederer RL, Singh-Grewal D, Tay-Kearney ML, Wells JM, Zagora SL, Australian and New Zealand Juvenile Idiopathic Arthritis-Uveitis Working Group, McCluskey PJ. Recommendations for the management of childhood juvenile idiopathic arthritis-type chronic anterior uveitis. *Clin Exp Ophthalmol* 2021;49(1):38–45.
8. Jabs DA, Nussenblatt BB, Rosenbaum JT. Standardization of uveitis nomenclature for reporting clinical data. Results of the first international workshop. *Am J Ophthalmol* 2005;140(3):509–16.
9. Ma T, Sims JL, Bennett S, Chew S, Niederer RL. High rate of conversion from ocular hypertension to glaucoma in subjects with uveitis. *Br J Ophthalmol* 2021;in press. doi: 10.1136/bjophthalmol-2021-318809.
10. Morais LNA, David JPF, Peres Lima JV, Demachki S, Diniz DG, Almeida EF. Acquired acoria and iris pearls in leprosy: case report. *Eur J Ophthalmol* 2021;in press. doi: 10.1177/11206721211024057.
11. Nusssenblatt RB, Whipcup SM. Uveitis: Fundamentals and Clinical Practice (4th edition). Philadelphia, PA: Elsevier, 2010.
12. Nussenblatt RB, Palestine AG, Chan CC, *et al.* Standardization of vitreal inflammatory activity in intermediate and posterior uveitis. *Ophthalmology* 1985;94(4):467–71.
13. Rosenbaum JT, Sibley CH, Lin P. Retinal vasculitis. *Curr Opin Rheumatol* 2016;28(3):228–35.
14. Jap A, Sivakumar M, Chee S-P. Is Posner Schlossman syndrome benign? *Ophthalmology* 2001;108:913–8.

15. Sen HN, Drye LT, Goldstein DA, Larson TA, Merrill PT, Pavan PR, Sheppard JD, Burke A, Srivastava SK, Jabs DA, Multicenter Uveitis Steroid Treatment (MUST) Trial Research Group. Hypotony in patients with uveitis: the Multicenter Uveitis Steroid Treatment (MUST) trial. *Ocul Immunol Inflamm* 2012;20(2):104–12.
16. Kiss S, Damico FM, Young LH. Ocular manifestations and treatment of syphilis. *Semin Ophthalmol* 2005;20(3):161–7.

https://doi.org/10.1142/9789811251474_0003

Chapter 3

Imaging in Uveitis

François Pépin, Lilian Koh*†

Imaging technologies have evolved rapidly in the last three decades. In modern day ophthalmology practice, imaging occupies a central role and is heavily relied upon in the evaluation of a patient with uveitis. It is important to know when to order and how to interpret all these different tests. They all have different functions and can be used for a variety of reasons including diagnostic purposes, assessment of disease progression, detection of complications and monitoring response to treatment.

3.1 Anterior Segment Photography

Anterior segment photos can be used for monitoring anterior segment pathology. In uveitis practice, it can be used to document keratic precipitates, evolution of posterior synechia (Figure 3.1), iris nodules or other signs of anterior uveitis and its complications.

Photos can be used for evaluation of progression and response to treatment in anterior segment pathologies like herpetic keratouveitis (Figure 3.2), iris granulomas (Figure 3.3) or iris atrophy (Figure 3.4). They can also have academic purposes for teaching or scientific publications and for patient education.

*CHU de Québec — Université Laval, Quebec, Canada

†Department of Ophthalmology, Woodlands Health, National Healthcare Group Eye Institute, Singapore

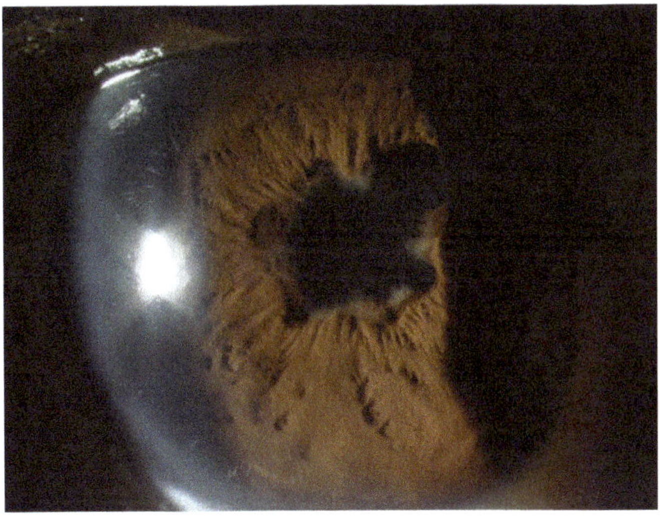

Figure 3.1. Posterior synechiae.

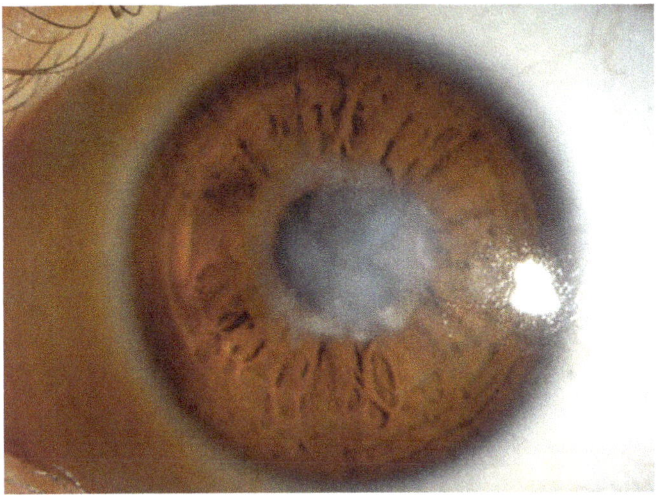

Figure 3.2. Herpetic disciform keratitis.

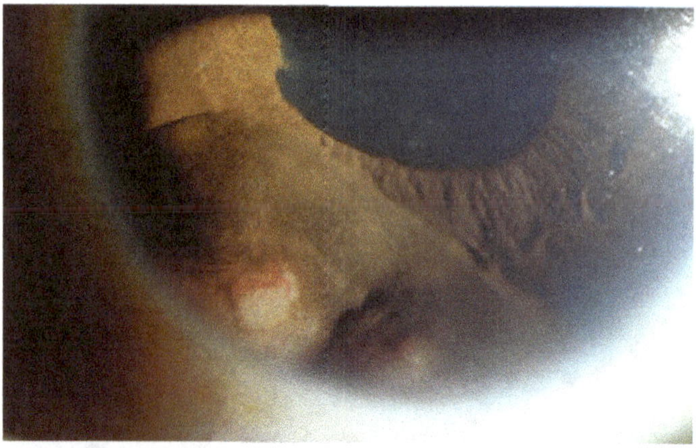

Figure 3.3. Iris granuloma related to sarcoidosis.

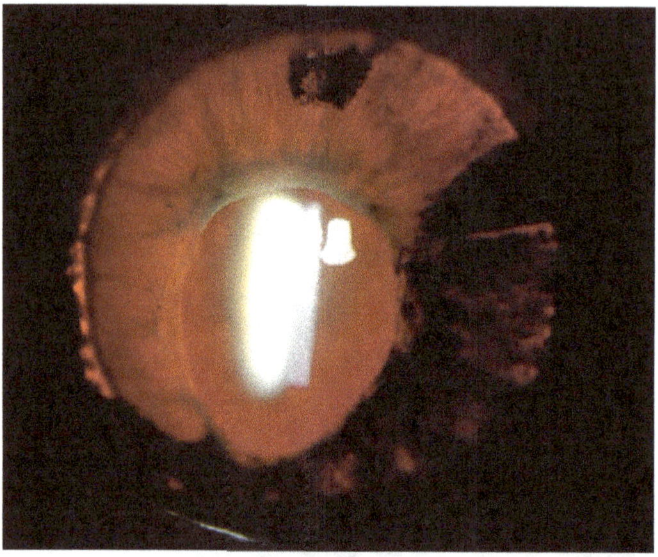

Figure 3.4. Iris atrophy in herpetic uveitis.

3.2 Fundus Photography and Widefield Imaging

The use of widefield imaging, defined as imaging beyond the posterior pole but posterior to vortex vein ampulla, and ultra-widefield (UWF) imaging capturing over 100 degrees of retina with a single image or a montage of images, have become increasingly performed since the 1980s. The Optos camera (Optos, UK) with pseudo-color images captures up to 200 degrees of retina in a single photo and further increases the utility of fundus photography in uveitis.[1]

UWF imaging in uveitis has multiple uses. It is particularly helpful in patients with challenging fundal examination (children, small pupils and photophobic patients). It also allows ophthalmologists to have a view of nearly all the retina and choroid at once to appreciate the global appearance of the fundus. This is essential in diseases like birdshot chorioretinitis (BCR) where the diagnosis can be less evident when you look at different parts of the retina separately (Figure 3.5). Moreover, it is very useful to evaluate and monitor vascular sheathing by comparing images side by side, which may otherwise be hard to see and monitor only with clinical examination, especially if the sheathing is mild and segmental.

Fundus photography can also be used to correlate presence of lesions on other imaging (optical coherence tomography (OCT), fundus autofluorescence (FAF) or angiography) and can be used in cases with choroidal and/or retinal lesions for diagnosis, follow-up and monitoring of response to treatment. The degree of vitreous haze can also be easily compared from visit to visit in an objective manner.

Optos photos may produce a limited view of the superior and inferior retina because of the eyelid, but gaze-directed image acquisition is possible, and peripheral areas can be photographed if needed.

3.3 Fundus Autofluorescence (FAF)

This is a non-invasive imaging technique first used in humans in 1995[2] that utilizes fluorescent properties of lipofuscin in the retinal pigment epithelium (RPE) when excited by a specific light wavelength. Different machines use slightly different wavelengths to stimulate the RPE, such as blue light (488 nm) used in Spectralis (Heidelberg, CA) and green light (514 nm) used in Optos.[3] Images taken by different machines cannot be used for direct comparison. This is due to differences in autofluorescence wavelength, as blue light is more strongly absorbed by the macula pigments compared to green light.

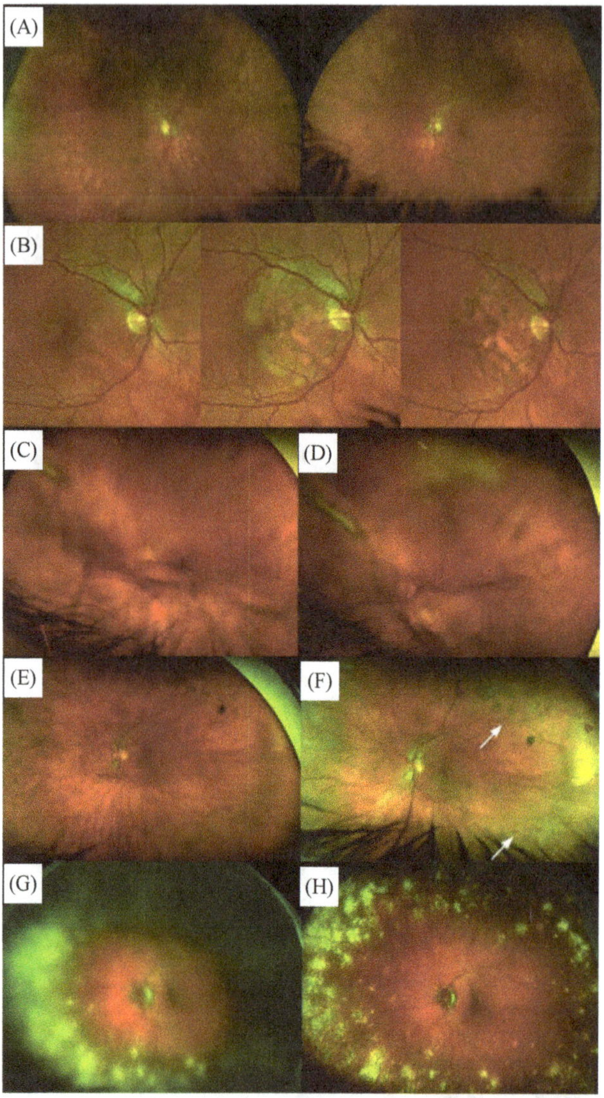

Figure 3.5. (A) Patient with bilateral birdshot chorioretinitis. (B) Patient with right eye serpiginous choroidopathy showing evolution over time (left to right). (C) Patient with acute retinal necrosis. (D) Superior peripheral necrotic lesions in the same patient as C, imaged with gaze-directed image acquisition. (E) Patient with retinal vasculitis showing progression in lesions over 2 months (F). (G) Patient with multifocal choroiditis and panuveitis, showing resolution of vitritis after 1 month of immunosuppressive drugs (H).

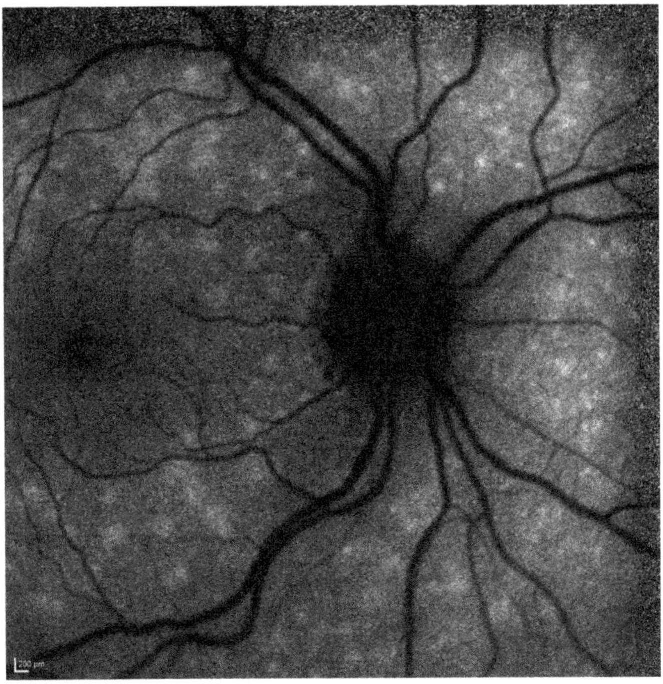

Figure 3.6. Blue autofluorescence in multiple evanescent white dot syndrome (MEWDS).

Increased RPE lipofuscin related to RPE dysfunction would result in hyperautofluorescence. In uveitis, FAF is mainly used to evaluate activity of inflammatory lesions such as in syphilitic retinitis, sarcoidosis panuveitis, Vogt-Koyanagi-Harada (VKH) and white dot syndromes (WDS) such as serpiginous choroidopathy (SC), multiple evanescent white dot syndrome (MEWDS) (Figure 3.6), punctate inner choroidopathy (PIC)/multifocal choroiditis (MFC) and panuveitis spectrum, BCR and acute zonal occult outer retinopathy (AZOOR).[4,5]

Active lesions generally show up as white hyperautofluorescent areas or have hyperautofluorescent borders, while inactive lesions show up as dark hypoautofluorescent lesions associated with RPE loss (Figure 3.7). Lesions which are healing can have mixed hyper- and hypoautofluorescence. Autoimmune retinopathy also typically has anomalies on fundus autofluorescence (Figure 3.8) and AZOOR typically shows the trizonal pattern[6] with autofluorescence anomalies corresponding to a visual field defect. Primary vitreoretinal lymphoma can show leopard skin-like changes[7] (Figure 3.9).

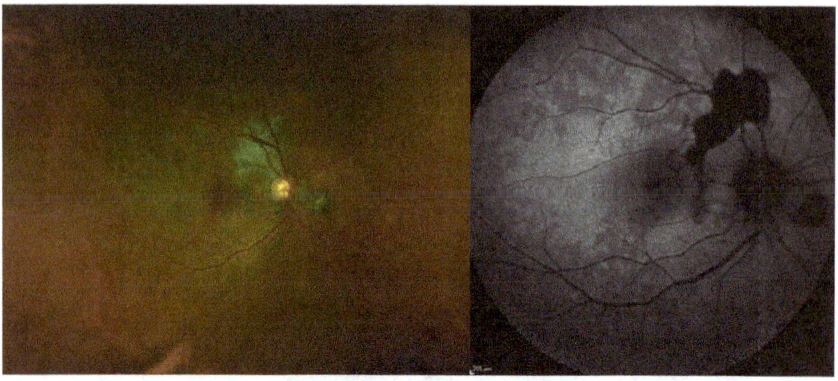

Figure 3.7. Optos fundus photo (left) and green fundus autofluorescence (right) of a patient with tuberculosis choroiditis. On FAF, hypoautofluorescent areas relate to an old scar and multifocal hyperautofluorescent lesions relate to active choroiditis.

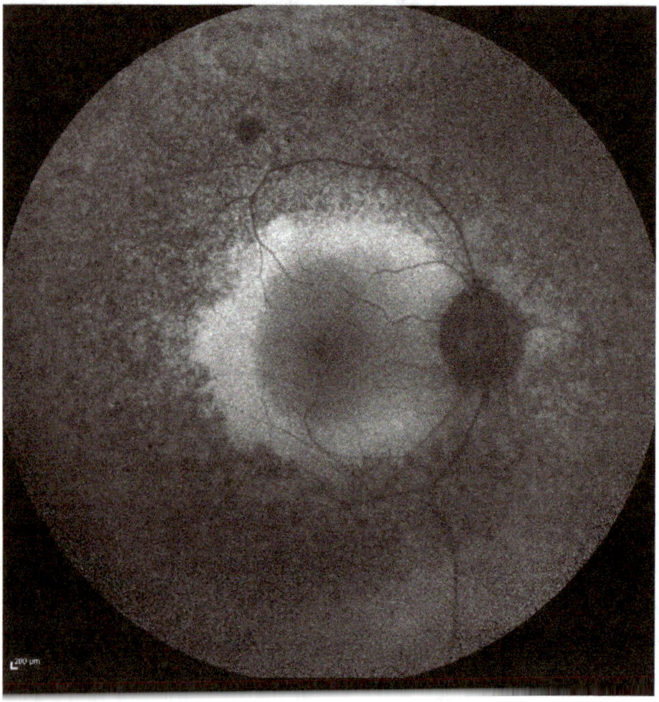

Figure 3.8. Autoimmune retinopathy is often associated with a ring of hyperautofluorescence in the macular area.

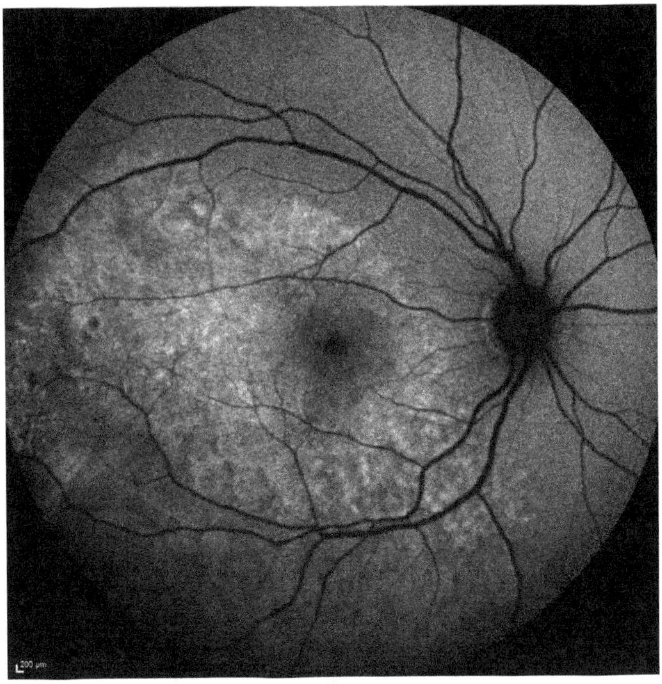

Figure 3.9. Primary intraocular lymphoma.

3.4 Fundus Fluorescein Angiography (FFA)

FFA was first described in 1961[8] and has a wide range of utility in patients with uveitis for diagnosis, monitoring for complications and assessing response to treatment.[9] Sodium fluorescein is injected intravenously, and the retinal fluorescence of unbound fluorescein molecules is captured in a series of images. This allows for the evaluation of the retinal circulation, perfusion and integrity of the blood-retinal barrier (BRB). Uveitis may affect tissues normally protected by the BRB, including retinitis, retinal vasculitis, retinochoroiditis and optic neuritis.[10]

Hyperfluorescence in FFA can occur due to leakage, staining, pooling or in window transmission defects.

Leakage is often an indication of ongoing inflammation and activity. A patient with active ocular inflammation may have optic disc leakage and diffuse capillary hyperpermeability described as capillary ferning (Figure 3.10). Leakage can also occur in retinal vasculitis (Figures 3.11 and

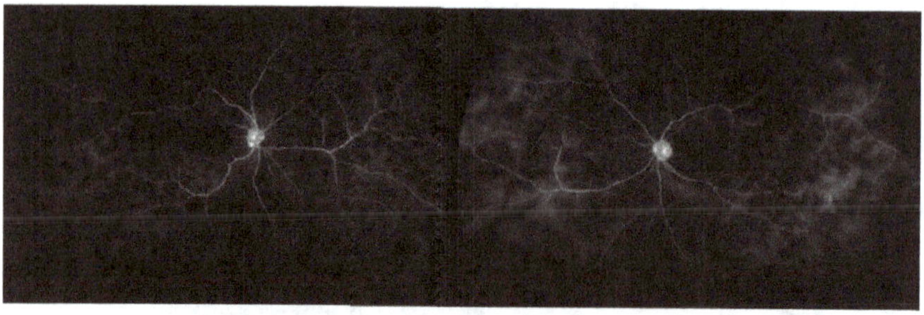

Figure 3.10. Fluorescein angiography showing diffuse capillary hyperpermeability or "ferning" in a patient with intermediate uveitis.

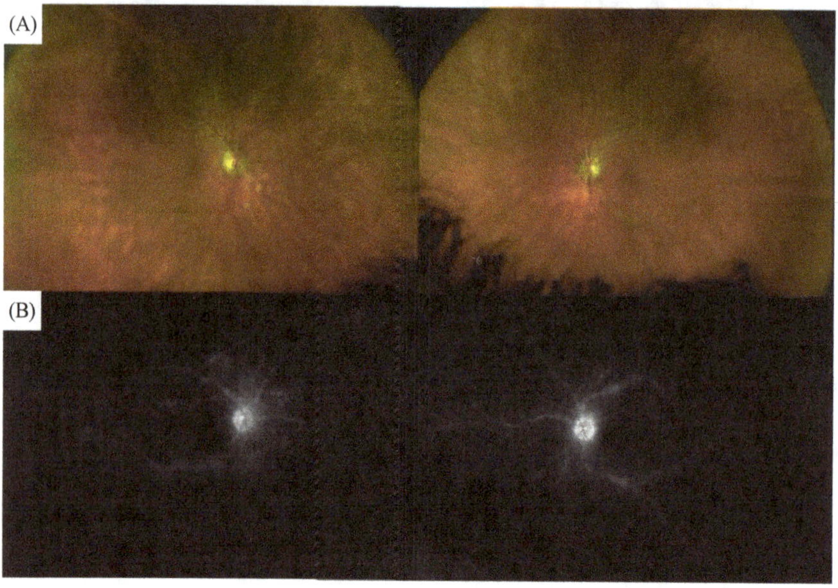

Figure 3.11. (A) Patient diagnosed with bilateral birdshot chorioretinitis with (B) disc leakage and retinal vasculitis on fluorescein angiography. Note dye leaking from the retinal vessels.

3.12), and FFA helps to differentiate active vasculitis with leakage from old inactive vascular sheathing. FFA is also useful for evaluating the development of uveitic complications such as secondary choroidal neovascularization and angiographic cystoid macula edema.

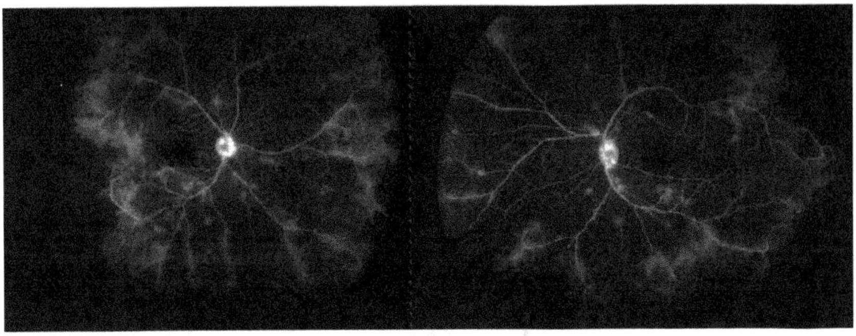

Figure 3.12. FFA of a patient with idiopathic retinitis, vasculitis, aneurysms and neuroretinitis (IRVAN) showing occlusive vasculitis and capillary non-perfusion.

Hypofluorescence can occur either due to a blocking effect or from filling defects. This is particularly useful in diagnosing patients with occlusive vasculitis, enabling the mapping out of areas of retinal ischemia. Occlusive vasculitis usually carries a poorer prognosis with a higher risk of complications secondary to ischemia and is associated with certain conditions such as Behçet's disease (Figure 3.13), systemic lupus erythematosus or tuberculosis (Figure 3.14), helping to narrow down the differential diagnosis.

In some patients where it may be difficult to assess for clinical response after initiation of treatment, it is helpful to assess for improvement on follow-up FFA. The presence of leakage may reveal ongoing inflammatory activity despite a relatively quiet clinical picture. Low-grade inflammation which is left untreated may lead to further complications such as chronic cystoid macula edema, resulting in loss of vision.

The increasing use of UWF FFA enables the evaluation and detection of very peripheral pathology that was previously not possible, including peripheral vasculitis, neovascularization and capillary non-perfusion (Figure 3.14).

3.5 Indocyanine Green Angiography (ICGA)

Indocyanine green is a larger molecule compared to fluorescein dye. It is largely protein bound and fluoresces at near-infrared wavelengths (806 nm). These properties allow for better imaging of the deeper choroidal

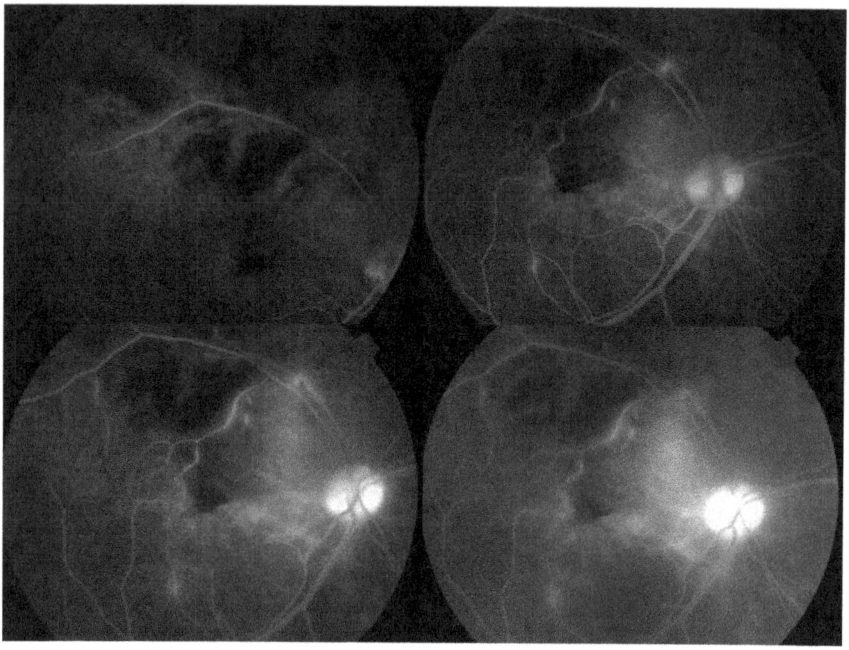

Figure 3.13. Fundus fluorescein angiogram of occlusive vasculitis in Behçet's disease.

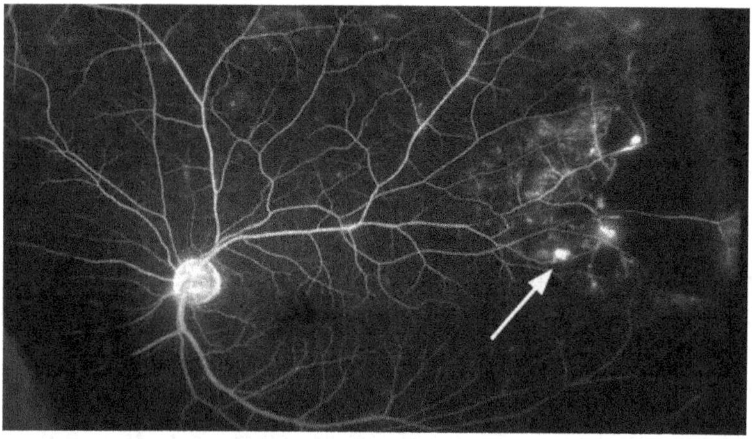

Figure 3.14. Fundus fluorescein angiography of occlusive vasculitis and neovascularization (arrow) due to tuberculosis.

vasculature, with images captured at the early, mid and late phases up to 10 minutes after injection of the dye.

The choroid is the starting point of many diseases in posterior uveitis. The features seen on ICGA can vary depending on the primary location of inflammation, and differentiation of these can help to clinch the diagnosis. ICGA can also detect subclinical disease otherwise undetected on fundal examination, help monitor progression and guide treatment.[11]

In primary inflammatory choriocapillaropathies (such as in white dot syndromes), choriocapillaris non-perfusion or hypoperfusion manifests as ICGA hypofluorescence. This may be more clearly visible on late frames and often corresponds to areas of hyperfluorescence on FFA.

Inflammatory (often granulomatous) foci may be present in the choroid, which will also appear as hypofluorescent spots on ICGA. The distribution of such foci may also be telling, being more evenly sized and regularly distributed in primary choroiditis such as VKH, sympathetic ophthalmia and BCR (Figures 3.15 and 3.16), compared to other conditions

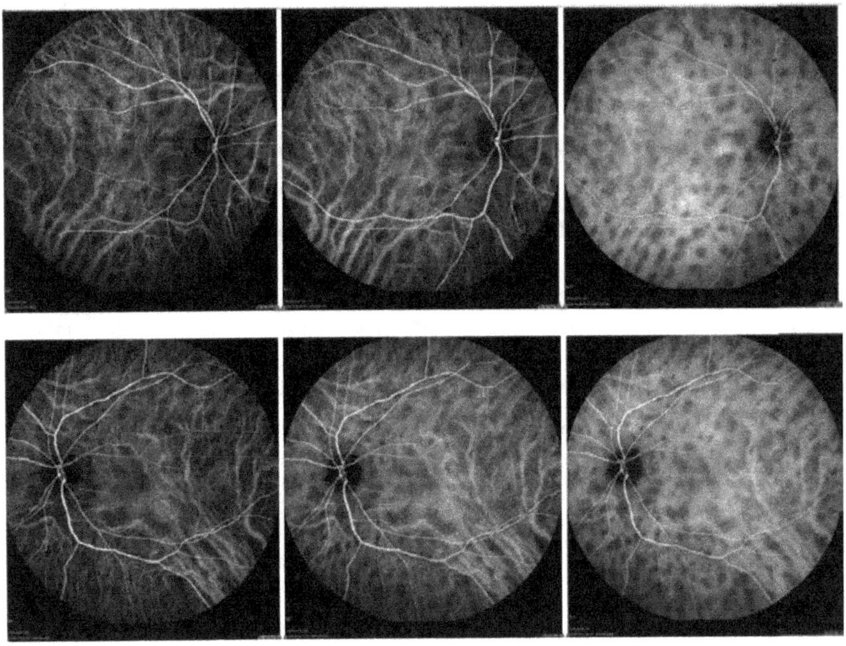

Figure 3.15. Patient with birdshot chorioretinitis, with ICGA captured at early, mid and late frames (top row right eye, bottom row left eye), revealing multiple hypofluorescent dark dots in the choroid representative of inflammatory foci, likely granulomas.

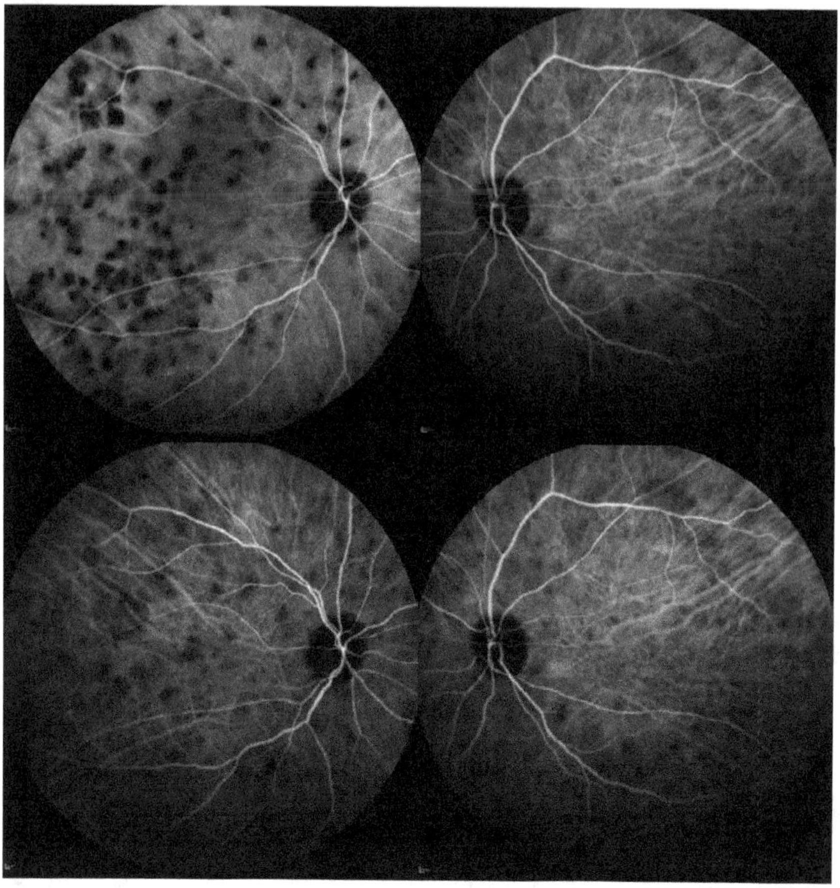

Figure 3.16. Top: VKH subclinical activity detected by ICGA. Immunosuppression therapy was adjusted. Bottom: ICGA was repeated 6 months later showing decreased activity.

that may also involve the choroid such as sarcoidosis (Figure 3.17) and tuberculosis. There may be an associated inflammation of the larger non-fenestrated stromal vessels appearing “fuzzy” in the intermediate phase followed by diffuse late choroidal hyperfluoresence.[12]

3.6 Optical Coherence Tomography (OCT)

The advent of time-domain OCT in 1991[13] revolutionized ophthalmology, allowing a non-invasive cross-sectional exam of the retina, where pathology

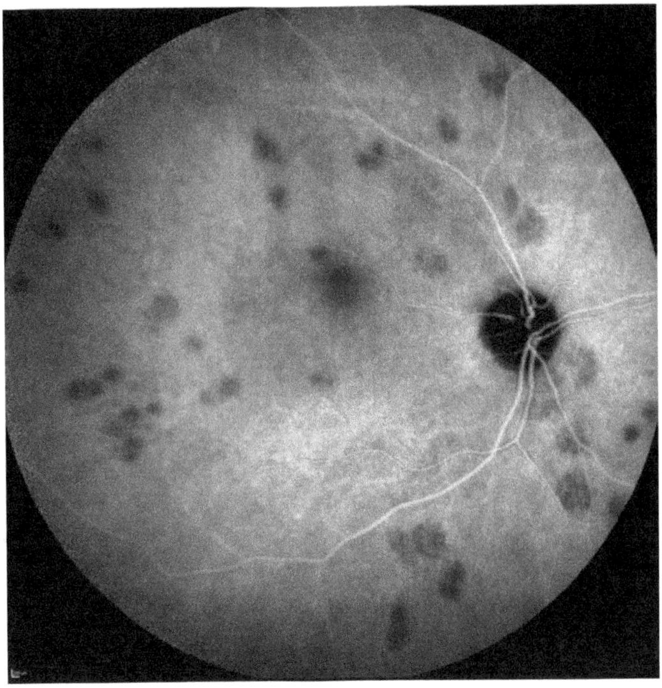

Figure 3.17. Indocyanine green angiography of choroidal granulomas in sarcoidosis.

which is previously difficult to see on fundal exam could be easily imaged. Today, two types of OCTs are commonly used, which are spectral-domain OCT[14] and swept-source OCT.[15]

In inflammatory conditions, OCT helps to evaluate and monitor retinal structural involvement (disruption, infiltration or atrophy of the inner, outer or entire retina) and is therefore a helpful diagnostic and monitoring tool in posterior uveitis for pathologies like toxoplasmosis chorioretinitis, sarcoid posterior uveitis, PIC/MFC, AZOOR or acute posterior multifocal placoid pigment epitheliopathy (APMPPE) (Figures 3.18 and 3.19).[12] OCT is very useful to ascertain the exact layer of the retina affected by the disease, and also provide objective evidence of resolution. Presence of vitritis may also be visible on the OCT. OCT is useful to detect and monitor complications of uveitis like cystoid macular edema (Figure 3.20), subretinal fluid related to inflammatory choroidal neovascular membrane (CNVM) (Figure 3.21) or central serous chorioretinopathy (CSCR), epiretinal membrane (ERM) and retinal atrophy.

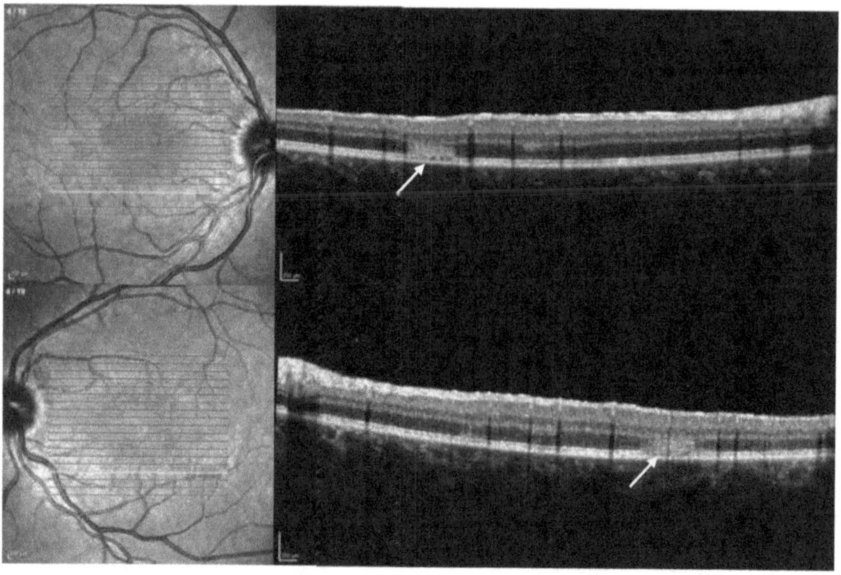

Figure 3.18. Patient with APMPPE and classical hyperreflective lesions of the outer retina (arrows).

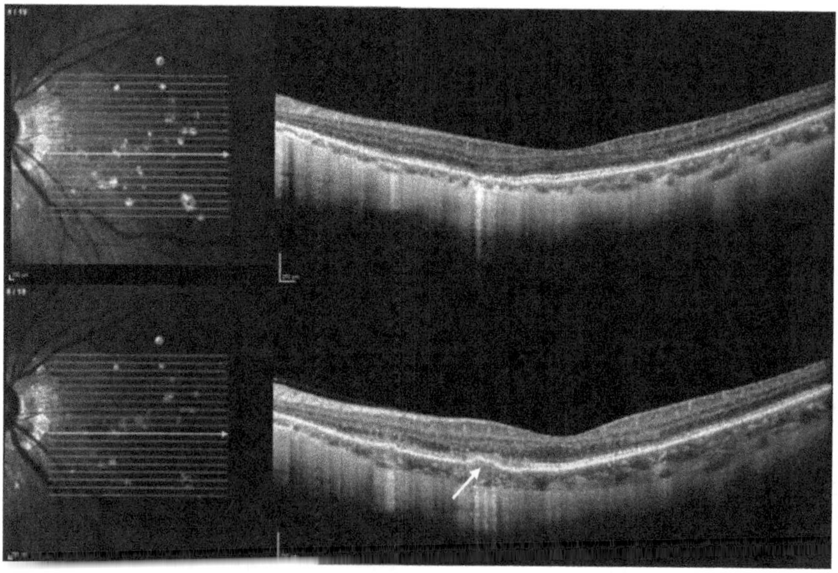

Figure 3.19. Patient with punctate inner choroiditis (top image), showing reactivation of PIC lesion 2 months later (bottom image, arrow).

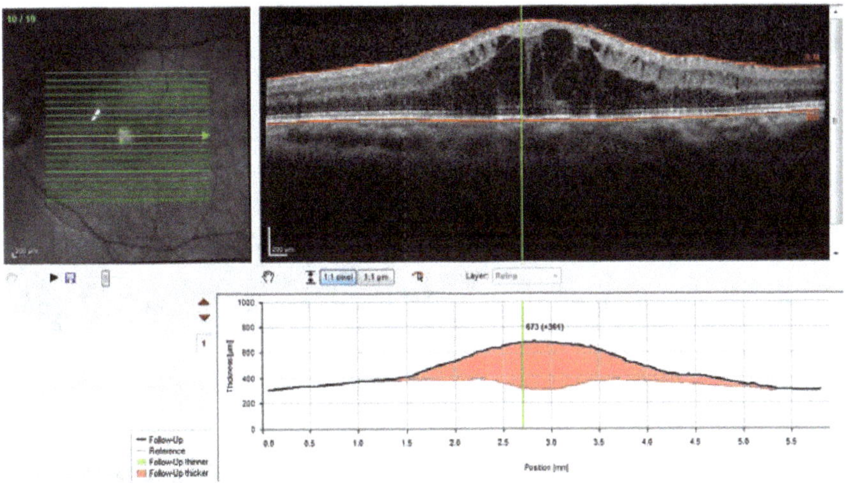

Figure 3.20. **Cystoid macular edema in a patient with HLA-B27 anterior uveitis.**

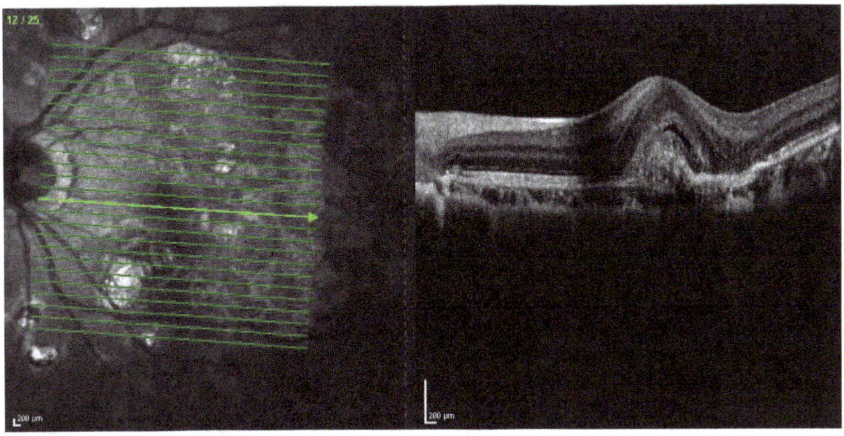

Figure 3.21. **Choroidal neovascular membrane in tuberculosis multifocal choroiditis.**

3.7 Enhanced Depth Imaging (EDI)-OCT

EDI-OCT is a modified technique of image acquisition to better see the choroid.[16] In uveitis, this is particularly helpful to evaluate choroidal thickness (Figure 3.22). In certain pathologies like VKH, sympathetic ophthalmia, BCR, sarcoidosis and tuberculosis, a thickened choroid is

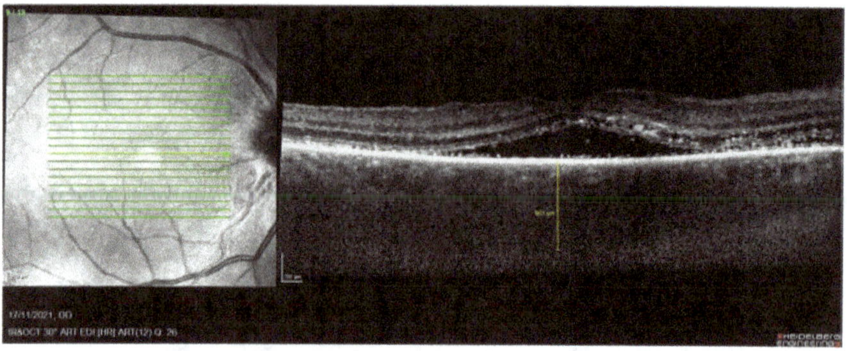

Figure 3.22. Patient with VKH showing an increased choroidal thickness of 600 μm in the right eye.

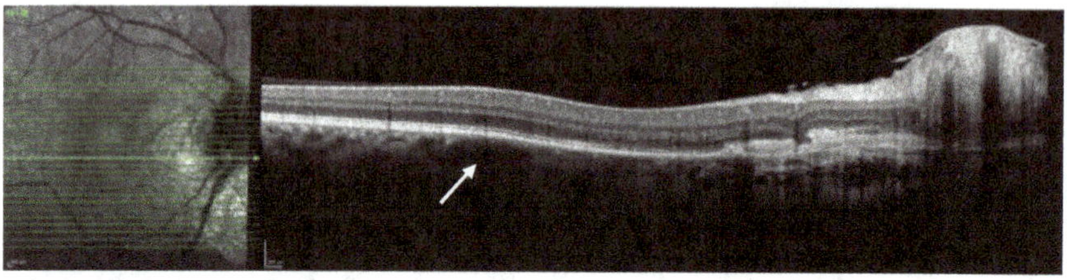

Figure 3.23. EDI-OCT enabling the visualization of a choroidal granuloma (arrow) in a patient with sarcoidosis uveitis.

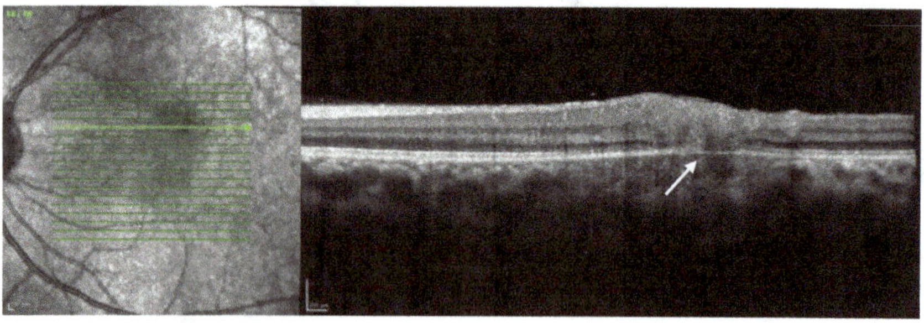

Figure 3.24. Left eye toxoplasmosis retinochoroiditis recurrence at an area of previous chorioretinal scar.

generally associated with active inflammation[17] and quiescent disease is generally associated with normal or thinned choroid. Choroidal lesions like granulomas can also sometimes be seen on EDI-OCT and allows for monitoring of disease activity or response to treatment[18] (Figures 3.23 and 3.24).

3.8 OCT-Angiography (OCT-A)

The first clinical studies using OCT-A were published in 2013.[19] This technology allows imaging of the microvasculature of the retina and the choroid without intravenous dye. The primary use in uveitis patients would be to evaluate for the presence of inflammatory CNVM, which may occur especially in patients with PIC or MFC[20] (Figure 3.25). It has several advantages over conventional fluorescein angiography including high spatial resolution (lateral resolution of 5.7 μm per pixel), shorter test time compared to FFA, non-invasive nature of the test, no obscuring of the signal by leakage from retinal blood vessels, and the ability to image non-exudative CNVM and differentiate them from inflammatory lesions. However, it is limited by the small area it can image (typically up to 20°×20°), it is unable to image peripheral retinal pathologies, it cannot demonstrate blood-retinal barrier disruption and leakage from inflamed vessels, it is very sensitive to movement artefacts, and it has a considerable acquisition time (several minutes). See Table 3.1 for a comparison of FFA and OCT-A.

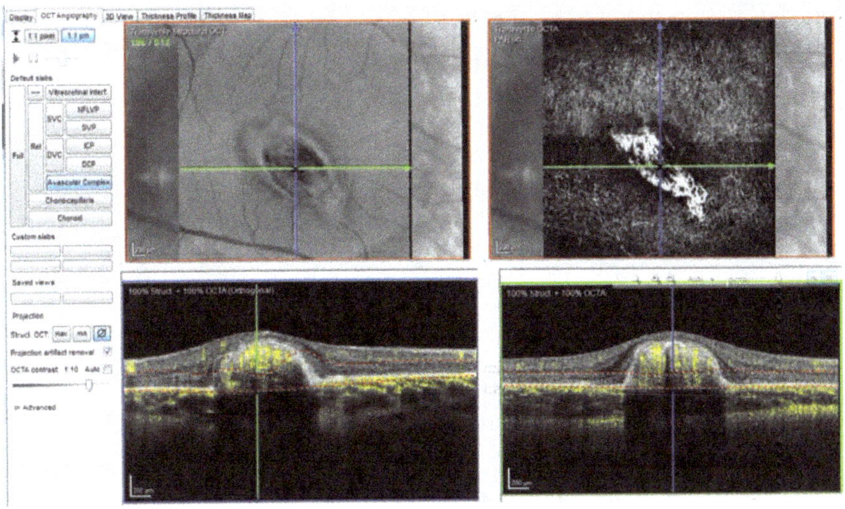

Figure 3.25. Non-exudative prominent inflammatory CNVM in a patient with PIC.

Table 3.1. Comparison between OCT-A and FFA.

	OCT-A	FFA
Resolution	High resolution demonstrating capillaries at different levels	Lower resolution
Non-invasive	+	–
Capillary non-perfusion	+	+
Vascular leakage	–	+
Distinguish between early CNVM and inflammatory lesion	+	–
Retinal periphery	–	+
Movement artefacts	++	+/–

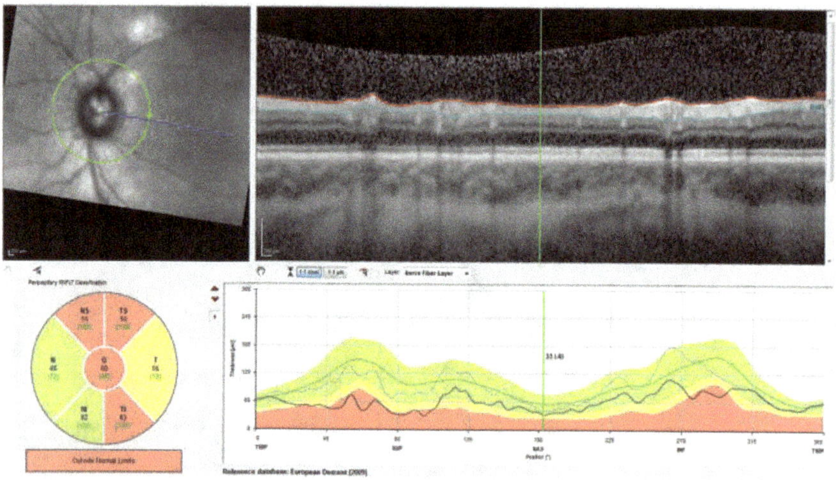

Figure 3.26. Uveitic glaucoma in a patient with chronic anterior uveitis.

3.9 OCT of the Retinal Nerve Fibre Layer (RNFL)

This imaging modality is useful in patients with uveitic glaucoma to diagnose and monitor progression of disease (Figure 3.26).[21] It is also useful in patients with optic nerve swelling related to inflammation to ascertain baseline measurements and to monitor its evolution (Figure 3.27).

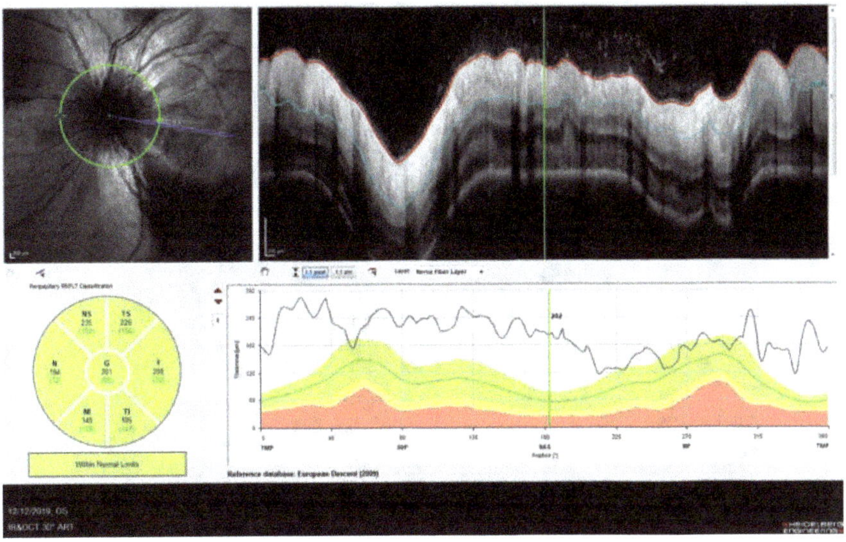

Figure 3.27. Optic nerve swelling in Vogt-Koyanagi-Harada syndrome.

Oftentimes an early recurrence of optic nerve swelling can be subtle on clinical examination but can be detected early using OCT RNFL.

3.10 Ophthalmic Ultrasound

B-scan ultrasound is useful to evaluate the posterior segment when there is no view on fundal exam, as with severe anterior uveitis or with significant media opacities. However, information given by the B-scan is limited. The main things that can be seen in the context of ocular inflammation are presence of vitritis, exudative retinal detachment (Figure 3.28), ocular masses and thickened choroid. For vitritis and choroidal thickening, we recommend comparing with the other eye if inflammation is unilateral because it is not always evident to determine if vitreous or choroid are abnormal on the B-scan. Another important purpose of the B-scan ultrasound is to evaluate for the presence of a T-sign (Figure 3.29), indicating fluid in the sub-Tenon's space in posterior scleritis.[22] Finally, B-scan can also be useful to rule out masquerades like retinoblastoma with a pseudo-hypopyon or dilated episcleral vessels caused by ciliary body melanoma (B-scan or ultrasound biomicroscopy).

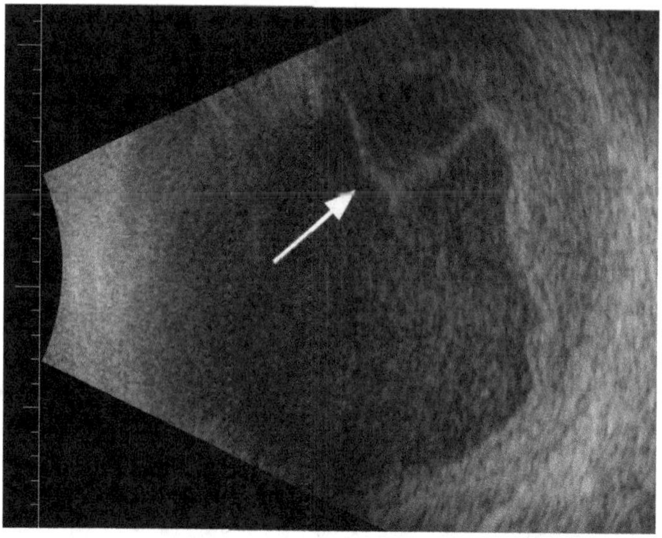

Figure 3.28. B-scan demonstrating vitritis and exudative retinal detachments (arrow) in panuveitis.

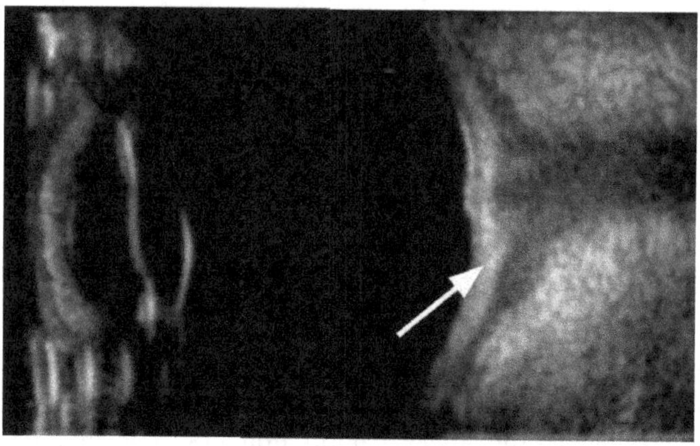

Figure 3.29. B-scan ultrasonography demonstrating T-sign (arrow).

Ultrasound biomicroscopy (UBM) is another type of ultrasound with higher frequency to image the anterior segment of the eye. Its use in uveitis is limited but it can be useful in suspected cases of uveitis-glaucoma-hyphema (UGH) syndrome to determine the position of the haptics of the

IOL or to evaluate the presence of ciliary processes fibrosis/membranes in uveitis patients with hypotonic eyes (see Chapter 11, Figure 11.4). It can also evaluate and monitor the extent of snowbanking in pars planitis.

3.11 Multimodal Imaging

Armed with a wide-ranging number of imaging modalities available to the ophthalmologist, each with its own utility, the practice of multimodal imaging has become commonplace. It is described as an approach to diagnose disease by combining different imaging modalities. Each test provides specific information, and the combination of these information allows for the development of an accurate compositive picture. This is helpful for diagnosis and monitoring (Figure 3.30). For example, in punctate inner choroidopathy, serial fundus photography is very useful to monitor for new lesions, while both OCT and FAF are useful to look for signs of activity.

In conclusion, access to a wide range of imaging modalities greatly enhances the ability to effectively diagnose a patient with uveitis, accurately

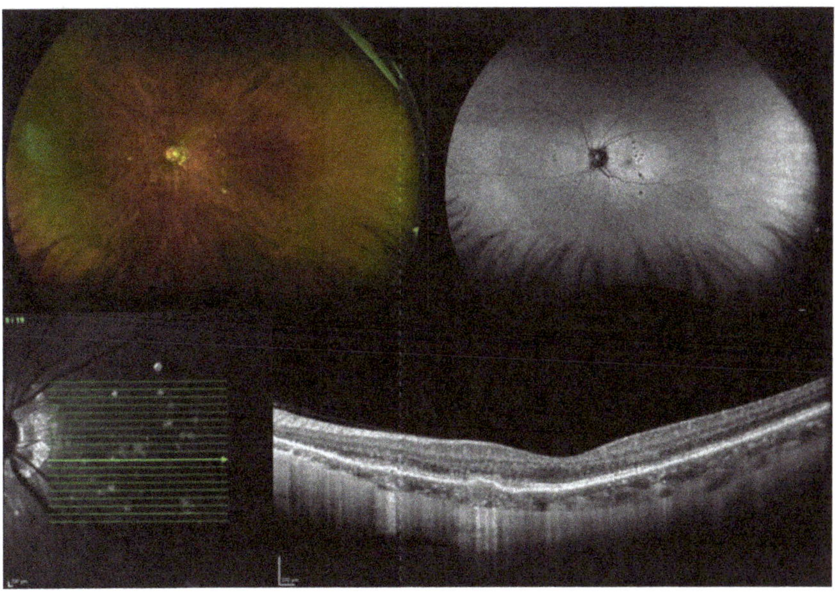

Figure 3.30. Multimodal imaging used in the evaluation of punctate inner choroiditis.

monitor progression, and allows for early detection of recurrences and complications.

Teaching Points

- Ultra-widefield imaging is very useful in uveitis to visualize the entire retina and choroid and demonstrate peripheral disease. It also facilitates easy objective comparison with previous visits.
- Fundus autofluorescence can be used to monitor the activity and progression of inflammatory lesions in uveitis. Changes in lesion size and areas of hyperautofluorescence suggest active disease.
- Fundus fluorescein angiography and particularly ultra-widefield studies provide valuable information regarding maculopathy, peripheral retinal disease, vasculitis and areas of retinal ischemia. Repeat studies are used to determine response to treatment.
- Indocyanine green angiography captures more detailed images of the choroidal vasculature. It is valuable in the diagnosis of choroiditis and cases of posterior uveitis like birdshot chorioretinitis, where it demonstrates more widespread lesions than can be seen on fluorescein.
- OCT is used for identifying the specific retinal layer affected by the disease, maculopathies like macular edema, epiretinal membranes and macular scarring. It is also very useful for monitoring progression or resolution. OCT angiography is useful for early detection of inflammatory CNVM.

References

1. Patel SN, Shi A, Wibbelsman TD, Klufas MA. Ultra-widefield retinal imaging: an update on recent advances. *Ther Adv Ophthalmol* 2020;12: 2515841419899495.
2. Delori FC, Dorey CK, Staurenghi G, Arend O, Goger DG, Weiter JJ. In vivo fluorescence of the ocular fundus exhibits retinal pigment epithelium lipofuscin characteristics. *Invest Ophthalmol Vis Sci* 1995;36(3):718–29.
3. Bittencourt MG, Hassan M, Halim MS, *et al.* Blue light versus green light fundus autofluorescence in normal subjects and in patients with retinochoroidopathy secondary to retinal and uveitic diseases. *J Ophthalmic Inflamm Infect* 2019;9(1):1.

4. Meleth AD, Sen HN. Use of fundus autofluorescence in the diagnosis and management of uveitis. *Int Ophthalmol Clin* 2012;52(4):45–54.
5. Samy A, Lightman S, Ismetova F, Talat L, Tomkins-Netzer O. Role of autofluorescence in inflammatory/infective diseases of the retina and choroid. *J Ophthalmol* 2014;2014:418193.
6. Mrejen S, Khan S, Gallego-Pinazo R, Jampol LM, Yannuzzi LA. Acute zonal occult outer retinopathy: a classification based on multimodal imaging. *JAMA Ophthalmol* 2014;132(9):1089–98.
7. Casady M, Faia L, Nazemzadeh M, Nussenblatt R, Chan CC, Sen HN. Fundus autofluorescence patterns in primary intraocular lymphoma. *Retina* 2014;34(2):366–72.
8. Novotny HR, Alvis DL. A method of photographing fluorescence in circulating blood in the human retina. *Circulation* 1961;24:82–6.
9. Campbell JP, Leder HA, Sepah YJ, *et al.* Wide-field retinal imaging in the management of noninfectious posterior uveitis. *Am J Ophthalmol* 2012;154(5):908–11.e2.
10. Forrester JV, Kuffova L, Dick AD. Autoimmunity, autoinflammation, and infection in uveitis. *Am J Ophthalmol* 2018;189:77–85.
11. Herbort C. Fluorescein and indocyanine green angiography for uveitis. *Middle East Afr J Ophthalmol* 2009;16(4):168–87.
12. Thomas AS, Lin P. Multimodal imaging in infectious and noninfectious intermediate, posterior and panuveitis. *Curr Opin Ophthalmol* 2021;32(3):169–82.
13. Huang D, Swanson EA, Lin CP, *et al.* Optical coherence tomography. *Science* 1991;254(5035):1178–81.
14. Wojtkowski M, Bajraszewski T, Gorczy. ska I, *et al.* Ophthalmic imaging by spectral optical coherence tomography. *Am J Ophthalmol* 2004;138(3):412–9.
15. Adhi M, Liu JJ, Qavi AH, *et al.* Choroidal analysis in healthy eyes using swept-source optical coherence tomography compared to spectral domain optical coherence tomography. *Am J Ophthalmol* 2014;157(6):1272–81.e1.
16. Spaide RF, Koizumi H, Pozzoni MC. Enhanced depth imaging spectral-domain optical coherence tomography. *Am J Ophthalmol* 2008;146(4):496–500.
17. Nakayama M, Keino H, Okada AA, *et al.* Enhanced depth imaging optical coherence tomography of the choroid in Vogt-Koyanagi-Harada disease. *Retina* 2012;32(10):2061–9.
18. Invernizzi A, Agarwal A, Mapelli C, Nguyen QD, Staurenghi G, Viola F. Longitudinal follow-up of choroidal granulomas using enhanced depth imaging optical coherence tomography. *Retina* 2017;37(1):144–53.

19. Kim DY, Fingler J, Zawadzki RJ, *et al.* Optical imaging of the chorioretinal vasculature in the living human eye. *Proc Natl Acad Sci USA* 2013;110(35): 14354–9.
20. Niederer RL, Gilbert R, Lightman S, Tomkins-Netzer O. Risk factors for developing choroidal neovascular membrane and visual loss in punctate inner choroidopathy. *Ophthalmology* 2018;125(2):288–94.
21. Din NM, Talat L, Isa H, Tomkins-Netzer O, Barton K, Lightman S. Difference in glaucoma progression between the first and second eye after consecutive bilateral glaucoma surgery in patients with bilateral uveitic glaucoma. *Graefes Arch Clin Exp Ophthalmol* 2016;254(12):2439–48.
22. Rochels R, Reis G. [Echography in posterior scleritis (author's transl)]. *Klin Monbl Augenheilkd* 1980;177(5):611–3.

https://doi.org/10.1142/9789811251474_0004

Chapter 4 Systemic Investigations in Uveitis

*Lazha Sharief**

Uveitis can be associated with a diverse range of systemic infectious, non-infectious or masquerade conditions. Occasionally uveitis is the first presenting symptom indicating a systemic disorder, including life-threatening conditions. A systematic approach to identifying such connections can optimize the uveitis treatment, as well as lead to systemic diagnoses and prevention of further morbidity. While the diagnosis of uveitis is primarily based on clinical symptoms and signs, the utilization of systemic investigations can provide indispensable support for the diagnosis of possible etiologic conditions.

Arranging for specific systemic investigations is based on correlations between ocular findings and specific systemic diseases.[1] Ordering a wide range of tests in the hope that they provide some guidance to a diagnosis results in many cases in very low specificity without advancing clinical management. The positive predictive value of the angiotensin-converting enzyme (ACE), when used as a routine screening in any case of uveitis, is only 18%.[2] Recognising correlations between clinical findings and possible systemic diseases is the basis for conducting focused investigations, increasing the likelihood of a meaningful result and establishing a firm diagnosis.

Systemic investigations should be based on the type and characteristics of uveitis, the patient ocular and medical history as well as geographic and environmental factors. Unilateral uveitis can be associated with an underlying infectious disease such as herpes simplex virus, varicella zoster virus, *Toxocara canis* or *Toxoplasma gondii*, but can also be associated with non-infectious diseases such as HLA-B27-associated uveitis. The presence of non-ocular signs also aids in directing the type of investigations ordered:

*Ophthalmology Department, King's College Hospital NHS Foundation Trust, London, UK

uveitis associated with a palmar or plantar rash may indicate disease secondary to syphilis; musculoskeletal signs such as chronic joint pain may direct us toward ordering tests to rule out arthritis; respiratory symptoms, mainly chronic cough, may indicate testing for tuberculosis or sarcoidosis.

The Standardization of Uveitis Nomenclature (SUN) project developed specific criteria for the diagnosis and description of 26 common uveitis entities (see Chapter 1, Table 1.5).[3–27] These are based on combinations of clinical signs and ancillary tests. A practical approach to arranging systemic investigations for uveitis is according to the SUN anatomical classification of uveitis and uveitis characteristics (Table 4.1).

Table 4.1. Systemic screening workout for uveitis patients based on SUN anatomical classification and characteristics of uveitis.

Uveitis SUN classification	Uveitis characteristics	Blood test workup	Additional investigations if indicated
Anterior uveitis	Unilateral Non-granulomatous	HLA-B27, syphilis serology	—
	Bilateral recurrent/ chronic Non-granulomatous	Syphilis serology, ACE/ lysozyme, RFT, IGRA, PPD	If RFT abnormal, then order urine β-microglobulin
	Granulomatous	Syphilis serology, ACE/ lysozyme, IGRA, PPD, LFT	CXR +/– CT scan Lyme ELISA
	Children (<16 years old)	RF, ANA, HLA-B27, ACE/ lysozyme, IGRA, PPD	+/– CXR
Intermediate uveitis	With neurological manifestations	CBC, LFT, RFT, syphilis serology, ACE/lysozyme	CXR, consider referring to neurologist for brain MRI and to rule out demyelinating diseases
	Lack neurological manifestations	CBC, LFT, RFT, syphilis serology, ACE/ lysozyme, IGRA, PPD, HLA-B27	CXR
Posterior/ panuveitis	Mainly retinitis	CBC, CRP, LFT, RFT, syphilis serology, toxoplasmosis ELISA, IGRA, PPD, HIV	CT scan brain in HIV with toxoplasmosis If Behçet's disease suspected, refer to rheumatologist for investigation

Table 4.1. (*Continued*)

Uveitis SUN classification	Uveitis characteristics	Blood test workup	Additional investigations if indicated
	Mainly multifocal choroiditis	CBC, CRP/ESR, LFT, RFT, syphilis serology, IGRA, PPD, ACE/lysozyme, HLA-A29	CXR ± CT scan
	Choroidal granuloma	CBC, CRP/ESR, LFT, RFT, IGRA, PPD, ACE/ lysozyme, Toxocara serology (unilateral cases)	CXR ± CT scan
Papillitis		CBC, CRP/ESR, syphilis serology, ACE/ lysozyme, toxoplasmosis ELISA, Bartonella ELISA or IFA, IGRA, PPD	Lyme ELISA, consider brain MRI
Retinal vasculitis		CBC, CRP/ESR, IGRA, PPD, syphilis serology, ACE/lysozyme, ANCA, anti-dsDNA Abs, anticardiolipin Abs	CXR

Ab = antibodies; ACE = angiotensin-converting enzyme; ANA = anti-nuclear antibody; CBC = complete blood count; CRP = C-reactive protein; CT = computed tomography; CXR = chest X-ray; dsDNA = double-stranded deoxyribonucleic acid; ELISA = enzyme-linked immunosorbent assay; ESR = erythrocyte sedimentation rate; HIV = human immunodeficiency virus; HLA = human leukocyte antigen; IFA = immunofluorescence assay; IGRA = interferon-gamma release assay; LFT = liver function test; PPD = purified protein derivative (a type of tuberculin skin test); RF = rheumatic factor; RFT = renal function test

4.1 Anterior Uveitis

Anterior uveitis (AU) is the most common form of uveitis and accounts for up to half of the cases,[1] with two-thirds idiopathic. For most cases of first episode of acute, unilateral AU, systemic investigations are not warranted, as they are non-specific and seldom lead to a clear etiology.[28] In cases of recurrent, chronic, bilateral AU, or in the presence of additional signs, systemic investigations are used. Around 25% of AU cases can be associated with a systemic condition that warrants a further investigation.

4.1.1 Tests for HLA-B27-Associated Diseases

HLA-B27-associated acute AU is the most common systemic association with anterior uveitis.[29] Testing for the HLA-B27 serotype is indicated in patients presenting with AU, especially when characterized as being unilateral, non granulomatous, severe, painful with or without anterior chamber fibrin, hypopyon and synechiae (Figure 4.1). The diagnosis of HLA-B27-associated uveitis aids in establishing the ocular prognosis and increases patient awareness regarding relapses. It also raises patient awareness of the risk of systemic manifestations that can be associated with the HLA-B27 serotype, including inflammatory bowel disease, psoriasis, reactive arthritis and the 50% probability of developing spondyloarthropathy during a patient's lifetime.[30]

4.1.2 Tests for Sarcoidosis

Granulomatous uveitis should raise suspicion of an underlying systemic granulomatous disease, such as sarcoidosis. According to the International Workshop on Ocular Sarcoidosis (IWOC) which set the international criteria for the diagnosis of ocular sarcoidosis, a combination of laboratory

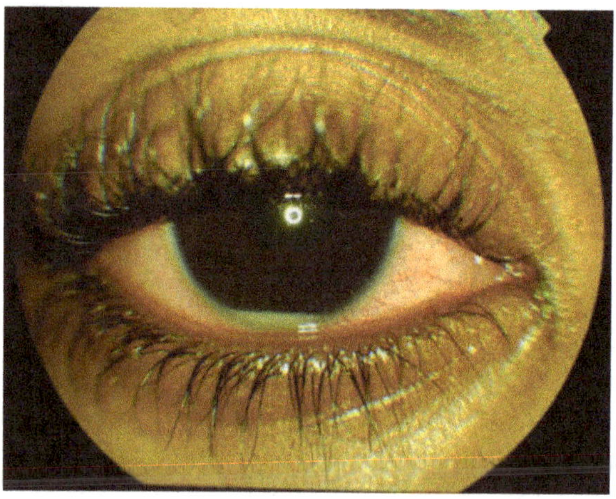

Figure 4.1. Anterior uveitis in a patient with HLA-B27-associated uveitis. Note the conjunctival hyperemia and hypopyon.

and systemic imaging studies are used together with specific ocular findings to diagnose ocular sarcoidosis (Table 4.2).[31,32] A normal chest X-ray does not rule out sarcoidosis due to low sensitivity and in the presence of a high clinical suspicion (Figure 4.2),[33] the ophthalmologist should consider

Table 4.2. International Workshop on Ocular Sarcoidosis revised diagnostic criteria.

Clinical signs

1. Mutton-fat keratic precipitates (large and small) and/or iris nodules at pupillary margin (Koeppe) or in stroma (Busacca).
2. Trabecular meshwork nodules and/or tent-shaped peripheral anterior synechia.
3. Snowballs/string of pearls vitreous opacities.
4. Multiple chorioretinal peripheral lesions (active and/or atrophic).
5. Nodular and/or segmental periphlebitis (± candlewax drippings) and/or retinal macroaneurysm in an inflamed eye.
6. Optic disc nodule(s)/granulomas and/or solitary choroidal nodule.
7. Bilaterality.

Systemic investigations

1. Bilateral hilar lymphadenopathy (BHL) by chest X-ray and/or chest-computed CT scan.
2. Negative tuberculin test or interferon-gamma releasing assays.
3. Elevated serum ACE.
4. Elevated serum lysozyme.
5. Elevated CD4/CD8 ratio (>3.5) in bronchoalveolar lavage fluid.
6. Abnormal accumulation of gallium-67 scintigraphy or 18F-fluorodeoxyglucose positron emission tomography imaging.
7. Lymphopenia.
8. Parenchymal lung changes consistent with sarcoidosis, as determined by pulmonologists or radiologists.

Diagnostic criteria

Definite: diagnosis supported by biopsy with compatible uveitis.

Presumed: diagnosis not supported by biopsy, but BHL present with two intraocular signs.

Probable: diagnosis not supported by biopsy and BHL absent, but three intraocular signs and two systemic investigations (selected from two to eight above) are present.

Adapted from Mochizuki M, Smith JR, Takase H, *et al.* Revised criteria of International Workshop on Ocular Sarcoidosis (IWOS) for the diagnosis of ocular sarcoidosis. Br J Ophthalmol 2019;103(10): 1418–22.[32]

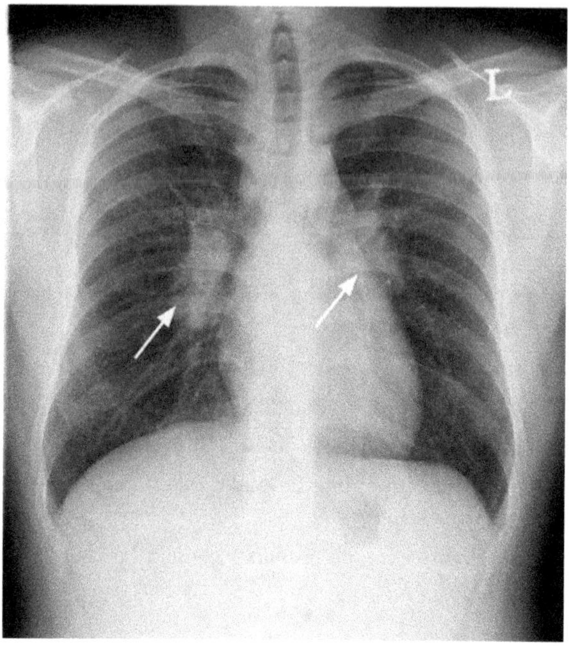

Figure 4.2. **Chest X-ray with bilateral hilar lymphadenopathy (arrows).**

referring for a high-resolution computed tomography (CT) chest scan with gallium and possible biopsy (Figure 4.3).

Serum ACE level are elevated in 50–80% of patients with sarcoidosis, with serum levels >65 IU/L suggestive of active sarcoidosis.[34] However, the serum ACE level should not be used as the only means to establish a diagnosis and should be interpreted together with clinical findings. In a large cohort study involving 1,035 subjects with uveitis an elevated ACE level (>65 IU/L) was found in approximately 19% of cases, but less than half of these cases were eventually considered to have sarcoidosis, resulting in a true positive rate of 77%.[35] The test had a sensitivity of 78% with a specificity of 90%, with a high negative predictive value of 97%. Lymphopenia occurs in up to 50% of patients with sarcoidosis and is associated with chronic disease. Based on the ocular signs and systemic investigations (Table 4.2) the revised IWOC suggested three levels of certainty for the diagnosis of ocular sarcoidosis: (1) Definite ocular sarcoidosis; (2) Presumed ocular sarcoidosis; (3) Probable ocular sarcoidosis.[32]

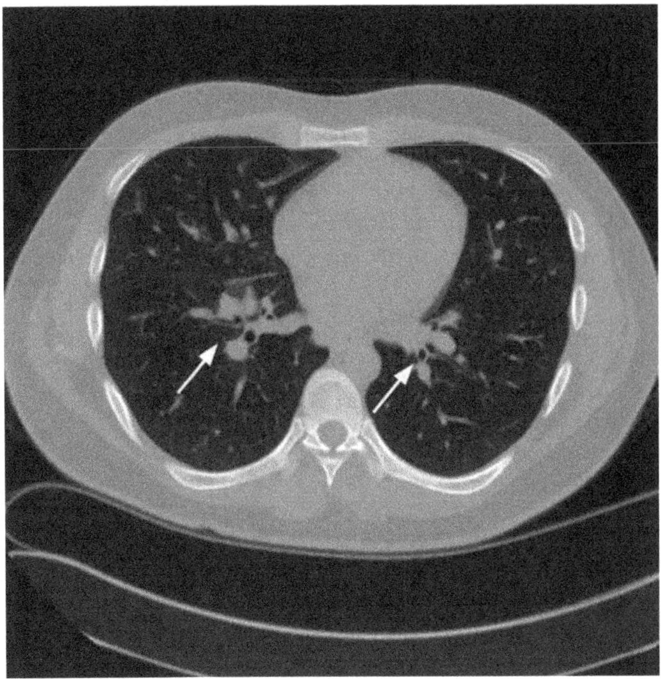

Figure 4.3. **High-resolution CT demonstrating bilateral hilar lymphadenopathy (arrows).**

4.1.3 *Tests for Treponema Pallidum*

In cases presenting with recurrent or chronic AU, serology testing for *Treponema pallidum* is indicated. Testing should also be considered in the presence of risk factors for syphilis, or if there is presence of rash over palms and soles. The two types of antibody-based serology assays used in the diagnosis of syphilis infection are non-treponemal and treponemal tests. The non-treponemal tests include Rapid Plasma Reagin (RPR) and the Venereal Disease Research Laboratory (VDRL) tests. These tests have the advantage of reflecting disease activity and response to treatment, but with the disadvantage of having low sensitivity to syphilis.[36] Treponemal tests have the advantage of being highly sensitive as well as specific to syphilis. Examples of treponemal tests include Fluorescent Treponemal Antibody Absorption (FTA-ABS), *Treponema pallidum* particle agglutination (TPPA), and *Treponema pallidum* hemagglutination (TPHA). One should also consider the small possibility of false positive results which may occur

Table 4.3. SUN classification criteria for syphilitic uveitis.

Criteria: 1 and 2

1. Uveitis with a compatible uveitic presentation, including
   a. Anterior uveitis **OR**
   b. Intermediate uveitis or anterior/intermediate uveitis **OR**
   c. Posterior uveitis or panuveitis with 1 of the following presentations:
      i. Placoid inflammation of the retinal pigment epithelium **OR**
      ii. Multifocal inflammation of the retina/retinal pigment epithelium **OR**
      iii. Necrotizing retinitis **OR**
      iv. Retinal vasculitis

AND

2. Evidence of infection with *Treponema pallidum*, either
   a. Positive treponemal test and nontreponemal test **OR**
   b. Positive treponemal test with 2 different treponemal tests

Exclusions:

1. History of adequate treatment for syphilitic uveitis

Adapted from The Standardization of Uveitis Nomenclature (SUN) Working Group. Classification criteria for syphilitic uveitis. Am J Ophthalmol 2021;228:182–91.[9]

in older patients or with underlying collagen vascular diseases such as rheumatoid arthritis or systemic lupus erythematosus, or in subjects from tropical regions a non-specific positive test due to previous Yaws infection.[37] When a patient is positive for syphilis, additional testing for human immune deficiency virus (HIV) infection should follow as they are often associated. A referral to an infectious disease specialist or sexually transmitted disease clinic should also be arranged for further investigations to rule out neurological syphilis as well as testing for other sexually transmitted infections. The SUN criteria incorporated treponemal and non-treponemal tests into the diagnostic criteria for syphilitic uveitis (Table 4.3).[9]

4.1.4 *Tests for Mycobacterium Tuberculosis*

In cases of chronic AU (particularly granulomatous), or if posterior involvement is seen, testing for previous exposure to *Mycobacterium tuberculosis* (TB) may be required. Tests include chest X-ray to rule out pulmonary lesions (Figure 4.4) and direct TB tests, such as Interferon-Gamma Release Assays (IGRA-QuantiFERON TB gold and T-SPOT tests) or the tuberculin skin test (PPD) test. These tests may even be considered during initial workup assessment if the uveitis patient resides or travelled to TB-endemic

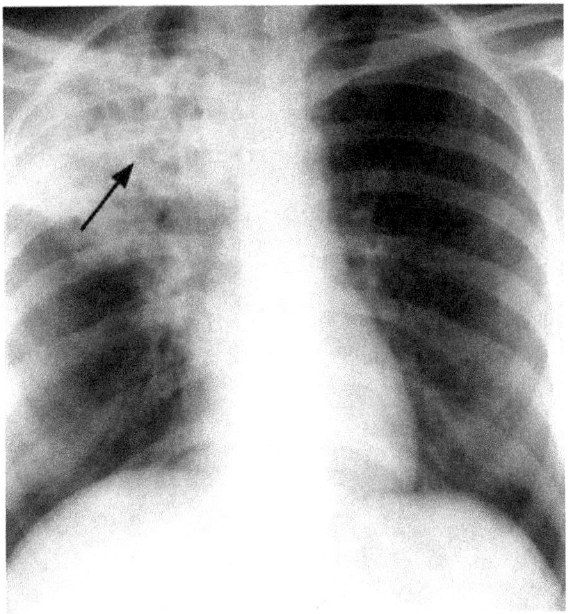

Figure 4.4. **Chest X-ray of patient with tuberculosis demonstrating consolidation in the upper right lobe (arrow).**

regions or has a known contact history with an active TB patient. While there is no significant difference in the sensitivity of the tests in detecting TB exposure, the IGRA tests are more specific with a lower false-positive rate when testing patients previously immunized with the Bacillus Calmette-Guérin (BCG) vaccine.[38,39] The SUN criteria included IGRA and PPD tests in the diagnostic criteria for tubercular uveitis (Table 4.4).

4.1.5 *Tests for Borrelia Burgdorferi*

Lyme disease can be associated with any form of uveitis, including severe granulomatous AU. The disease has a variable prevalence and is more common in northwestern states of the USA and Canada, as well as most of Europe. Because of its variable presentation, serology testing is based more on geographic location and less on specific signs and symptoms, with testing in regions of low disease prevalence limited to patients with a high clinical suspicion, such as a history of tick bite. The presence of cutaneous erythema chronicum migrans in a patient with uveitis can be considered diagnostic

Table 4.4. SUN classification criteria for tubercular uveitis.

Criteria: 1 and 2

1. Evidence of a tubercular uveitis compatible uveitic syndrome
   a. Anterior uveitis with iris nodules
   b. Serpiginous-like tubercular choroiditis
   c. Choroidal nodule (i.e., tuberculoma)
   d. In individuals with active systemic tuberculosis, multifocal choroiditis
   e. Occlusive retinal vasculitis

AND

2. Evidence of infection with *Mycobacterium tuberculosis*, either
   a. Histologically or microbiologically confirmed infection with *Mycobacterium tuberculosis*[a] **OR**
   b. Positive IGRA[b] **OR**
   c. Positive tuberculin skin test[c]

Exclusions:

1. Positive serology for syphilis using a treponemal test
2. Positive biopsy for sarcoidosis (and therefore an absence of histologic or microbiologic confirmation of infection with *Mycobacterium tuberculosis*)
3. Uveitic syndrome compatible with either sarcoidosis-associated uveitis or tubercular uveitis, and bilateral hilar adenopathy on chest imaging without histologic or microbiologic confirmation of the diagnosis of infection with *Mycobacterium tuberculosis*[d]

IGRA = interferon-gamma release assay.

[a]For example, biopsy, fluorochrome stain, culture, or polymerase chain reaction-based assay.

[b]For example, QuantiFERON gold or T-spot.

[c]For example, purified protein derivative skin test; a positive result should be >10 mm in duration. However, a positive skin test and a negative IGRA should be taken as evidence of atypical mycobacterial infection and not tuberculosis.

[d]In patients with a uveitic syndrome compatible either with sarcoidosis-associated uveitis or with tubercular uveitis, bilateral hilar adenopathy, and evidence of latent tuberculosis (e.g., positive tuberculin skin test or IGRA), the classification requires histologic or microbiologic confirmation of the diagnosis (i.e., classification cannot be made without such confirmation).

Adapted from The Standardization of Uveitis Nomenclature (SUN) Working Group. Classification criteria for tubercular uveitis. Am J Ophthalmol 2021;228:142–51.[14]

for Lyme disease. However, in the absence of this cutaneous sign, laboratory criteria for the diagnosis of Lyme disease are used, which consist of isolating *Borrelia burgdorferi* from tissue biopsies (mainly skin) or a positive serum serology test to *Borrelia burgdorferi.* During the acute stage of the disease the serology test may be negative as it takes around 2 weeks for IgM to become positive, with peak levels at 2 months. Therefore, repeating the test a few weeks after the initial presentation is recommended when clinical suspicion is high. Once positive, IgG and IgM response may persist for months to years.[40] In cases with positive IgM and/or IgG, a positive Western blot test is required to confirm the diagnosis of underlying Lyme disease.

4.1.6 *Pediatric Uveitis Tests*

For children under the age of 16 who present with AU, standard testing includes antinuclear antibody (ANA) and HLA-B27. These help in the early diagnosis of juvenile idiopathic arthritis (JIA-ANA test) or seropositive arthropathies (HLA-B27), both of which can present as uveitis. AU affects up to 20% of JIA patients and over a third of ankylosing spondylitis patients.[41–44] Early diagnosis can lead to disease control and prevention of developing systemic complications.

Tubulointerstitial nephritis and uveitis (TINU) is a rare cause of AU, more prevalent in children, accounting for <0.1% to 2% of uveitis cases.[45] The SUN Working Group suggested diagnostic criteria for TINU to include the presence of AU, with or without an associated vitritis, choroiditis or retinal vasculitis, together with evidence of tubulointerstitial nephritis (positive renal biopsy OR elevated urine β-microglobulin and either abnormal urine analysis or elevated serum creatinine). It is recommended to test for elevated urine β-microglobulin levels in patients with elevated serum creatinine.[3] In case of a positive result, patients should be referred to a nephrologist for further evaluations and treatment.

4.2 Intermediate Uveitis

Around 16% of cases with intermediate uveitis (IU) are associated with underlying systemic diagnosis.[29] The most common associations with intermediate uveitis include infectious diseases such as syphilis, tuberculosis and Lyme disease, and non-infectious etiologies such as sarcoidosis and multiple sclerosis.

4.2.1 *Multiple Sclerosis*

Multiple sclerosis (MS) is found in 0.9–3.1% of all uveitis cases, but between 5–11% of those with IU.[1,5] Lack of neurological signs at the time of IU presentation and complexity of MS diagnosis are a challenge in the initial management of these patients. In some patients evidence of MS can develop even years after presentation with IU. The SUN Working Group suggested that a diagnosis of MS-associated IU can be made based on the presence of IU (vitreous cells and haze with no evidence of retinitis or choroiditis) together with evidence of MS using the revised 2017 McDonald diagnostic criteria (Tables 4.5 & 4.6).[46] However, exclusion of other etiologies (syphilis, Lyme disease, sarcoidosis) is required before such a diagnosis can be made.[5] In cases of IU patients with no past history of MS, consider referring to a neurologist for further investigations including brain magnetic resonance imaging (MRI).[46] Screening for MS of patients who are scheduled to begin treatment with anti-tumor necrosis factor-α (anti-TNF-α) agents should be considered and a brain MRI scan performed. Presence of white matter lesions is considered a contraindication for starting treatment and patients should be referred to a neurologist (Figure 4.5).[46,47]

4.2.2 *Others*

Other less common systemic associations with IU should be considered in cases with specific demographic risk factors or non-ocular signs and symptoms. Patients with IU associated with gastrointestinal complaints should be tested for HLA-B27 and referred to a gastroenterologist to rule out

Table 4.5. SUN classification criteria for multiple sclerosis-associated intermediate uveitis.

Criteria: 1 and 2

1. Evidence of intermediate uveitis
   a. Vitreous cells or vitreous haze or both;
   b. If anterior chamber cells are present, anterior chamber inflammation is less than that of vitreous;
   c. No evidence of retinitis or choroiditis;

AND

2. Evidence of multiple sclerosis using the revised McDonald diagnostic criteria[6]

Exclusions:

1. Serology positive for syphilis, using a treponemal test;
2. Evidence of sarcoidosis (either bilateral hilar adenopathy on chest imaging or tissue biopsy demonstrating noncaseating granulomata);
3. Serology positive for Lyme disease; either IgG or IgM (e.g., positive ELISA and Western blot results, with the requisite number of bands for assay used).

Adapted from The Standardization of Uveitis Nomenclature (SUN) Working Group. Classification criteria for multiple sclerosis-associated intermediate uveitis. Am J Ophthalmol 2021;228:72–9.[5]

Table 4.6. The 2017 McDonald criteria for diagnosis of multiple sclerosis in patients with an attack at onset.

	Number of lesions with objective clinical evidence	Additional data needed for a diagnosis of multiple sclerosis
≥2 clinical attacks	≥2	None
	1 (as well as clear-cut historical evidence of a previous attack involving a lesion in a distinct anatomical location)	None
≥2 clinical attacks	1	Dissemination in space demonstrated by an additional clinical attack implicating a different CNS site or by MRI
1 clinical attack	≥2	Dissemination in time demonstrated by an additional clinical attack or by MRI OR demonstration of CSF-specific oligoclonal bands
1 clinical attack	1	Dissemination in space demonstrated by an additional clinical attack implicating a different CNS site or by MRI AND Dissemination in time demonstrated by an additional clinical attack or by MRI OR demonstration of CSF-specific oligoclonal bands

Adapted from Thompson AJ, *et al.* Diagnosis of multiple sclerosis: 2017 revisions of the McDonald criteria. *Lancet Neurol* 2018;17(2):162–73.[48]

an inflammatory bowel disease or Whipple's disease. Patients from areas endemic with HTLV-1 infection, such as Japan, the Caribbean islands, part of Central Africa and South America, should undergo serologic testing for HTLV-1.[49] In elderly patients (typically 5th to 6th decade) presenting with vitritis, in the absence of evidence of other systemic disease (sarcoidosis, MS, syphilis, Lyme disease or TB), intraocular lymphoma should be considered. A prompt vitreous biopsy for cytologic analysis, IL-10:IL-6 cytokine ratio (if available) and IgH rearrangement should be performed before treatment is initiated. In cases of a positive diagnosis referral to an oncologist should not be delayed.[50]

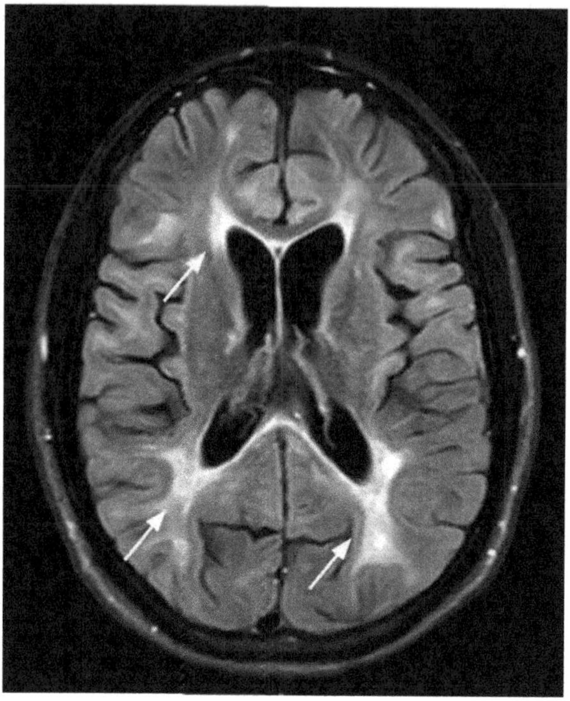

Figure 4.5. Brain MRI fluid attenuated inversion recovery scan demonstrating periventricular white matter lesions in a patient with multiple sclerosis (arrows).

4.3 Posterior and Panuveitis

Systemic investigation in cases of posterior or panuveitis are primarily based on the site of involvement, lesion appearance and additional systemic signs and symptoms.

4.3.1 *Tests for Toxoplasma Gondii*

Infection with *Toxoplasma gondii* is the most common cause of posterior uveitis and serologic testing should be performed in patients presenting with retinitis and/or papillitis. Presence of a typical area of focal retinitis adjacent to an old pigmented chorioretinal scar is extremely suggestive of the diagnosis (Figure 4.6) and is confirmed in the presence of positive IgG serology. In primary toxoplasmosis there may be only focal or paucifocal necrotizing retinitis and no visible chorioretinal scar. The diagnosis is

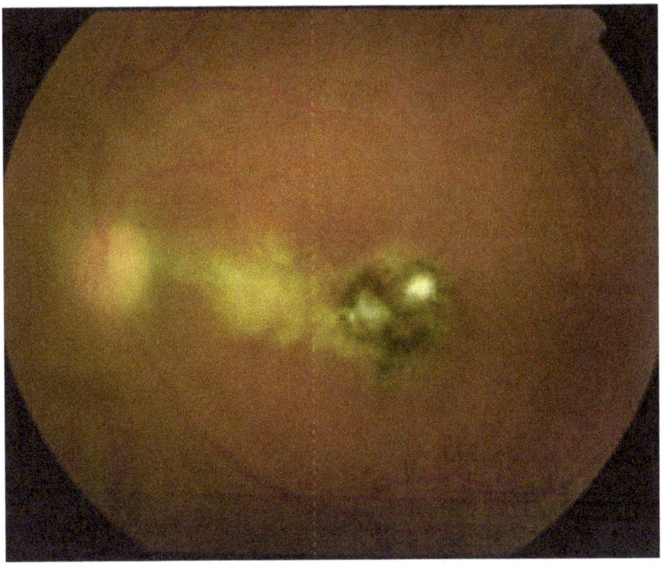

Figure 4.6. Classic appearance of toxoplasma chorioretinitis reactivation along the border of an old scar in a 12-year-old boy.

then based on a positive IgM test or a positive PCR for *Toxoplasma gondii* from either the aqueous or vitreous.[51,52] In primary toxoplasmosis an elevated IgM and a negative IgG is typically seen during the first few weeks following infection. In cases with a dense vitritis (which only occurs in reactivation lesions, not primary infection) that precludes a clear visualization of the retina, the chorioretinal lesion may not be visible and the diagnosis may need to be based initially on serology and a positive PCR, but the latter is only positive in about 40% of cases. Because seroprevalence differs globally, diagnosis is primarily based on suggestive clinical findings, with serology only supporting the diagnosis.[53] However, a negative combined IgG and IgM serology test would rule out a diagnosis of toxoplasmosis in unclear cases but may be negative in patients with congenital toxoplasmosis or in patients who are immunocompromised.[54] The role of vitreous or aqueous biopsy and PCR testing for *Toxoplasma gondii* is debatable, with a low positive rate even in clinically obvious lesions. A negative PCR result in a patient with suggestive clinical signs with or without positive serology should not rule out the diagnosis or affect treatment. Severe, bilateral, multifocal or atypical presentation of retinitis would require further investigation such as a complete blood

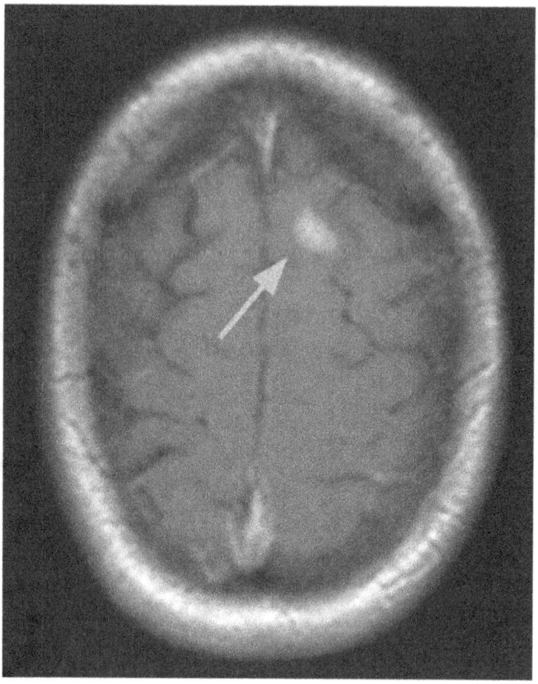

Figure 4.7. Brain computed tomography demonstrating cerebral toxoplasma granuloma (arrow).

count (CBC) and serology for human immunodeficiency virus (HIV) to rule out an underlying immunocompromised status. Patients with HIV presenting with active ocular toxoplasmosis require a brain CT scan to rule out cerebral involvement (Figure 4.7).

4.3.2 *Tests for Herpesviridae*

Retinitis due to herpes simplex virus or varicella zoster virus manifests as focal or confluent areas of retinitis often with severe vitritis and anterior chamber cells, that result in retinal necrosis followed by scarring (Figure 4.8). It can occur in patients with a normal immune system or those who are immunocompromised. Vitritis and/or anterior chamber cells may be less in immunocompromised patients. Serology testing for viruses of the *Herpesviridae* family is of limited value due to the high rate of seropositivity in the healthy general population. However, a negative serology result can help rule out these viruses as a causative agent if the patient is not immunocompromised. For all patients a vitreous biopsy with PCR testing for her-

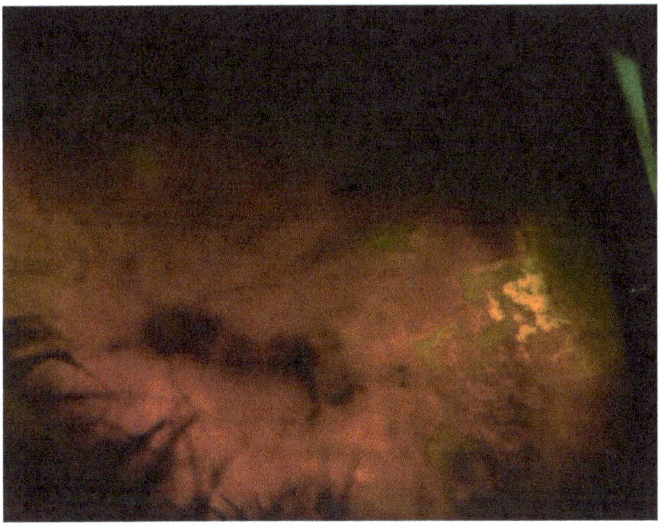

Figure 4.8. Acute retinal necrosis secondary to infection by herpes simplex virus with confluent retinitis and dense vitritis.

pes simplex virus or varicella zoster virus is usually useful in establishing a diagnosis. When the clinical findings are suggestive of herpes simplex virus, varicella zoster virus or cytomegalovirus retinitis, systemic investigations for immunocompromised status are required, including HIV testing.

4.3.3 *Tests for Behçet's Disease*

Non-infectious diseases that can manifest as retinitis include Behçet's disease (BD). Typically, areas of retinitis can be accompanied by ischemic vasculitis and retinal hemorrhages (Figure 4.9). Systemic evaluation by a rheumatologist should be conducted to identify systemic signs and symptoms, including painful oral or genital aphthous ulcers, skin rashes, arthritis and a positive pathergy test. A positive HLA-B51 test may be supportive but is not included in the diagnostic criteria.[55]

Vasculitis is a common finding in many posterior and panuveitis and can be either occlusive or non-occlusive. Retinal involvement with TB can manifest as an occlusive peripheral vasculitis and similar findings are seen along areas of retinal necrosis in acute retinal necrosis (ARN). Non-infectious diseases related to vasculitis include BD, sarcoidosis or systemic lupus erythematosus (SLE). A distinguishing feature of vasculitis related to SLE is vascular occlusion with no vitritis. This leads to changes in vascular structure (tortuous vessels,

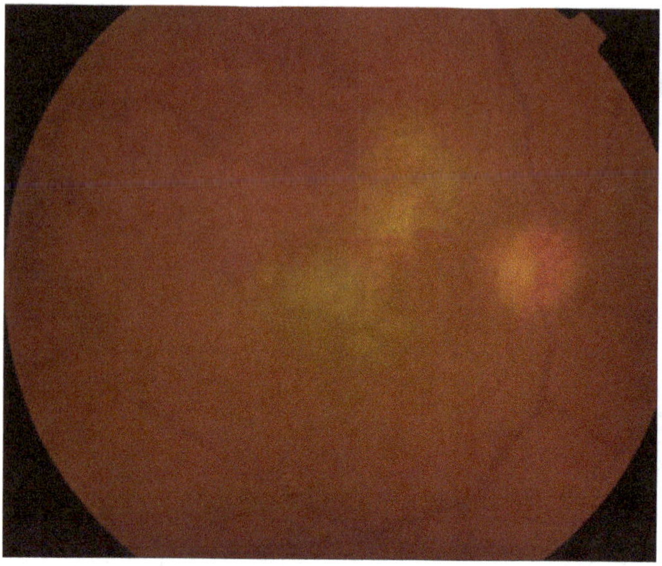

Figure 4.9. Behçet's disease involving the right eye of a 22-year-old man. Note the area of retinitis and adjacent hemorrhages due to a branch retinal vein occlusion.

telangiectasia, microaneurysms), as well as vascular occlusion and ghost vessels (Figure 4.10). Diagnosis is based on a positive ANA test at a dilution greater than 1:160, together with systemic clinical findings including arthritis, typical skin rashes and blood cell abnormalities.

A hyperemic optic disc with macular edema and exudation in a macular star pattern reflects neuroretinitis and should prompt serology testing for *Bartonella henselae* (Figure 4.11).

Patients presenting with multifocal choroidal lesions, primarily oval and yellow, should have an HLA-A29 test which can be positive in 90% of cases with birdshot chorioretinitis.[56] For many conditions such as presumed ocular histoplasmosis (POHS), punctate inner choroidopathy (PIC), Vogt-Koyanagi-Harada syndrome or sympathetic ophthalmia, there is no specific test to confirm the diagnosis. Diagnosis and treatment are based on clinical findings and exclusion of other possible etiologies.

Finally, in any form of uveitis where long-term systemic immunosuppression is planned, baseline tests should include CBC, liver and renal function as well as TB tests and hepatitis serology. Before treatment with anti-TNF-α agents is initiated, screening must include serology for hepatitis B virus, hepatitis C virus, TB and in case of neurologic symptoms (or undifferentiated intermediate uveitis) a neurologic evaluation including a brain MRI.

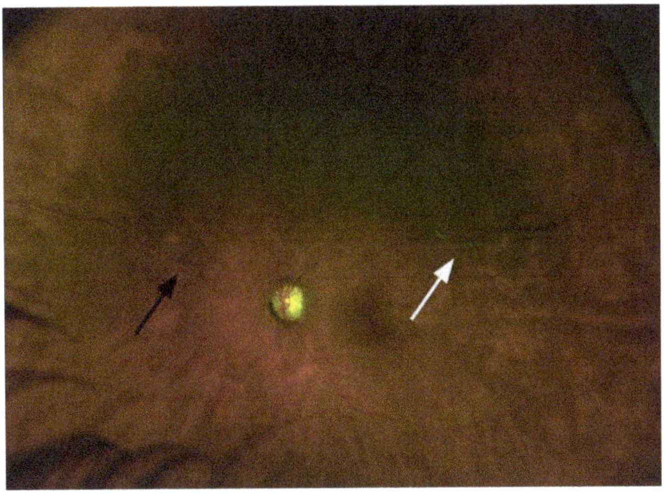

Figure 4.10. Vascular occlusion related to SLE. Note the ghost vessels along the superior and inferior arcades (white arrow), as well as tortuous vessels nasal to the optic disc (black arrow).

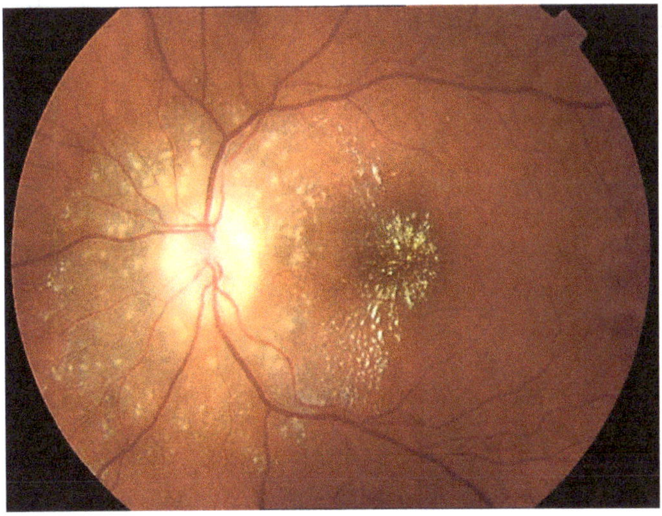

Figure 4.11. *Bartonella henselae* neuroretinitis.

Teaching Points

- Serum ACE is elevated in only 50–80% of patients with sarcoidosis, but is useful to rule it out with a negative predictive value of 97%.
- There is no significant difference in the sensitivity of the tests for detecting TB exposure (IGRA or PPD), but the IGRA tests are more

specific with a lower false-positive rate when testing patients previously immunized with the BCG vaccine.

- For children under the age of 16 who present with anterior uveitis, standard testing includes ANA and HLA-B27.
- Suspect TINU in cases of anterior uveitis if there is elevated urine β-microglobulin and either abnormal urine analysis or elevated serum creatinine.
- In cases of intermediate uveitis in patients with no past history of MS, consider referring to a neurologist for further investigations including brain MRI.
- In primary toxoplasmosis an elevated IgM and a negative IgG are typically seen during the first few weeks following infection.
- A positive HLA-B51 test may be supportive of a diagnosis of Behçet's disease, but is not included in the diagnostic criteria.
- HLA-A29 test can be positive in 90% of cases with birdshot chorioretinitis.

References

1. Tomkins-Netzer O, Talat L, Bar A, *et al.* Long-term clinical outcome and causes of vision loss in patients with uveitis. *Ophthalmology* 2014;121(12): 2387–92.
2. Zamecki KJ, Jabs DA. HLA typing in uveitis: use and misuse. *Am J Ophthalmol* 2010;149(2):189–93 e2.
3. Standardization of Uveitis Nomenclature Working G. Classification criteria for tubulointerstitial nephritis with uveitis syndrome. *Am J Ophthalmol* 2021;228:255–61.
4. Standardization of Uveitis Nomenclature Working G. Classification criteria for multiple evanescent white dot syndrome. *Am J Ophthalmol* 2021;228: 198–204.
5. Standardization of Uveitis Nomenclature Working G. Classification criteria for multiple sclerosis-associated intermediate uveitis. *Am J Ophthalmol* 2021;228:72–9.
6. Standardization of Uveitis Nomenclature Working G. Development of classification criteria for the uveitides. *Am J Ophthalmol* 2021;228:96–105.
7. Standardization of Uveitis Nomenclature Working G. Classification criteria for acute posterior multifocal placoid pigment epitheliopathy. *Am J Ophthalmol* 2021;228:174–81.
8. Standardization of Uveitis Nomenclature Working G. Classification criteria for juvenile idiopathic arthritis-associated chronic anterior uveitis. *Am J Ophthalmol* 2021;228:192–7.

9. Standardization of Uveitis Nomenclature Working G. Classification criteria for syphilitic uveitis. *Am J Ophthalmol* 2021;228:182–91.
10. Standardization of Uveitis Nomenclature Working G. Classification criteria for cytomegalovirus anterior uveitis. *Am J Ophthalmol* 2021;228:89–95.
11. Standardization of Uveitis Nomenclature Working G. Classification criteria for Vogt-Koyanagi-Harada disease. *Am J Ophthalmol* 2021;228:205–11.
12. Standardization of Uveitis Nomenclature Working G. Classification criteria for multifocal choroiditis with panuveitis. *Am J Ophthalmol* 2021;228:152–8.
13. Standardization of Uveitis Nomenclature Working G. Classification criteria for cytomegalovirus retinitis. *Am J Ophthalmol* 2021;228:245–54.
14. Standardization of Uveitis Nomenclature Working G. Classification criteria for tubercular uveitis. *Am J Ophthalmol* 2021;228:142–51.
15. Standardization of Uveitis Nomenclature Working G. Classification criteria for serpiginous choroiditis. *Am J Ophthalmol* 2021;228:126–33.
16. Standardization of Uveitis Nomenclature Working G. Classification criteria for acute retinal necrosis syndrome. *Am J Ophthalmol* 2021;228:237–44.
17. Standardization of Uveitis Nomenclature Working G. Classification criteria for punctate inner choroiditis. *Am J Ophthalmol* 2021;228:275–80.
18. Standardization of Uveitis Nomenclature Working G. Classification criteria for varicella zoster virus anterior uveitis. *Am J Ophthalmol* 2021;228:165–73.
19. Standardization of Uveitis Nomenclature Working G. Classification criteria for herpes simplex virus anterior uveitis. *Am J Ophthalmol* 2021;228:231–6.
20. Standardization of Uveitis Nomenclature Working G. Classification criteria for Behcet disease uveitis. *Am J Ophthalmol* 2021;228:80–8.
21. Standardization of Uveitis Nomenclature Working G. Classification criteria for Fuchs uveitis syndrome. *Am J Ophthalmol* 2021;228:262–7.
22. Standardization of Uveitis Nomenclature Working G. Classification criteria for pars planitis. *Am J Ophthalmol* 2021;228:268–74.
23. Standardization of Uveitis Nomenclature Working G. Classification criteria for sympathetic ophthalmia. *Am J Ophthalmol* 2021;228:212–9.
24. Standardization of Uveitis Nomenclature Working G. Classification criteria for spondyloarthritis/HLA-B27-associated anterior uveitis. *Am J Ophthalmol* 2021;228:117–25.
25. Standardization of Uveitis Nomenclature Working G. Classification criteria for birdshot chorioretinitis. *Am J Ophthalmol* 2021;228:65–71.
26. Standardization of Uveitis Nomenclature Working G. Classification criteria for sarcoidosis-associated uveitis. *Am J Ophthalmol* 2021;228:220–30.
27. Standardization of Uveitis Nomenclature Working G. Classification criteria for intermediate uveitis, non-pars planitis type. *Am J Ophthalmol* 2021;228:159–64.

28. Noble J, Hollands H, Forooghian F, *et al.* Evaluating the cost-effectiveness of anterior uveitis investigation by Canadian ophthalmologists. *Can J Ophthalmol* 2008;43(6):652–7.
29. Rothova A, Buitenhuis HJ, Meenken C, *et al.* Uveitis and systemic disease. *Br J Ophthalmol* 1992;76(3):137–41.
30. Wakefield D, Chang JH, Amjadi S, *et al.* What is new HLA-B27 acute anterior uveitis? *Ocul Immunol Inflamm* 2011;19(2):139–44.
31. Herbort CP, Rao NA, Mochizuki M, members of Scientific Committee of First International Workshop on Ocular S. International criteria for the diagnosis of ocular sarcoidosis: results of the first International Workshop On Ocular Sarcoidosis (IWOS). *Ocul Immunol Inflamm* 2009;17(3):160–9.
32. Mochizuki M, Smith JR, Takase H, *et al.* Revised criteria of International Workshop on Ocular Sarcoidosis (IWOS) for the diagnosis of ocular sarcoidosis. *Br J Ophthalmol* 2019;103(10):1418–22.
33. Niederer RL, Sims JL. Utility of screening investigations for systemic sarcoidosis in undifferentiated uveitis. *Am J Ophthalmol* 2019;206:149–53.
34. Sequeira W, Stinar D. Serum angiotensin-converting enzyme levels in sarcoid arthritis. *Arch Intern Med* 1986;146(1):125–7.
35. Niederer RL, Al-Janabi A, Lightman S, Tomkins-Netzer O. Serum angiotensin-converting enzyme has a high negative predictive value in the investigation for systemic sarcoidosis. *Am J Ophthalmol* 2018;194:82–7.
36. Backhouse JL, Nesteroff SI. Treponema pallidum western blot: comparison with the FTA-ABS test as a confirmatory test for syphilis. *Diagn Microbiol Infect Dis* 2001;39(1):9–14.
37. Gill H, Danesh-Meyer HV, Sims JL, *et al.* Ocular syphilis in Pacific peoples-are we making misdiagnoses secondary to yaws? *N Z Med J* 2020;133(1513):53–60.
38. Ang M, Htoon HM, Chee SP. Diagnosis of tuberculous uveitis: clinical application of an interferon-gamma release assay. *Ophthalmology* 2009;116(7):1391–6.
39. Ang M, Wong WL, Kiew SY, *et al.* Prospective head-to-head study comparing 2 commercial interferon gamma release assays for the diagnosis of tuberculous uveitis. *Am J Ophthalmol* 2014;157(6):1306–14; 14 e1–4.
40. Kalish RA, McHugh G, Granquist J, *et al.* Persistence of immunoglobulin M or immunoglobulin G antibody responses to Borrelia burgdorferi 10–20 years after active Lyme disease. *Clin Infect Dis* 2001;33(6):780–5.
41. Heiligenhaus A, Niewerth M, Mingels A, *et al.* [Epidemiology of uveitis in juvenile idiopathic arthritis from a national paediatric rheumatologic and ophthalmologic database]. *Klin Monbl Augenheilkd* 2005;222(12):993–1001.
42. Heiligenhaus A, Niewerth M, Ganser G, *et al.* Prevalence and complications of uveitis in juvenile idiopathic arthritis in a population-based nation-wide study in Germany: suggested modification of the current screening guidelines. *Rheumatology (Oxford)* 2007;46(6):1015–9.

43. Haroon M, Ahmad M, Baig MN, *et al.* Inflammatory back pain in psoriatic arthritis is significantly more responsive to corticosteroids compared to back pain in ankylosing spondylitis: a prospective, open-labelled, controlled pilot study. *Arthritis Res Ther* 2018;20(1):73.
44. Juanola X, Loza Santamaria E, Cordero-Coma M, Group SW. Description and prevalence of spondyloarthritis in patients with anterior uveitis: The SENTINEL Interdisciplinary Collaborative Project. *Ophthalmology* 2016;123(8):1632–6.
45. Okafor LO, Hewins P, Murray PI, Denniston AK. Tubulointerstitial nephritis and uveitis (TINU) syndrome: a systematic review of its epidemiology, demographics and risk factors. *Orphanet J Rare Dis* 2017;12(1):128.
46. Abraham A, Nicholson L, Dick A, *et al.* Intermediate uveitis associated with MS: Diagnosis, clinical features, pathogenic mechanisms, and recommendations for management. *Neurol Neuroimmunol Neuroinflamm* 2021;8(1):e909.
47. Petrushkin H, Kidd D, Pavesio C. Intermediate uveitis and multiple sclerosis: to scan or not to scan. *Br J Ophthalmol* 2015;99(12):1591–3.
48. Thompson AJ, *et al.* Diagnosis of multiple sclerosis: 2017 revisions of the McDonald criteria. *Lancet Neurol* 2018;17(2):162–73.
49. Takahashi T, Takase H, Urano T, *et al.* Clinical features of human T-lymphotropic virus type 1 uveitis: a long-term follow-up. *Ocul Immunol Inflamm* 2000;8(4):235–41.
50. Hearne E, Tomkins-Netzer O, Lightman S. Learning points in intraocular lymphoma. *Eye (Lond)* 2021;35(7):1815–7.
51. Moshfeghi DM, Dodds EM, Couto CA, *et al.* Diagnostic approaches to severe, atypical toxoplasmosis mimicking acute retinal necrosis. *Ophthalmology* 2004;111(4):716–25.
52. Crosson JN, Laird PW, Grossniklaus HE, Hendrick AM. Toxoplasma chorioretinitis diagnosed by histopathology in a patient with AIDS. *Retin Cases Brief Rep* 2015;9(2):162–3.
53. Pappas G, Roussos N, Falagas ME. Toxoplasmosis snapshots: global status of Toxoplasma gondii seroprevalence and implications for pregnancy and congenital toxoplasmosis. *Int J Parasitol* 2009;39(12):1385–94.
54. Standardization of Uveitis Nomenclature Working G. Classification criteria for toxoplasmic retinitis. *Am J Ophthalmol* 2021;228:134–41.
55. International Team for the Revision of the International Criteria for Behcet's D. The International Criteria for Behcet's Disease (ICBD): a collaborative study of 27 countries on the sensitivity and specificity of the new criteria. *J Eur Acad Dermatol Venereol* 2014;28(3):338–47.
56. Tomkins-Netzer O, Taylor SR, Lightman S. Long-term clinical and anatomic outcome of birdshot chorioretinopathy. *JAMA Ophthalmol* 2014;132(1):57–62.

https://doi.org/10.1142/9789811251474_0005

Chapter 5

Non-Infectious Uveitis

Yael Sharon,[*,†] *Michal Kramer*[*,†]

Non-infectious uveitis (NIU) refers to intraocular inflammation in which infectious and masquerade causes have been ruled out. It encompasses a heterogeneous group of diseases and can be classified based on the primary anatomical location of inflammation: anterior, intermediate, posterior or panuveitis.[1,2] Anatomic diagnostic approach guides physicians in the process of differential diagnosis establishment, employing ancillary tests, disease identification, and selecting the appropriate treatment.

NIU includes either diseases that are limited to the eye or associated with systemic autoimmune disorders.[3] Diagnosis can be challenging, since in most cases it is made by clinical findings which can overlap between entities.[4] Furthermore, there is no specific test for each disease and the etiology is often unknown.

Clinical approach is facilitated by embedding the Standardization of Uveitis Nomenclature (SUN) classification into real life.[5] By using this classification method, the clinician defines the anatomic location and kinetics of the disease. Additional valuable demographic characteristics include age, geography and ethnic origin. These parameters help to design the strategy for the relevant differential diagnosis, targeted workup and treatment.

5.1 Anterior Uveitis

Anterior uveitis constitutes the majority of cases, presenting in approximately 80% of NIU patients.[1,6] Abrupt onset anterior uveitis typically presents with eye redness, pain, photophobia and tearing. Signs include

* Department of Ophthalmology, Rabin Medical Center, Petah-Tikva, Israel
† Sackler Faculty of Medicine, Tel Aviv University, Tel Aviv, Israel

anterior chamber cells and flare, keratic precipitates (KPs), pupillary miosis, hypopyon (Figure 5.1) and fibrinous reaction in more severe cases (Figure 5.2). Posterior synechia (Figure 5.3) may occur early or suggest a previous episode. Iris nodules are typical of granulomatous etiologies (Figure 5.4). Visual acuity may be normal or decreased. Intraocular pressure (IOP) may be low, normal or elevated.

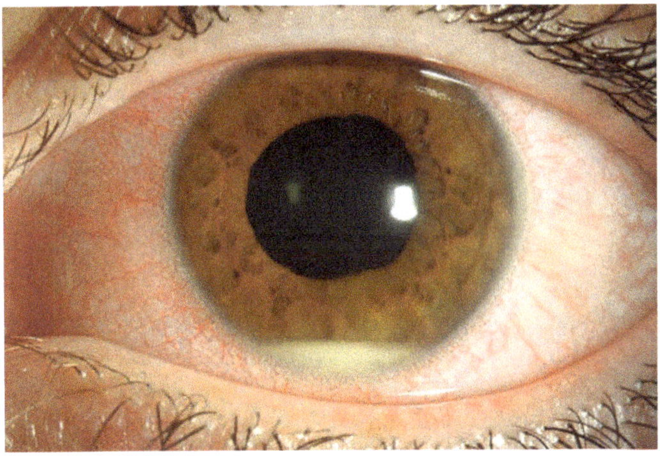

Figure 5.1. Hypopyon uveitis.

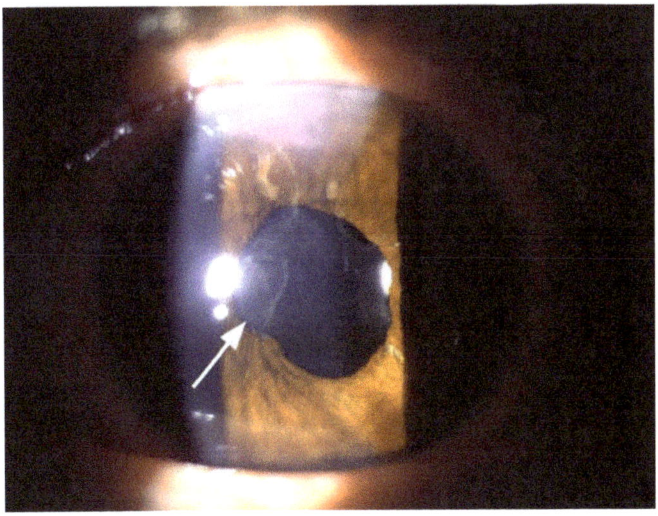

Figure 5.2. Fibrin in anterior chamber (arrow).

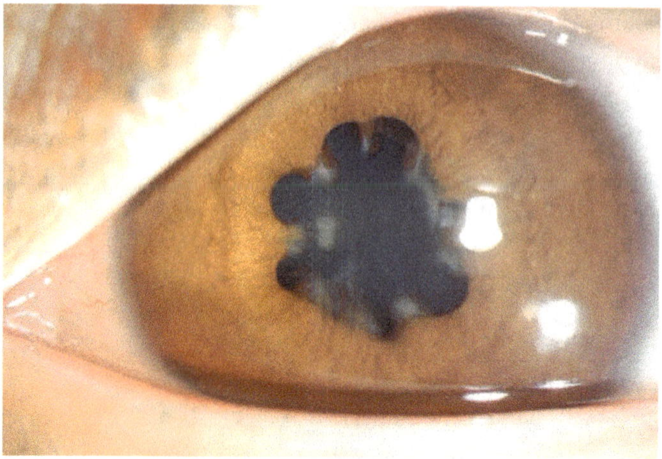

Figure 5.3. Posterior synechia.

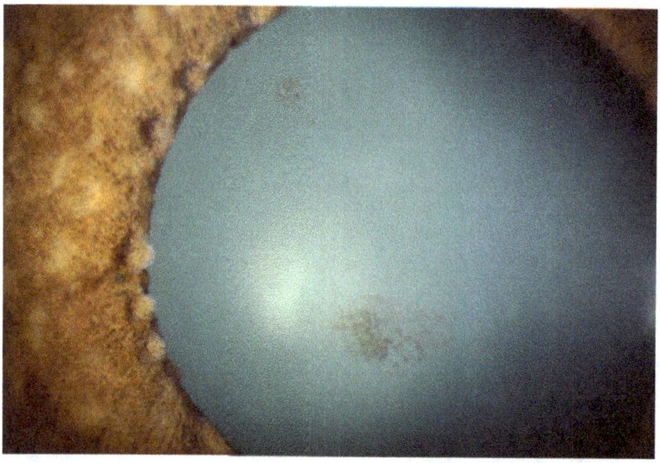

Figure 5.4. Koeppe iris nodules along the pupil margin.

The various etiologies can practically be categorized by the kinetics of inflammation, which includes the onset, duration and time course of the disease (see Chapter 1, Table 1.2). Anterior uveitis that manifests abruptly guides us to different etiologies than uveitis that is insidious at presentation.

When anterior uveitis is recurrent or granulomatous, suggested laboratory and imaging workup includes complete blood count (CBC), blood chemistry, C-reactive protein (CRP), erythrocyte sedimentation rate (ESR), angiotensin-converting enzyme (ACE) and lysozyme levels, chest X-ray (CXR), human leukocyte antigen B27 (HLA-B27) antigen tests for tuberculosis and syphilis testing. Other testing should be performed based on clinical suspicion for various diseases.

Sub-categorization can be made by additional clinical features including laterality (unilateral, simultaneous bilateral and alternating), severity (mild, moderate and severe), and age at presentation (children, young adults, adults and elderly).

5.1.1 *Acute Anterior Uveitis*

5.1.1.1 *Idiopathic Anterior Uveitis*

Kinetics: Acute, sudden, and limited non-granulomatous anterior uveitis.

Laterality: Unilateral or simultaneous bilateral.

Severity: Usually mild to moderate anterior inflammation accompanied by KPs, anterior chamber cells and flare.

Age at presentation: Varies, 30–60 years.

Clinical features: Accounts for 50% of cases. May have seasonal variations.

Diagnostic techniques: The first episode of abrupt onset non-granulomatous, unilateral anterior uveitis, with no accompanying systemic symptoms and signs, does not usually require further systemic workup.

Treatment and prognosis: Topical corticosteroids and cycloplegics. Usually resolves in less than 3 months.

5.1.1.2 *Tubulointerstitial Nephritis and Uveitis Syndrome (TINU)*

Kinetics: Acute, sudden, and limited non-granulomatous anterior uveitis. Intermediate uveitis in 40%.[7,8]

Laterality: Bilateral.

Severity: Mild to moderate anterior inflammation.

Age at presentation: 10–30 years.

Clinical features: Preceding systemic signs and symptoms including abnormal renal function tests and associated systemic illnesses consisting of fever, weight loss, fatigue, anorexia and arthralgia are present.[9]

Diagnostic techniques: Diagnosis is made clinically with supporting laboratory tests. Common laboratory abnormalities include elevated serum creatinine level, elevated ESR and abnormal urinalysis findings such as elevated urinary beta-2-microglobulin levels.[10]

Treatment and prognosis: Topical and systemic corticosteroids. The visual prognosis appears to be favorable.

5.1.2 Recurrent Anterior Uveitis

5.1.2.1 HLA-B27-associated Uveitis

Kinetics: Recurrent, sudden, and limited non-granulomatous anterior uveitis.[11]

Laterality: Bilateral and alternating.

Severity: Severe anterior inflammation accompanied by KPs, anterior chamber cells and flare, fibrinous reaction, hypopyon and the formation of posterior synechia.[12,13]

Age at presentation: 20–40 years.

Clinical features: Approximately 40–50% of patients with acute anterior uveitis are HLA-B27 positive.[14] There is a strong systemic association with the seronegative spondyloarthropathies, particularly ankylosing spondylitis (Figure 5.5).[12]

Diagnostic techniques: A comprehensive history taking and review of systems to look for joint, skin or bowel involvement, blood tests for autoimmune and infectious etiologies, HLA-B27 serotyping, X-ray and magnetic resonance imaging (MRI) of sacroiliac joint (Figures 5.5 and 5.6), and consider rheumatology referral for further workup.[12,15]

Treatment and prognosis: Consists of topical cycloplegic agents and corticosteroids. In severe cases, periocular or systemic corticosteroids may be required. Each episode usually lasts less than 3 months.

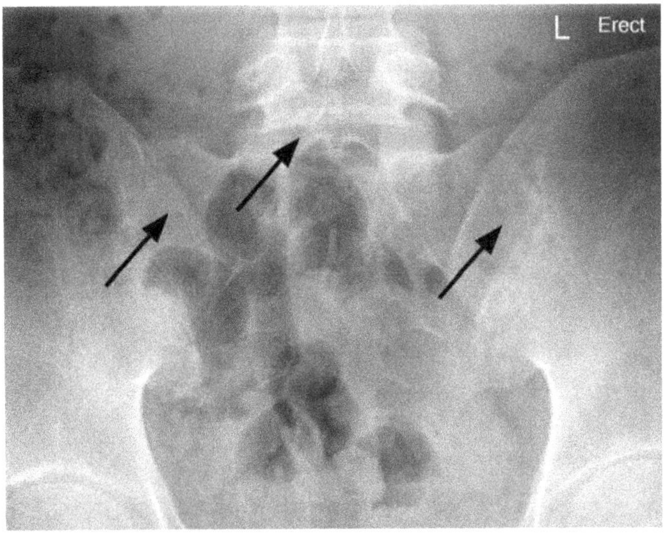

Figure 5.5. Ankylosing spondylitis on X-ray of lumbar spine and sacroiliac joint (fusion of lumbar and sacroiliac joints, arrows).

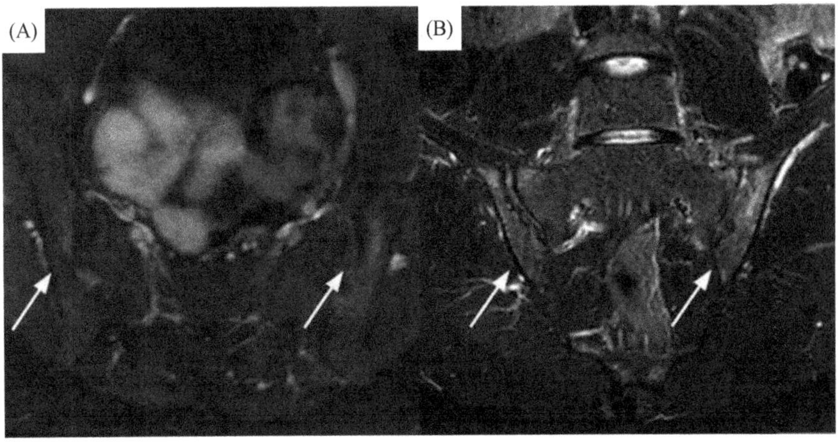

Figure 5.6. Lumbar MRI scan of a 32-year-old man with ankylosing spondylitis. (A) Coronal STIR MR image demonstrates bilateral subchondral bone marrow edema of the sacroiliac joints (arrows). (B) T1-fat-saturated post-gadolinium MR image showing bilateral focal enhancing bone marrow edema lesions of the sacroiliac joints (arrows).

5.1.2.2 *Posner-Schlossman Syndrome*

Kinetics: Recurrent, sudden and limited non-granulomatous anterior uveitis.

Laterality: Unilateral.

Severity: Mild inflammation with markedly elevated IOP.

Age at presentation: 20–50 years.

Clinical features: Corneal edema, a few fine stellate KPs in central or inferior cornea, anterior chamber cells and flare and markedly elevated IOP. Episodes can last from several hours to several days, and recurrences are common.[16]

Diagnostic techniques: Diagnosis is made clinically. Recurrent cytomegalovirus (CMV) infection is suspected to be the leading cause of the disease. Aqueous and blood sampling for the identification of underlying infectious cause may be performed.[17]

Treatment and prognosis: Topical corticosteroids and anti-glaucoma therapies. Prognosis is good overall. Recurrent episodes can result in chronic secondary glaucoma.

5.1.3 Chronic Anterior Uveitis

5.1.3.1 *Fuchs' Uveitis Syndrome (Fuchs' Heterochromic Iridocyclitis)*

Kinetics: Chronic, insidious, persistent non-granulomatous anterior uveitis.

Laterality: Unilateral.

Severity: Mild and asymptomatic. Patients may report mild blurring of vision and floaters.

Age at presentation: 30–40 years.

Clinical features: Stellate KPs scattered diffusely (Figure 5.7), iris nodules, diffuse iris stromal atrophy or heterochromia (Figure 5.8), abnormal blood vessels bridging the angle, absence of synechia and vitreous cells are characteristic.[18-20]

Diagnostic techniques: Diagnosis is based on clinical findings. There is no serologic or laboratory testing to confirm diagnosis. Chronic rubella virus infection is implicated as a possible cause.[21,22] Anterior chamber sampling can be performed to rule out infectious etiology.

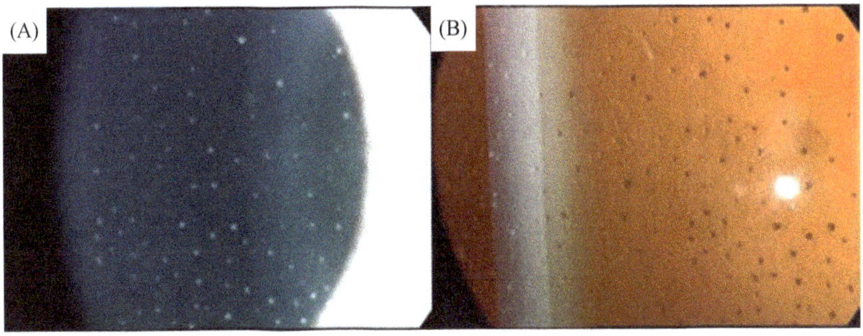

Figure 5.7. **(A) Slit lamp image and (B) retroillumination of Fuchs' uveitis syndrome showing stellate keratic precipitates crossing the horizontal midline.**

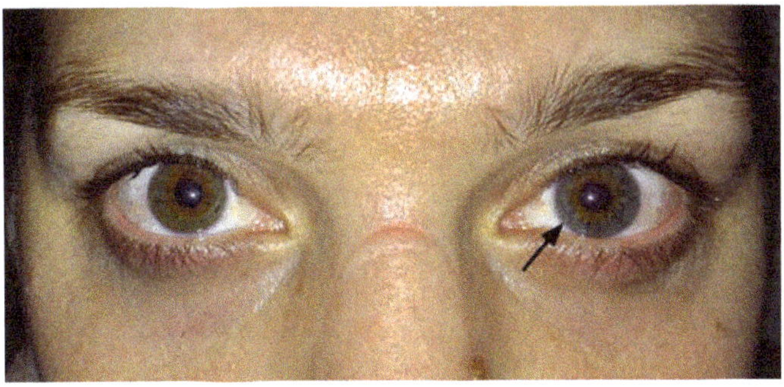

Figure 5.8. **Heterochromia in a patient with Fuchs' uveitis syndrome. Note the change in color of the iris in the left eye (arrow).**

Treatment and prognosis: Only few cases require topical corticosteroids. The prognosis is good in most cases. Development of cataract (Figure 5.9) and glaucoma can be seen.

5.1.3.2 *Juvenile Idiopathic Arthritis-Associated Uveitis*

Kinetics: Chronic, insidious, persistent non-granulomatous anterior uveitis.

Laterality: Bilateral.

Severity: Mild to moderate anterior inflammation.

Age at presentation: 3–12 years.

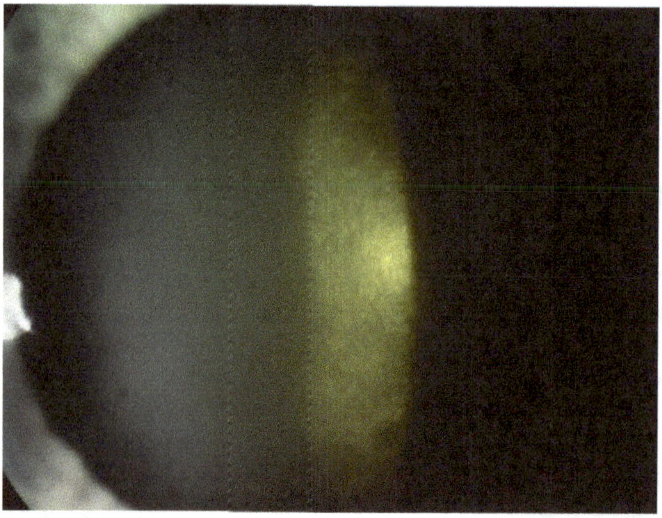

Figure 5.9. Posterior subcapsular lens opacification in Fuchs' uveitis syndrome. Note the absence of posterior synechia.

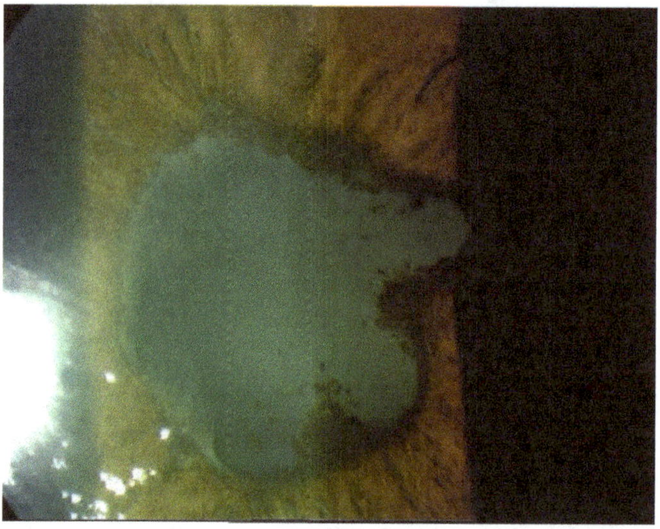

Figure 5.10. Posterior synechia in juvenile idiopathic arthritis-associated uveitis.

Clinical features: Usually asymptomatic and associated systemically with juvenile idiopathic arthritis (JIA) in the pediatric group.[23] In many cases eyes will have at presentation signs of previous episodes of active inflammation, such as posterior synechia (Figure 5.10), cataract and band

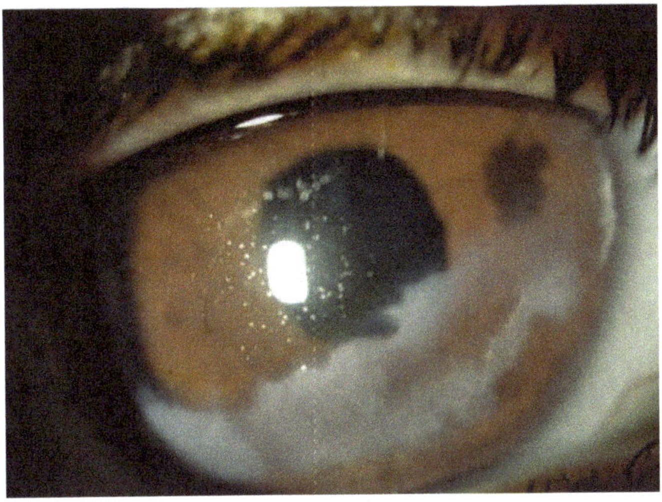

Figure 5.11. Band keratopathy in juvenile idiopathic arthritis-associated uveitis.

keratopathy (Figure 5.11). Despite evidence of previous episodes, parents state that eyes were never injected, and children did not complain of blurred vision, pain or photophobia. Risk factors include specific patterns of the systemic disease: female, oligoarticular-arthritis, positive antinuclear antibody (ANA), negative rheumatoid factor (RF) and age before 4 years old at onset of arthritis.[24]

Diagnostic techniques: Diagnosis is often made clinically during an ocular screening examination of patients with a diagnosis of JIA.[25] Alternatively, children are referred following an abnormal routine vision screening test.

Treatment and prognosis: Topical corticosteroids and early initiation of immunomodulatory therapy (IMT) are often used.[26] Prognosis depends on the extent of structural damage from ocular complications due to the asymptomatic nature of the disease.[27,28]

5.2 Intermediate Uveitis

Approximately 15–20% of uveitis cases present as intermediate uveitis. In intermediate uveitis, inflammation is predominantly located in the vitreous. The inflammation can be isolated to the eye or be associated with systemic diseases such as sarcoidosis, multiple sclerosis and various infections. The disease is commonly bilateral and asymmetric. Symptoms include

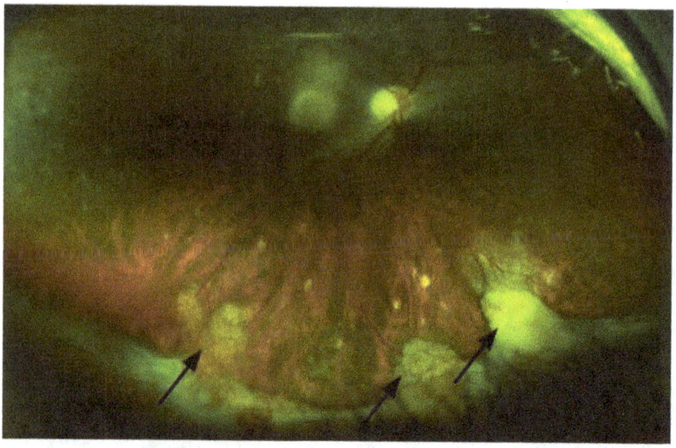

Figure 5.12. Vitreous snowballs and snowbank in intermediate uveitis. Note the neovascularization along the snowbank (arrows).

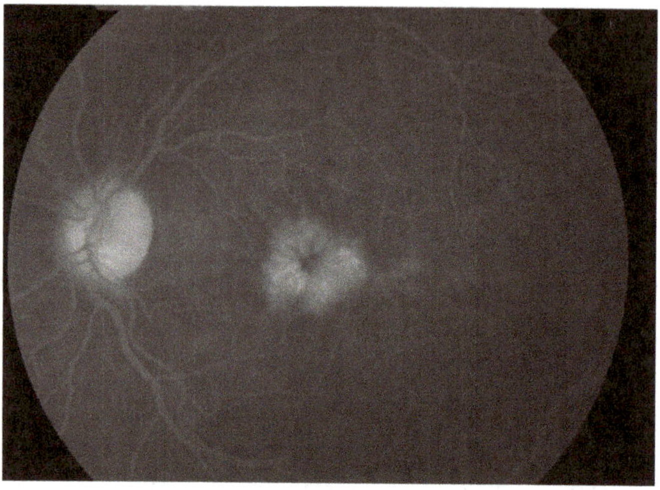

Figure 5.13. Fundus fluorescein angiography of cystoid macular edema in intermediate uveitis.

floaters and blurry vision. Ocular signs include vitreous cells, snowballs and snowbanks (Figure 5.12). There may also be associated peripheral retinal venous sheathing and macular edema (Figures 5.13 and 5.14).[29]

Intermediate uveitis can be caused by systemic autoimmune diseases including sarcoidosis and multiple sclerosis and by infectious causes such as syphilis, tuberculosis, toxoplasmosis and Lyme disease. Among the differential diagnosis of autoimmune and infectious causes, vitritis in

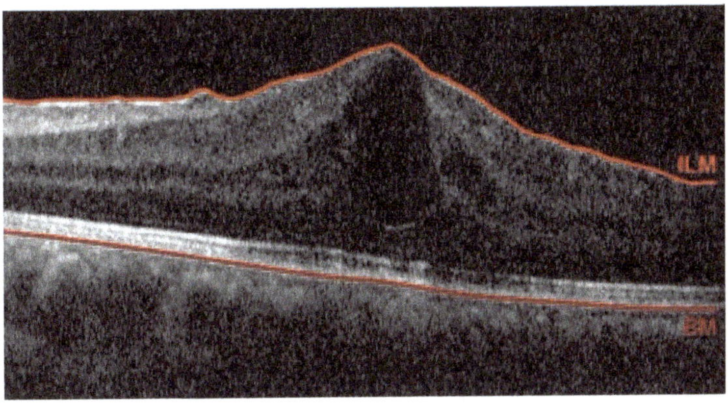

Figure 5.14. Optical coherence tomography of cystoid macular edema in intermediate uveitis. Note the hazy view of the retina, due to the vitritis.

elderly patients can be indicative of primary central nervous system (CNS) lymphoma and should be ruled out by diagnostic vitrectomy in some cases. The diagnosis is made according to classic clinical findings, supported by laboratory workup and systemic and ocular imaging tests. These include CBC and blood chemistry, ESR, CRP, serum ACE and lysozyme levels, syphilis testing, CXR, screening for tuberculosis and ocular imaging. Additional testing is performed based on the clinical circumstances.

5.2.1 *Pars Planitis*

Definition: Subset of intermediate uveitis, where chronic vitritis is found in the absence of underlying infectious or systemic disease.

Clinical features: Diffuse vitreous cells and haze, snowballs and snowbanks are characteristic findings. Predominantly affects children and adolescents.[30]

Diagnostic techniques: Etiology is unknown and is considered idiopathic. Diagnosis of idiopathic pars planitis is based on clinical findings.[31] There is no specific diagnostic laboratory test; however, systemic associations and mainly infectious causes need to be ruled out. Systemic investigations include autoimmune and infectious serology tests, CXR, screening for tuberculosis and brain MRI.[32]

Treatment and prognosis: A gradual approach is the most commonly used treatment strategy in patients with pars planitis. Oral or periocular corticosteroids usually constitute the first line of therapy, followed by immunosuppressive agents and biologic therapies. Surgical intervention such as pars plana vitrectomy and laser photocoagulation are seldom used. The clinical course is varied with 10% of cases who have a self-limited course, 30% with chronic course with few exacerbations and 60% who have prolonged course with exacerbations. In the chronic group, up to 70% of patients develop complications, such as cataract, macular edema, retinal phlebitis and optic disc edema leading to vision loss.[33]

5.2.2 Multiple Sclerosis-Associated Uveitis

Definition: Bilateral recurrent or chronic intermediate uveitis in patients with multiple sclerosis.

Clinical features: Vitreous cells and haze, snowballs and snowbanks are common findings as well as retinal phlebitis and concurrent granulomatous anterior chamber inflammation in young females (Figure 5.15).[34]

Diagnostic techniques: Brain and spine MRI with gadolinium and cerebrospinal fluid analysis. All to conform diagnosis of multiple sclerosis.[35]

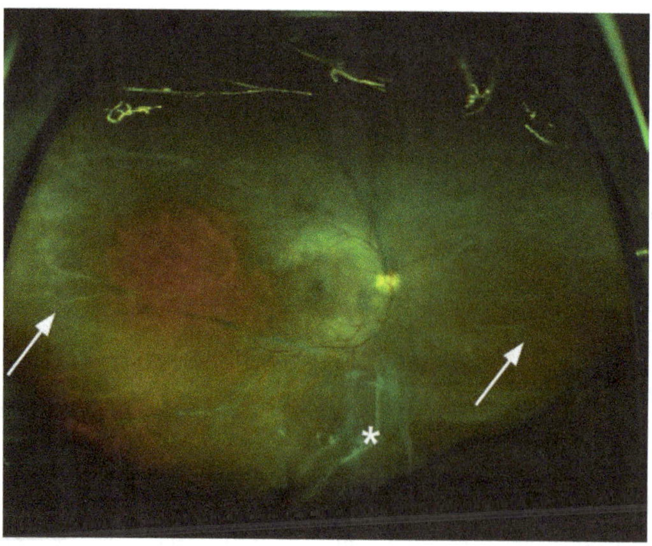

Figure 5.15. Intermediate uveitis and retinal vasculitis secondary to multiple sclerosis. Note the hazy view and vitreous opacities (asterisk) as well as peripheral vascular occlusion and ghost vessels (arrows).

Treatment and prognosis: Treatment includes periocular and systemic corticosteroids for the ocular inflammation as well as disease-modifying agents for their multiple sclerosis. Visual prognosis is good.

5.3 Posterior Uveitis

Posterior uveitis is inflammation that primarily involves the retina and/or choroid. As with anterior and intermediate uveitis, infectious, autoimmune and masquerading etiologies should be ruled out. Presence of posterior segment complications such as macular edema, retinal vasculitis, optic disc edema, neovascularization and retinal detachment are not considered in the diagnosis criteria of posterior uveitis. Presenting symptoms include blurred vision, floaters, photopsias, scotomas, metamorphopsia, nyctalopia and visual field loss.

Posterior uveitis can be associated with systemic autoimmune diseases or be limited to the eye.

Laboratory and systemic testing are usually done to exclude other etiologies on the differential diagnosis. Additional to CBC, blood chemistry, CRP, ESR, ACE and CXR, serologic testing for syphilis and antibodies for vasculitides are recommended in all patients, as well as screening for tuberculosis in patients with high risk for exposure. Ocular diagnostic testing may assist in the diagnosis with characteristic features evident on fundus fluorescein angiography (FFA), enhanced depth imaging optical coherence tomography (EDI-OCT), visual field testing, indocyanine green (ICG) angiography, fundus autofluorescence (FAF), and electroretinography (ERG) studies.

The inflammatory chorioretinopathies are a heterogeneous group of unknown cause that are confined to the eye. They all share similar clinical features of bilateral, discrete, multiple white lesions located at the level of the retina and choroid, typically seen in young, otherwise healthy adults. Whether they represent a clinical spectrum of the same disease entity or are separate diseases is debatable.

5.3.1 *Punctate Inner Choroiditis (PIC)*

Definition: Bilateral multifocal chorioretinal inflammation, affecting young healthy myopic women and characterized by small, punctate lesions of the inner choroid and retinal pigment epithelium (RPE).

Clinical features: The lesions are round, yellow-white, <200 μm in size, may have subretinal fluid, heal with atrophic scarring and become punched out (Figure 5.16).[36] They are commonly limited to the posterior pole. Choroidal neovascular membrane (CNVM) may be present.

Diagnostic techniques: Diagnosis is made clinically with complementary ocular imaging studies.[37] Optical coherence tomography (OCT) demonstrates hyperreflective RPE elevation with disruption of the inner and outer segment and choroidal thickening on EDI (Figure 5.17). On fluorescein angiography active lesions are hyperfluorescent and on autofluorescence they are hyperautofluorescent. On ICG angiography the lesions are

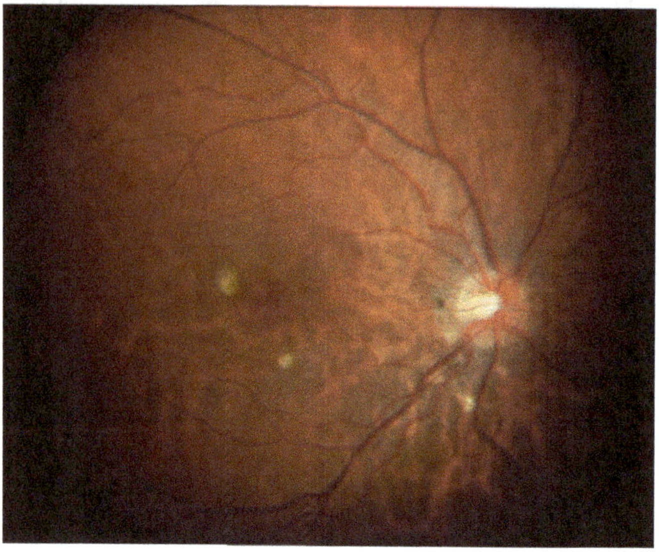

Figure 5.16. Punctate inner choroiditis.

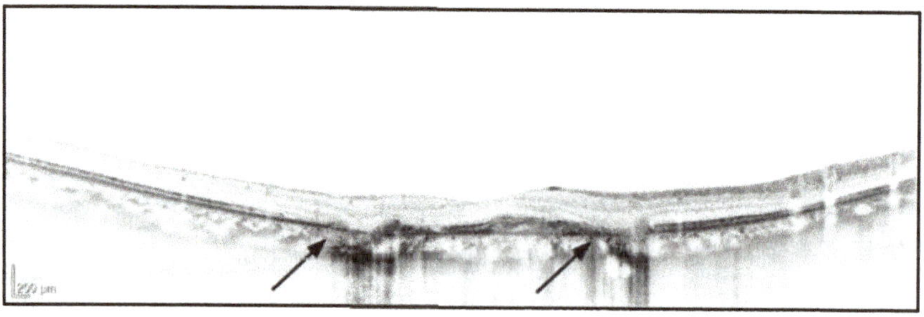

Figure 5.17. OCT demonstrating hyperreflective retinal pigment epithelium lesions in a patient with punctate inner choroiditis.

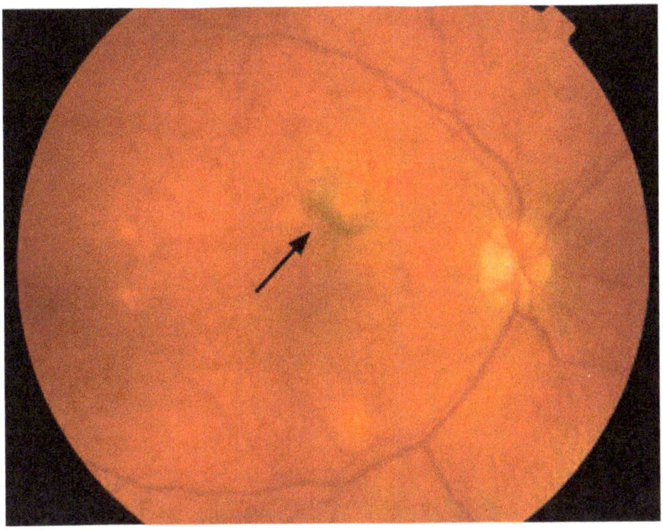

Figure 5.18. Punctate inner choroiditis with choroidal neovascular membrane. Note the subretinal and retinal hemorrhages over the neovascular membrane (arrow).

hypocyanescent. Anterior chamber and vitreous cells are typically absent. Choroidal neovascularization frequently develops (Figure 5.18). Sarcoidosis, syphilis, and tuberculosis need to be ruled out.

Treatment and prognosis: Treatment consists of systemic and regional corticosteroids and IMT for vision-threatening active lesions and for recurrent disease. Choroidal neovascular membranes can be effectively treated with intravitreal anti-vascular endothelial growth factor (VEGF) agents.[38] The course of disease is variable.

5.3.2 *Multifocal Choroiditis with Panuveitis (MFC-PU)*

Definition: Chronic bilateral inflammatory multifocal chorioretinal disorder in young healthy myopic women. PIC and MFC-PU are thought to belong on the clinical spectrum of the same entity.

Clinical features: The predominant lesions are multiple, yellow-gray at the level of the RPE, 50–350 μm in size in conjunction with multiple atrophic punched-out lesions.[39] They are located both in and outside the posterior pole with propensity to the peripapillary region (Figure 5.19). Anterior chamber and vitreous inflammation are often present.

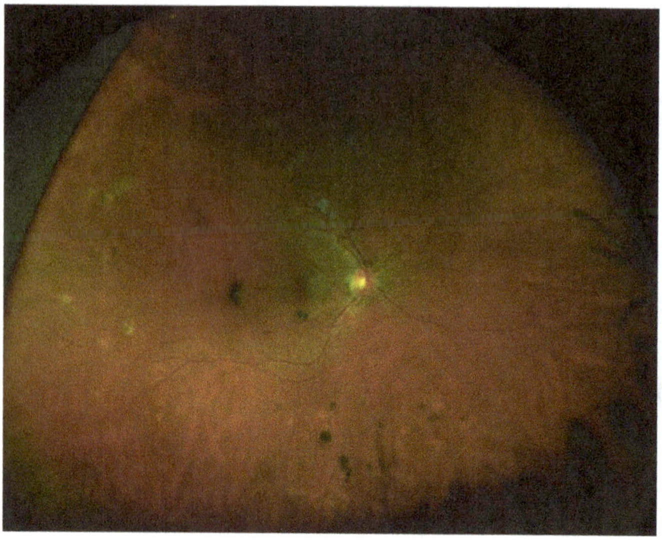

Figure 5.19. Multifocal choroiditis.

Diagnostic techniques: The diagnosis is of exclusion since sarcoidosis, syphilis, and tuberculosis may demonstrate similar appearing lesions. Supporting imaging studies are recommended including EDI-OCT, FFA, FAF, ICG and visual field testing. FAF may be useful in monitoring response to treatment.[40]

Treatment and prognosis: Systemic and periocular corticosteroids are used for short-term remission and IMT for long-term due to the chronic nature of the disease course. Intravitreal anti-VEGF agents are used as adjuncts for the treatment of CNVM. Visual prognosis is guarded. CNVM is the most common cause of vision loss (Figure 5.20), followed by macular edema and epiretinal membrane (ERM).[41]

5.3.3 *Multiple Evanescent White Dot Syndrome (MEWDS)*

Definition: Idiopathic acute, unilateral, self-limiting retinal inflammatory disorder, affecting otherwise healthy young females. Patients present with acute, unilateral decreased vision, photopsias, and central or paracentral scotoma following a viral prodrome.[42]

Clinical features: Clinical manifestations include multiple small transient gray-white lesions, 100–200 μm in size at the level of RPE and outer ret-

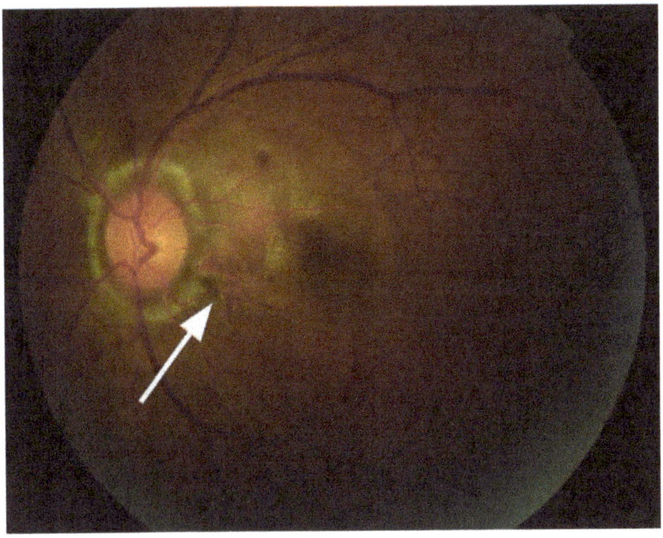

Figure 5.20. Multifocal choroiditis with choroidal neovascular membrane (arrow).

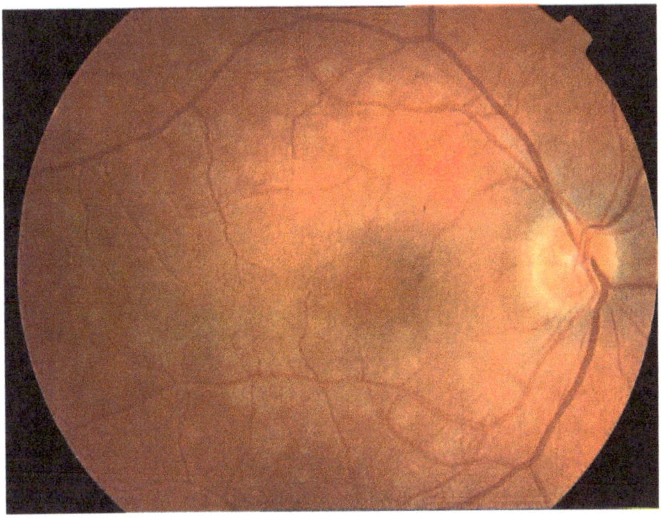

Figure 5.21. Multiple evanescent white dot syndrome.

ina, macular granularity, mild optic disc edema and minimal vitreous cells (Figure 5.21).[43] The retinal spots are transient and frequently missed.

Diagnostic techniques: Diagnosis is clinical; there are no specific lab tests. Infectious and autoimmune disorders should be ruled out. Imaging tests

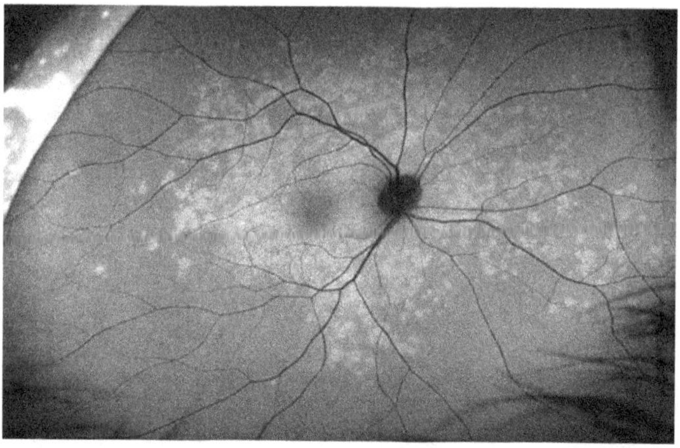

Figure 5.22. Fundus autofluorescence (wide-field imaging) of multiple evanescent white dot syndrome.

are complementary and include OCT, FFA, FAF, ICG and visual field testing. "Wreath-like" hyperfluorescent lesions are observed on FFA. OCT shows hyperreflective lesions extending from RPE through ellipsoid zone. FAF shows hyperfluorescent spots corresponding to and more numerous than those found on clinical examination (Figure 5.22). Visual field demonstrates enlargement of the blind spot. Absent to mild anterior chamber and vitreous cells are characteristic.

Treatment and prognosis: No treatment is needed. The disease is self-limiting (2–10 weeks) and visual prognosis is excellent.[42] In rare cases lesions can be complicated by the development of CNVM.

5.3.4 *Birdshot Chorioretinitis*

Definition: Chronic and bilateral multifocal chorioretinitis, characterized by vitritis, multiple, hypopigmented choroidal lesions and retinal vascular leakage, with a slight female predominance. Blurred vision, floaters, loss of peripheral vision, nyclatopia and disturbance of color vision are the presenting symptoms.

Clinical features: Cream colored choroidal spots emanating from the optic nerve, following the underlying choroidal vessels (Figure 5.23). There is absent to mild anterior chamber cells. HLA-A29 is highly specific and is complementary for the diagnosis.[44]

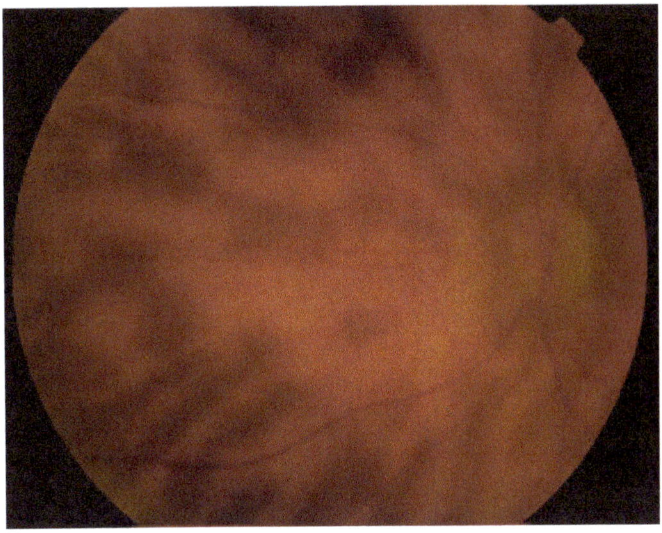

Figure 5.23. Birdshot chorioretinitis.

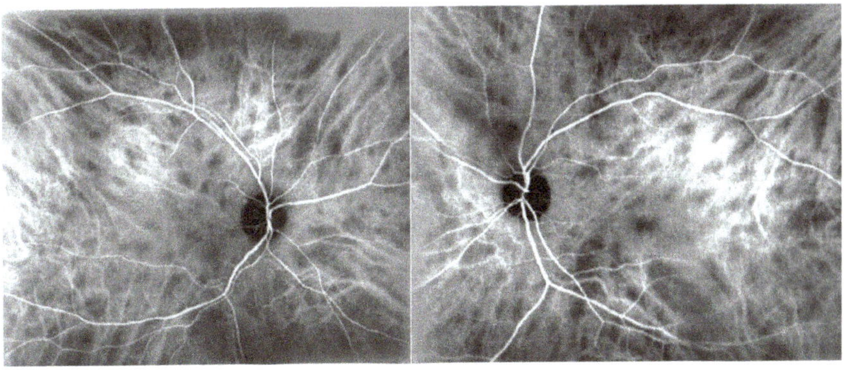

Figure 5.24. Indocyanine green in birdshot chorioretinitis, demonstrating multiple choroidal lesions in both eyes.

Diagnostic techniques: Diagnosis is made clinically with ancillary multimodal imaging and HLA-A29 gene testing. The diffuse retinal damage manifests as visual field loss or an abnormal ERG, particularly the 30 Hz flicker test. The choroidal lesions are best demonstrated on ICG as multifocal hypocyanescent spots and are typically more numerous than those detected on clinical examination or FFA (Figure 5.24). OCT may show macular edema and disruption of photoreceptors. ERG and visual field testing are used for disease monitoring and response to treatment.[45]

Treatment and prognosis: Treatment consists of systemic corticosteroids with early introduction of steroid-sparing IMT. Macular edema is the most common cause of reduced visual acuity. Even patients with good visual acuity may have diminished contrast sensitivity and decreased quality of vision.[46]

5.3.5 Acute Posterior Multifocal Placoid Pigment Epitheliopathy (APMPPE)

Definition: Bilateral acute disease manifesting as multifocal lesions, located around the posterior pole.[47] Patients complain of sudden painless blurred vision, photopsias and scotomas. The second eye may manifest concurrently or within several days. Neurologic manifestations may occur including cerebral vasculitis, aseptic meningitis, transient hearing loss, seizures and even cerebral ischemia.[48]

Clinical features: Multifocal yellowish-creamy, subretinal, placoid lesions appear around the posterior pole (Figure 5.25). On FFA lesions appear hypofluorescent during the early stages of the study, later becoming hyperfluorescent (Figure 5.26).[49] On OCT the placoid lesions appear as disruption of the outer retina with hyperreflective material at the level of the RPE (Figure 5.27). As the lesions resolve, the hyperreflectivity disappears with partial restoration of its appearance or areas of atrophy. FAF is used to follow patients and can demonstrate the stage of the disease, with active

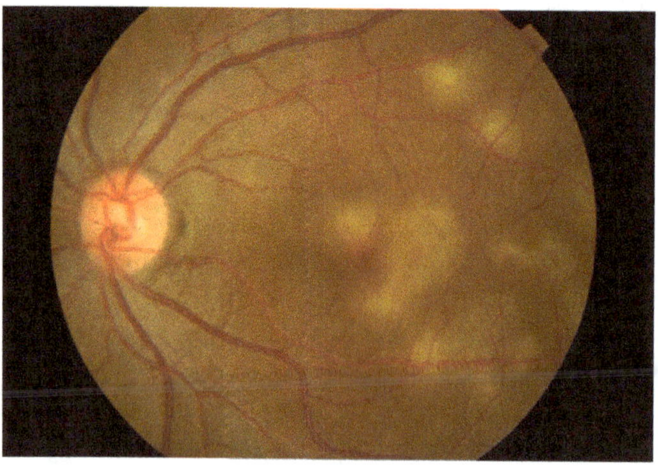

Figure 5.25. Acute posterior multifocal placoid pigment epitheliopathy.

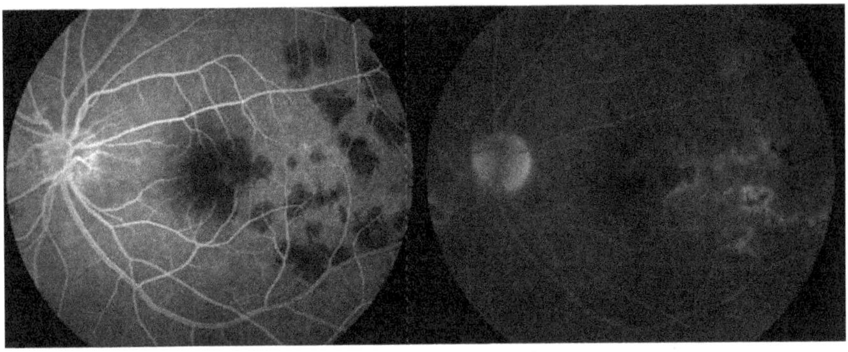

Figure 5.26. Fundus fluorescein angiography demonstrating lesions with the typical pattern of early blockage hypofluorescence (left) and late leakage hyperfluorescence (right).

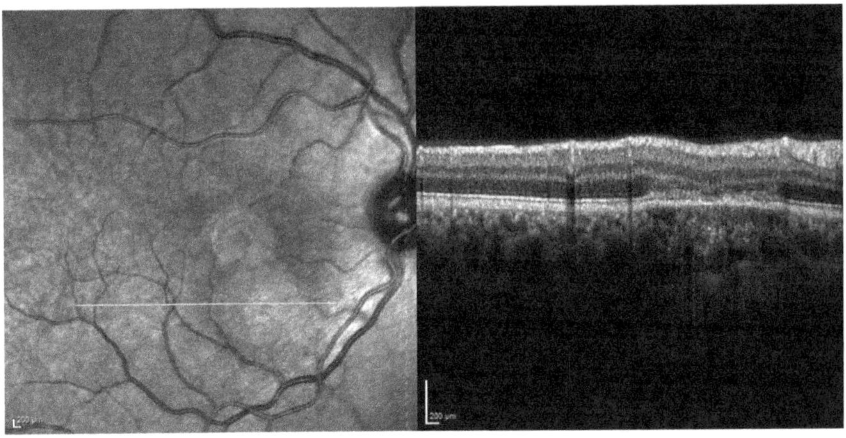

Figure 5.27. Optical coherence tomography (right) demonstrating hyperreflective material at the level of the outer retina of a lesion (left).

lesions appearing as hyperautofluorescence and resolved lesions speckled with hypoautofluorescence (Figure 5.28).[50]

Diagnostic techniques: Diagnosis is based on clinical and imaging findings. An infectious cause must be ruled out including syphilis and tuberculosis. An ACE test should be performed to rule out sarcoidosis. In case of any neurologic complaints, patients must be investigated with brain MRI and cerebral spinal fluid examination.

Treatment and prognosis: APMPPE is a self-limiting condition with a good prognosis, though it can recur with progressive visual loss.[51] During the

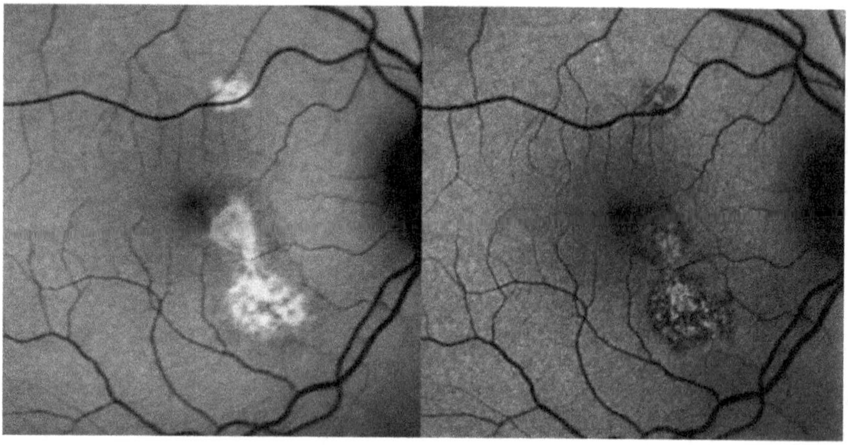

Figure 5.28. Fundus autofluorescence of active (left) and resolved (right) APMPPE lesions.

acute stage, treatment is recommended with systemic corticosteroids. In recurrent disease the use of steroid-sparing IMT is advocated.[47]

5.4 Panuveitis

Panuveitis represents ocular inflammation that is observed in the anterior, intermediate and posterior chambers. Diagnosis is established in the presence of choroidal or retinal inflammation, vitreous inflammation and presence of signs of anterior uveitis.

5.4.1 *Ocular Sarcoidosis*

Definition: Bilateral chronic granulomatous ocular inflammation in a patient with systemic manifestations suggestive of sarcoidosis (pulmonary, lymph nodes, skin, CNS, liver and joints). It is an important diagnostic consideration in elderly patients with new onset uveitis.[52]

Clinical features: Anterior uveitis with mutton fat KPs (Figure 5.29), broad-based peripheral anterior synechiae, and iris nodules or anterior segment granulomas are the most common ocular manifestations (Figure 5.30). Vitreous involvement presents with cells and snowballs as "string of pearls" (Figure 5.31), perivascular sheathing and periphlebitis ("candle wax drippings", Figure 5.32). Choroid is usually thickened and there may be multifocal choroidal granulomas (Figure 5.33).[53]

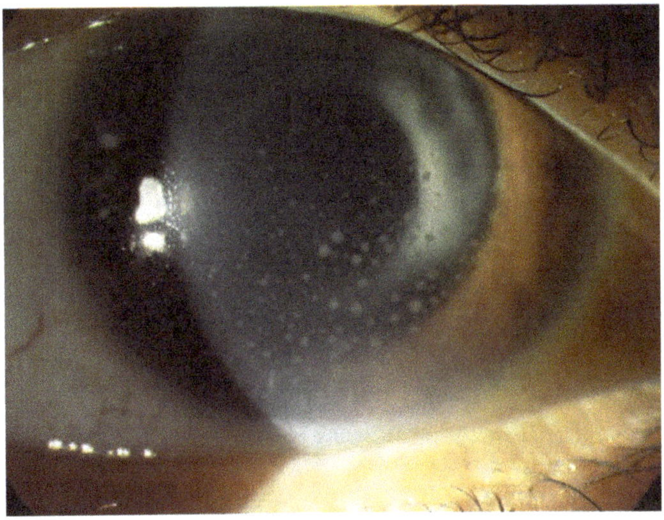

Figure 5.29. Sarcoid panuveitis with mutton fat keratic precipitates.

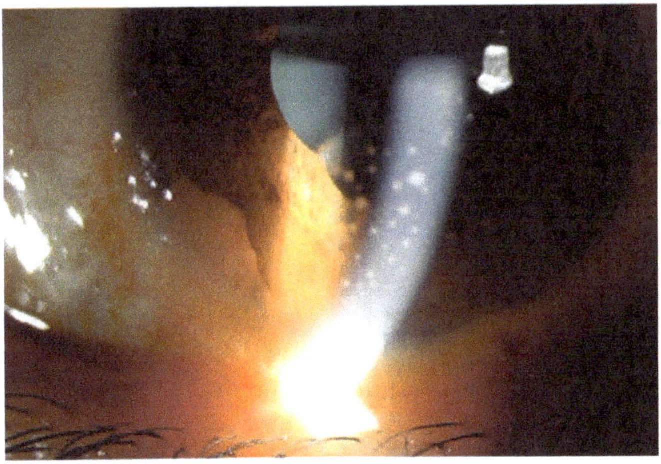

Figure 5.30. Anterior segment granuloma and mutton fat keratic precipitates in sarcoidosis.

Diagnostic techniques: Pulmonary manifestations such as hilar lymphadenopathy on CXR, elevated serum ACE and lysozyme levels, abnormal gallium scan and characteristics signs on chest computed tomography are helpful in diagnosing sarcoidosis (Figure 5.34). Clinical diagnosis is based

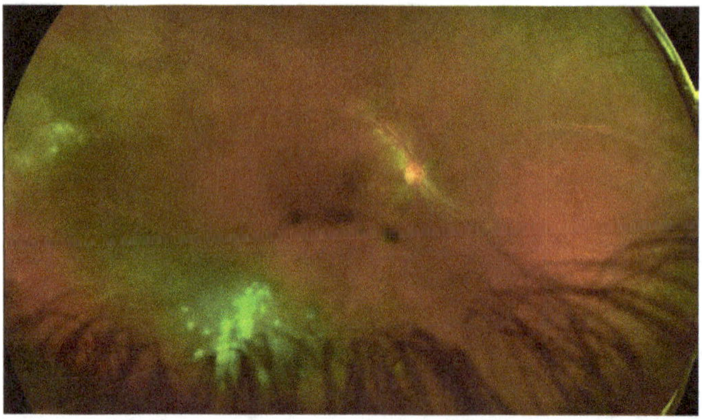

Figure 5.31. Ocular sarcoidosis with "string of pearls" snowballs in the vitreous and vascular sheathing.

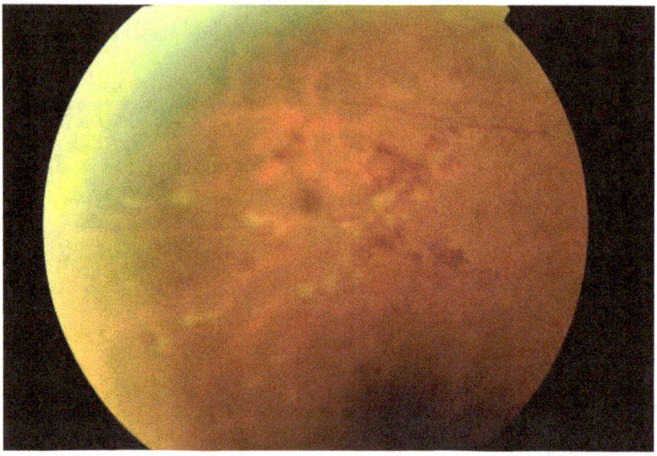

Figure 5.32. Ocular sarcoidosis with "candle wax dripping" vasculitis.

on a scoring system of combinations of ocular and systemic findings (see Chapter 4, Table 4.2).[52,54,55] Definite diagnosis is made with a compatible uveitis with positive biopsy.

Treatment and prognosis: Local and systemic corticosteroids, as well as IMT for chronic disease. Pulmonary disease is the major cause of morbidity. Sarcoid uveitis is associated with a favorable visual prognosis.[56]

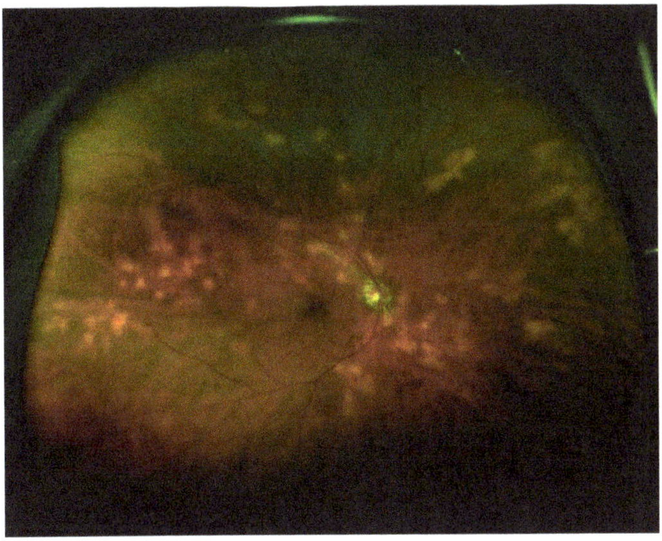

Figure 5.33. Multifocal choroidal granulomas in sarcoidosis.

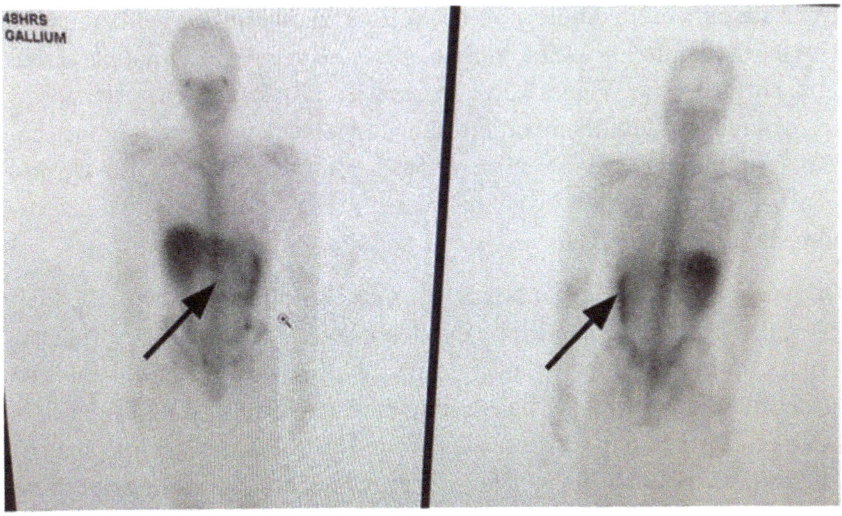

Figure 5.34. Gallium-67 scan of a patient with sarcoidosis demonstrating pulmonary uptake (arrow).

5.4.2 *Vogt-Koyanagi-Harada Disease (VKH)*

Definition: Chronic bilateral granulomatous panuveitis accompanied by auditory, neurologic and dermatologic manifestations. Typically occurs in young adults, more frequently in darkly pigmented ethnic groups.

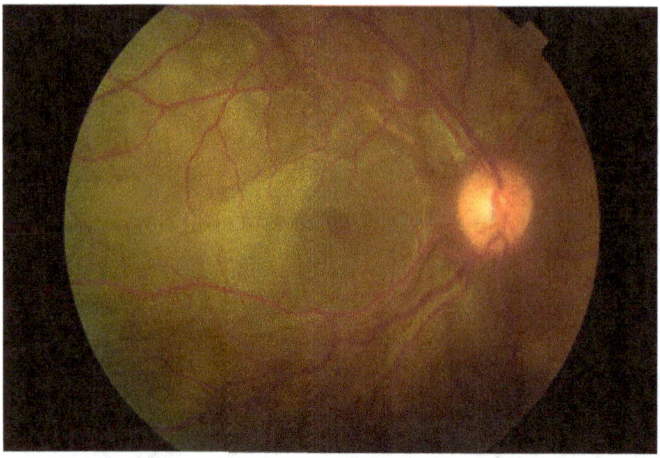

Figure 5.35. Vogt-Koyanagi-Harada syndrome.

Clinical features: There are four stages of the disease; prodromal with flu-like symptoms, acute uveitic, convalescent, and chronic recurrent.[57] In the acute uveitis stage there is a diffuse, non-necrotizing, granulomatous inflammation with bilateral anterior uveitis, vitritis, optic disc edema and multiple serous retinal detachments (Figure 5.35). The convalescent stage is characterized by non-granulomatous inflammation with gradual depigmentation of the choroid, resulting in the classic sunset-glow fundus (Figure 5.36). The chronic recurrent stage is marked by granulomatous anterior uveitis, with the development of KPs, posterior synechia, iris nodules, and stromal atrophy.[58]

Diagnostic techniques: Diagnosis is based on clinical features with the typical ocular signs, accompanied by the characteristic systemic signs (poliosis, vitiligo, alopecia, sensorineural hearing loss, tinnitus, vertigo).[59] Bilateral involvement, no history of penetrating ocular trauma and no evidence of other ocular or systemic disease are required criteria for diagnosis. Imaging studies (FFA, ICG, OCT, FAF), lumbar puncture, and ultrasonography may be useful.[57] FFA reveals numerous punctate hyperfluorescent dots, followed by pooling of dye in areas of neurosensory detachment and disc leakage ("starry sky" pattern) (Figure 5.37). ICG shows multiple hypocyanescent spots throughout the fundus (Figure 5.38). EDI-OCT demonstrates serous macular detachments and choroidal thickening (Figure 5.39).

Treatment and prognosis: Treatment includes systemic corticosteroids with slow tapering according to clinical response over 6–12 months. Consider initiating IMT early for steroid-sparing effect. Visual prognosis is fair.

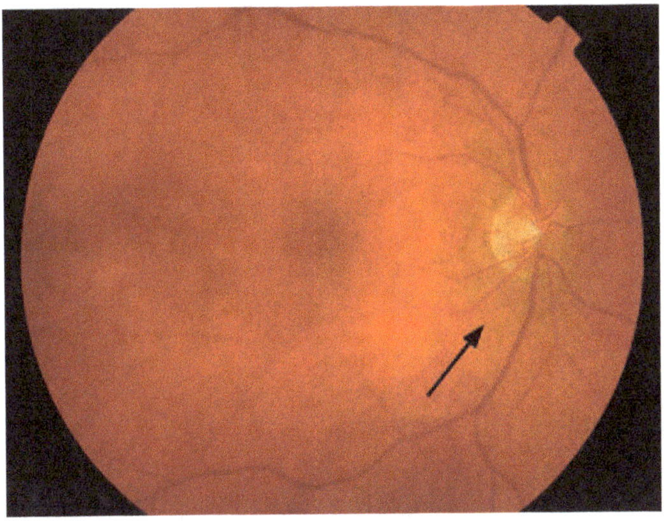

Figure 5.36. Sunset-glow fundus in Vogt-Koyanagi-Harada syndrome. Note the peripapillary discoloration.

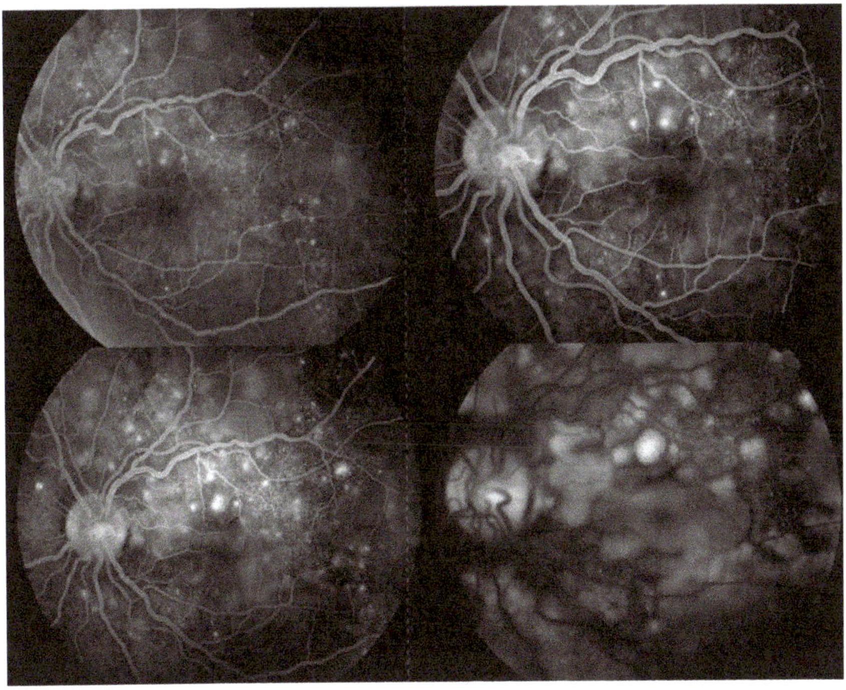

Figure 5.37. Fundus fluorescein angiography of Vogt-Koyanagi-Harada syndrome demonstrating the "starry sky" pattern.

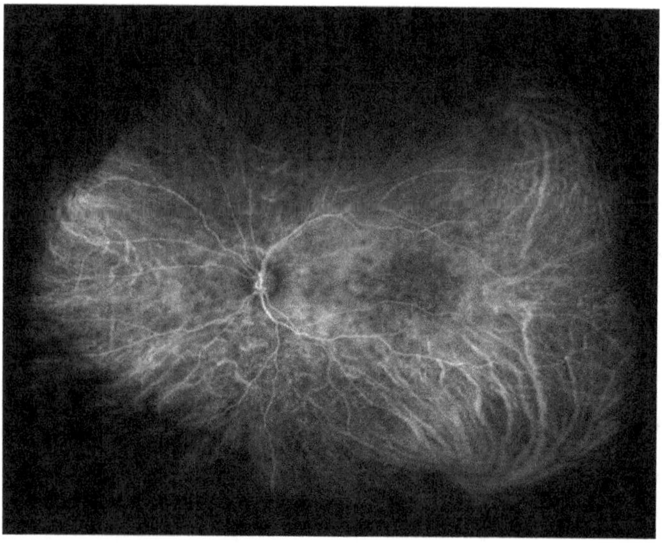

Figure 5.38. ICG scan with multiple hypocyanescent spots throughout the fundus in Vogt-Koyanagi-Harada syndrome.

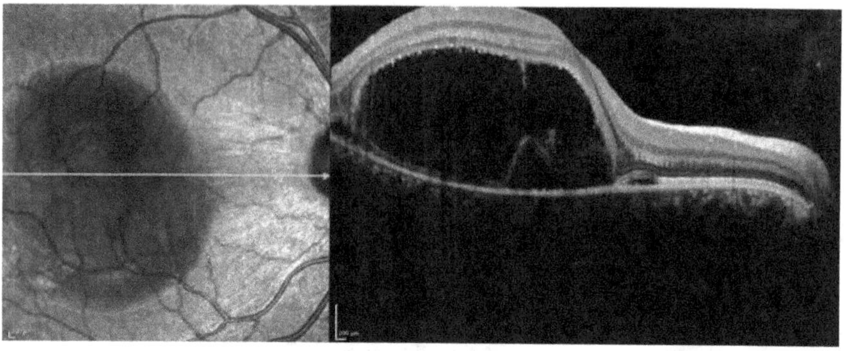

Figure 5.39. Optical coherence tomography demonstrating a large serous retinal detachment in a patient with Vogt-Koyanagi-Harada syndrome.

Ocular complications include cataract, glaucoma, CNVM and subretinal fibrosis (Figure 5.40).

5.4.3 *Behçet's Disease Uveitis*

Definition: A chronic recurrent multisystem inflammatory disorder, affecting mostly young men in countries along the ancient Silk Road. The disease constitutes a triad of mouth ulcers, genital ulcers, and uveitis.

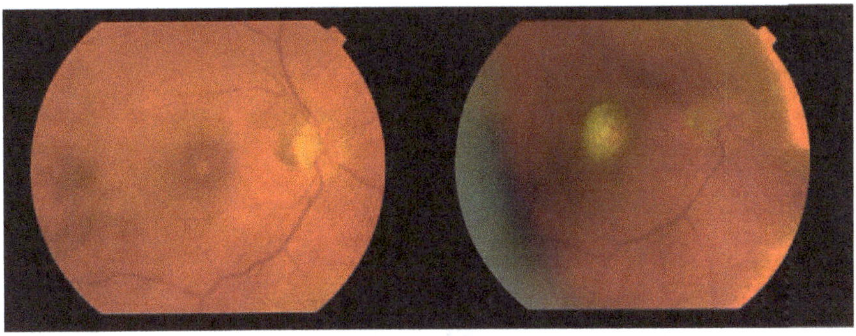

Figure 5.40. Progression of Vogt-Koyanagi-Harada syndrome over three years (left to right) showing development of sunset-glow fundus, choroidal neovascular membrane and fibrosis.

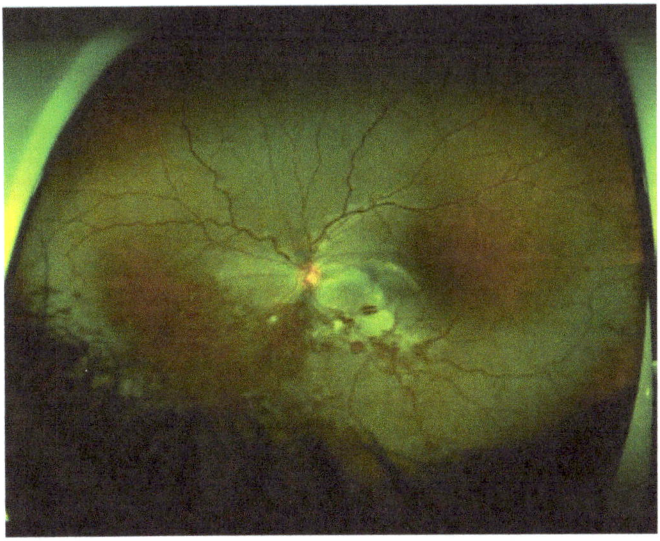

Figure 5.41. Behçet's disease with retinitis, retinal vasculitis and retinal hemorrhage.

Clinical features: Relapsing remitting panuveitis with occlusive retinal vasculitis and/or focal white infiltrates, affects both arteries and veins (Figures 5.41 and 5.42). May present with hypopyon in a white eye (Figure 5.43).

Diagnostic techniques: The diagnosis is performed by clinical criteria; recurrent oral ulcers plus 2 of recurrent genital ulcers, uveitis, skin lesions or positive pathergy test. There is also an association with HLA-B51.[60-62]

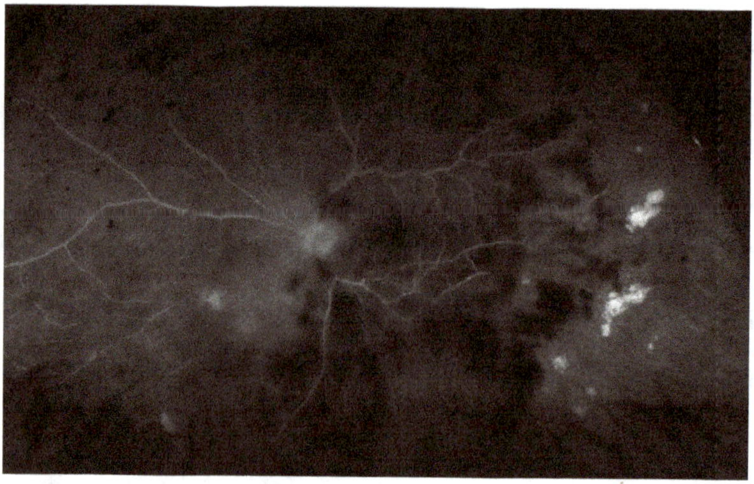

Figure 5.42. Fluorescein angiography in Behçet's disease. Note extensive retinal hemorrhages, ischemic vasculitis and peripheral ischemia in the inferior retina.

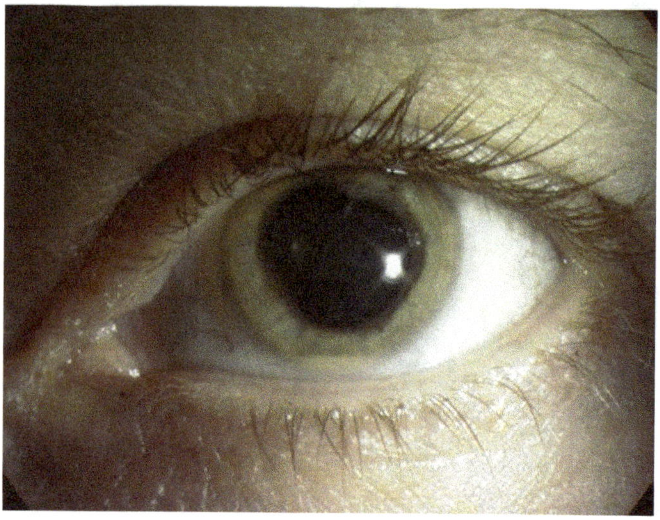

Figure 5.43. Hypopyon in an eye with Behçet's disease.

Treatment and prognosis: Systemic corticosteroids are not sufficiently effective for long-term remission, therefore early initiated IMT is warranted. Inflammation is particularly responsive to anti-tumor necrosis factor (TNF)-α agents.[63] Untreated, the uveitis has a poor prognosis, with high rates of blindness.

5.4.4 *Sympathetic Ophthalmia*

Definition: Diffuse granulomatous panuveitis that may arise following ocular trauma. Initially penetrating ocular trauma was the primary mechanism, but in recent years this has been superseded by iatrogenic trauma, in particular, vitreoretinal surgery.

Clinical features: Granulomatous anterior uveitis with mutton-fat KPs, vitritis, optic nerve swelling, multifocal exudative retinal detachments and choroidal granulomas appearing as Dalen-Fuchs' nodules (Figures 5.44 and 5.45).

Diagnostic techniques: Clinical diagnosis based on classic presentation and history of preceding trauma or surgery.

Treatment and prognosis: Adequate treatment is critical as the other eye usually has very poor vision secondary to trauma or previous recurrent retinal detachment. High dose corticosteroids (often intravenous methylprednisolone) will be used at treatment induction, followed by a long slow taper of oral prednisone, typically accompanied by IMT. Many cases will also benefit from the addition of anti-TNF treatment. With early aggressive treatment the prognosis can be good, but vision may be limited by complications such as subretinal fibrosis, optic nerve atrophy, glaucomatous optic neuropathy, epiretinal membrane and choroidal neovascular membrane.

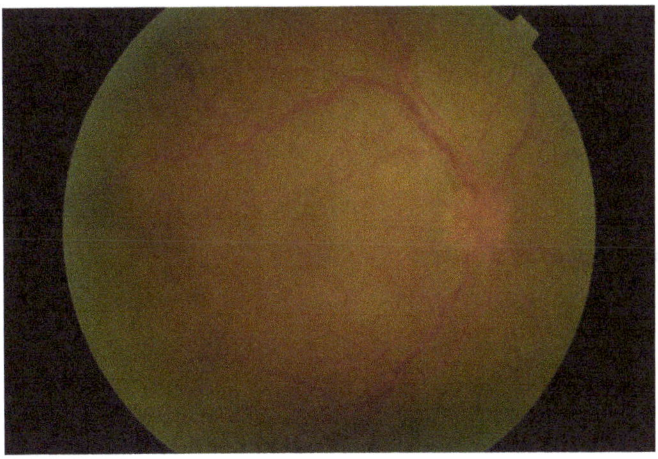

Figure 5.44. Sympathetic ophthalmia with optic nerve swelling and exudative retinal detachment.

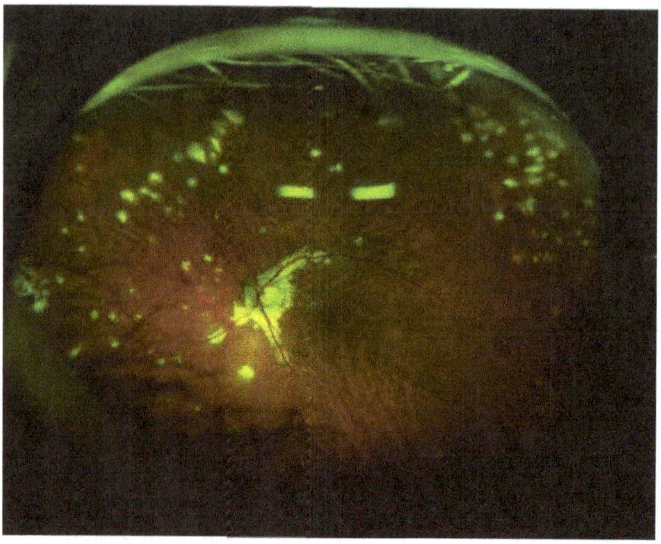

Figure 5.45. Late sequelae of sympathetic ophthalmia with chorioretinal atrophic scars.

Teaching Points

- Posner-Schlossman syndrome may be related to CMV infection, though use of antiviral treatment is not clear.
- Punctate inner choroiditis (PIC) and multifocal choroiditis with panuveitis (MFC-PU) have many similarities. These include: affecting young healthy myopic women, atrophic punched-out lesions and the complication of CNVM. Differences include PIC having yellow-white lesions while MFC-PU has yellow-gray lesions, peripheral retina lesions in MFC-PU, and absence of anterior chamber and vitreous cells in PIC whilst MFC-PU often displays anterior chamber and vitreous cells.
- Multiple evanescent white dot syndrome (MEWDS) is generally self-limiting (2–10 weeks), although in rare cases can develop CNVM.
- Acute posterior multifocal placoid pigment epitheliopathy (APMPPE) presents with sudden painless blurred vision, photopsias and scotomas, rarely neurological symptoms.
- Behçet's disease uveitis is associated with HLA-B51, however the diagnosis is made when there are recurrent oral ulcers plus 2 of recurrent genital ulcers, uveitis, skin lesions or a positive pathergy test.

References

1. Thorne JE, Suhler E, Skup M, *et al.* Prevalence of noninfectious uveitis in the United States: a claims-based analysis. *JAMA Ophthalmol* 2016;134(11):1237–45.
2. McCannel CA, Holland GN, Helm CJ, *et al.* Causes of uveitis in the general practice of ophthalmology. UCLA Community-Based Uveitis Study Group. *Am J Ophthalmol* 1996;121(1):35–46.
3. Acharya NR, Tham VM, Esterberg E, *et al.* Incidence and prevalence of uveitis: results from the Pacific Ocular Inflammation Study. *JAMA Ophthalmol* 2013;131(11):1405–12.
4. Rosenbaum JT, Bodaghi B, Couto C, *et al.* New observations and emerging ideas in diagnosis and management of non-infectious uveitis: A review. *Semin Arthritis Rheum* 2019;49(3):438–45.
5. Jabs DA, Nussenblatt RB, Rosenbaum JT. Standardization of uveitis nomenclature for reporting clinical data. Results of the First International Workshop. *Am J Ophthalmol* 2005;140(3):509–16.
6. Rodriguez A, Calonge M, Pedroza-Seres M, *et al.* Referral patterns of uveitis in a tertiary eye care center. *Arch Ophthalmol* 1996;114(5):593–9.
7. Mandeville JT, Levinson RD, Holland GN. The tubulointerstitial nephritis and uveitis syndrome. *Surv Ophthalmol* 2001;46(3):195–208.
8. Levinson RD, Mandeville JT, Holland GN, Rosenbaum JT. Tubulointerstitial nephritis and uveitis syndrome: recognizing the importance of an uncommon disease. *Am J Ophthalmol* 2000;129(6):798–9.
9. Mackensen F, Billing H. Tubulointerstitial nephritis and uveitis syndrome. *Curr Opin Ophthalmol* 2009;20(6):525–31.
10. Mackensen F, Smith JR, Rosenbaum JT. Enhanced recognition, treatment, and prognosis of tubulointerstitial nephritis and uveitis syndrome. *Ophthalmology* 2007;114(5):995–9.
11. Suhler EB, Martin TM, Rosenbaum JT. HLA-B27-associated uveitis: overview and current perspectives. *Curr Opin Ophthalmol* 2003;14(6):378–83.
12. Wakefield D, Clarke D, McCluskey P. Recent developments in HLA B27 anterior uveitis. *Front Immunol* 2020;11:608134.
13. Loh AR, Acharya NR. Incidence rates and risk factors for ocular complications and vision loss in HLA-B27-associated uveitis. *Am J Ophthalmol* 2010;150(4):534–42 e2.
14. Chang JH, McCluskey PJ, Wakefield D. Acute anterior uveitis and HLA-B27. *Surv Ophthalmol* 2005;50(4):364–88.
15. Standardization of Uveitis Nomenclature Working G. Classification criteria for spondyloarthritis/HLA-B27-associated anterior uveitis. *Am J Ophthalmol* 2021;228:117–25.

16. Shazly TA, Aljajeh M, Latina MA. Posner-Schlossman glaucomatocyclitic crisis. *Semin Ophthalmol* 2011;26(4–5):282–4.
17. Megaw R, Agarwal PK. Posner-Schlossman syndrome. *Surv Ophthalmol* 2017;62(3):277–85.
18. Standardization of Uveitis Nomenclature Working G. Classification criteria for Fuchs uveitis syndrome. *Am J Ophthalmol* 2021;228:262–7.
19. Rothova A, La Hey E, Baarsma GS, Breebaart AC. Iris nodules in Fuchs' heterochromic uveitis. *Am J Ophthalmol* 1994;118(3):338–42.
20. Velilla S, Dios E, Herreras JM, Calonge M. Fuchs' heterochromic iridocyclitis: a review of 26 cases. *Ocul Immunol Inflamm* 2001;9(3):169–75.
21. de Visser L, Braakenburg A, Rothova A, de Boer JH. Rubella virus-associated uveitis: clinical manifestations and visual prognosis. *Am J Ophthalmol* 2008;146(2):292–7.
22. de Groot-Mijnes JD, de Visser L, Rothova A, *et al.* Rubella virus is associated with Fuchs heterochromic iridocyclitis. *Am J Ophthalmol* 2006;141(1):212–4.
23. Clarke SL, Sen ES, Ramanan AV. Juvenile idiopathic arthritis-associated uveitis. *Pediatr Rheumatol Online J* 2016;14(1):27.
24. Standardization of Uveitis Nomenclature Working G. Classification criteria for juvenile idiopathic arthritis-associated chronic anterior uveitis. *Am J Ophthalmol* 2021;228:192–7.
25. Angeles-Han ST, Ringold S, Beukelman T, *et al.* 2019 American College of Rheumatology/Arthritis Foundation Guideline for the screening, monitoring, and treatment of juvenile idiopathic arthritis-associated uveitis. *Arthritis Care Res (Hoboken)* 2019;71(6):703–16.
26. Thorne JE, Woreta FA, Dunn JP, Jabs DA. Risk of cataract development among children with juvenile idiopathic arthritis-related uveitis treated with topical corticosteroids. *Ophthalmology* 2010;117(7):1436–41.
27. Hawkins MJ, Dick AD, Lee RJ, *et al.* Managing juvenile idiopathic arthritis-associated uveitis. *Surv Ophthalmol* 2016;61(2):197–210.
28. Thorne JE, Woreta F, Kedhar SR, *et al.* Juvenile idiopathic arthritis-associated uveitis: incidence of ocular complications and visual acuity loss. *Am J Ophthalmol* 2007;143(5):840–6.
29. Standardization of Uveitis Nomenclature Working G. Classification criteria for intermediate uveitis, non-pars planitis type. *Am J Ophthalmol* 2021; 228:159–64.
30. Ozdal PC, Berker N, Tugal-Tutkun I. Pars planitis: epidemiology, clinical characteristics, management and visual prognosis. *J Ophthalmic Vis Res* 2015;10(4):469–80.
31. Prieto JF, Dios E, Gutierrez JM, *et al.* Pars planitis: epidemiology, treatment, and association with multiple sclerosis. *Ocul Immunol Inflamm* 2001;9(2): 93–102.

32. Standardization of Uveitis Nomenclature Working G. Classification criteria for pars planitis. *Am J Ophthalmol* 2021;228:268–74.
33. Berker N, Sen E, Elgin U, *et al.* Analysis of clinical features and visual outcomes of pars planitis. *Int Ophthalmol* 2018;38(2):727–36.
34. Zein G, Berta A, Foster CS. Multiple sclerosis-associated uveitis. *Ocul Immunol Inflamm* 2004;12(2):137–42.
35. Standardization of Uveitis Nomenclature Working G. Classification criteria for multiple sclerosis-associated intermediate uveitis. *Am J Ophthalmol* 2021;228:72–9.
36. Gilbert RM, Niederer RL, Kramer M, *et al.* Differentiating multifocal choroiditis and punctate inner choroidopathy: a cluster analysis approach. *Am J Ophthalmol* 2020;213:244–51.
37. Standardization of Uveitis Nomenclature Working G. Classification criteria for punctate inner choroiditis. *Am J Ophthalmol* 2021;228:275–80.
38. Woronkowicz M, Niederer RL, Lightman S, Tomkins-Netzer O. Intravitreal anti-vascular endothelial growth factor treatment for inflammatory choroidal neovascularization in non-infectious uveitis. *Am J Ophthalmol* 2021;236:281–7.
39. Standardization of Uveitis Nomenclature Working G. Classification criteria for multifocal choroiditis with panuveitis. *Am J Ophthalmol* 2021;228:152–8.
40. Kedhar SR, Thorne JE, Wittenberg S, *et al.* Multifocal choroiditis with panuveitis and punctate inner choroidopathy: comparison of clinical characteristics at presentation. *Retina* 2007;27(9):1174–9.
41. Thorne JE, Wittenberg S, Jabs DA, *et al.* Multifocal choroiditis with panuveitis incidence of ocular complications and of loss of visual acuity. *Ophthalmology* 2006;113(12):2310–6.
42. Gross NE, Yannuzzi LA, Freund KB, *et al.* Multiple evanescent white dot syndrome. *Arch Ophthalmol* 2006;124(4):493–500.
43. Standardization of Uveitis Nomenclature Working G. Classification criteria for multiple evanescent white dot syndrome. *Am J Ophthalmol* 2021;228: 198–204.
44. Standardization of Uveitis Nomenclature Working G. Classification criteria for birdshot chorioretinitis. *Am J Ophthalmol* 2021;228:65–71.
45. Shah KH, Levinson RD, Yu F, *et al.* Birdshot chorioretinopathy. *Surv Ophthalmol* 2005;50(6):519–41.
46. Tomkins-Netzer O, Taylor SR, Lightman S. Long-term clinical and anatomic outcome of birdshot chorioretinopathy. *JAMA Ophthalmol* 2014;132(1): 57–62.
47. Testi I, Vermeirsch S, Pavesio C. Acute posterior multifocal placoid pigment epitheliopathy (APMPPE). *J Ophthalmic Inflamm Infect* 2021;11(1):31.

48. Brownlee WJ, Anderson NE, Sims J, Pereira JA. Neurological complications of acute multifocal placoid pigment epitheliopathy. *J Clin Neurosci* 2016;31: 76–80.
49. Dunn JP. Imaging in the white dot syndromes. *Int Ophthalmol Clin* 2016;56(4):175–201.
50. Souka AA, Hillenkamp J, Gora F, *et al.* Correlation between optical coherence tomography and autofluorescence in acute posterior multifocal placoid pigment epitheliopathy. *Graefes Arch Clin Exp Ophthalmol* 2006;244(10): 1219–23.
51. Thomas BC, Jacobi C, Korporal M, *et al.* Ocular outcome and frequency of neurological manifestations in patients with acute posterior multifocal placoid pigment epitheliopathy (APMPPE). *J Ophthalmic Inflamm Infect* 2012;2(3):125–31.
52. Standardization of Uveitis Nomenclature Working G. Classification criteria for sarcoidosis-associated uveitis. *Am J Ophthalmol* 2021;228:220–30.
53. Ma SP, Rogers SL, Hall AJ, *et al.* Sarcoidosis-related uveitis: clinical presentation, disease course, and rates of systemic disease progression after uveitis diagnosis. *Am J Ophthalmol* 2019;198:30–6.
54. Mochizuki M, Smith JR, Takase H, *et al.* Revised criteria of International Workshop on Ocular Sarcoidosis (IWOS) for the diagnosis of ocular sarcoidosis. *Br J Ophthalmol* 2019;103(10):1418–22.
55. Niederer RL, Ma SP, Wilsher ML, *et al.* Systemic associations of sarcoid uveitis: correlation with uveitis phenotype and ethnicity. *Am J Ophthalmol* 2021;229:169–75.
56. Hwang DK, Sheu SJ. An update on the diagnosis and management of ocular sarcoidosis. *Curr Opin Ophthalmol* 2020;31(6):521–31.
57. O'Keefe GA, Rao NA. Vogt-Koyanagi-Harada disease. *Surv Ophthalmol* 2017;62(1):1–25.
58. Read RW, Holland GN, Rao NA, *et al.* Revised diagnostic criteria for Vogt-Koyanagi-Harada disease: report of an international committee on nomenclature. *Am J Ophthalmol* 2001;131(5):647–52.
59. Standardization of Uveitis Nomenclature Working G. Classification criteria for Vogt-Koyanagi-Harada disease. *Am J Ophthalmol* 2021;228:205–11.
60. Standardization of Uveitis Nomenclature Working G. Classification criteria for Behcet disease uveitis. *Am J Ophthalmol* 2021;228:80–8.
61. Tugal-Tutkun I, Onal S, Altan-Yaycioglu R, *et al.* Uveitis in Behcet disease: an analysis of 880 patients. *Am J Ophthalmol* 2004;138(3):373–80.
62. Tugal-Tutkun I, Onal S, Stanford M, *et al.* An algorithm for the diagnosis of Behcet disease uveitis in adults. *Ocul Immunol Inflamm* 2021;29(6): 1154–63.

63. Al-Janabi A, El Nokrashy A, Sharief L, *et al.* Long-term outcomes of treatment with biological agents in eyes with refractory, active, noninfectious intermediate uveitis, posterior uveitis, or panuveitis. *Ophthalmology* 2020;127(3):410–6.

https://doi.org/10.1142/9789811251474_0006

Chapter 6

Infectious Uveitis

*Sophia L Zagora**

Uveitis due to infectious etiologies accounts for a significant proportion of the uveitis burden and vision loss worldwide.[1] At tertiary care referral centers, it represents an even higher proportion of uveitis cases, approximately 26–35%.[2] While infectious uveitis can affect various anatomic locations of the eye ranging from anterior to posterior uveitis, the most devastating cases are represented by those that cause posterior involvement such as acute retinal necrosis associated with herpes viruses, or toxoplasmosis retinochoroiditis. Infectious uveitis can often mimic immune-mediated uveitis. Recognizing an infectious cause of uveitis, and early aggressive treatment with appropriate antimicrobial agents, are of paramount importance for preserving vision. The clinical presentation of various types of infectious uveitis and appropriate use of molecular diagnostics to aid in identifying an infectious agent are crucial in the management of these conditions.

6.1 Viral Uveitis

6.1.1 *Keratouveitis*

Herpes Simplex Virus (HSV) and Varicella Zoster Virus (VZV) keratouveitis are very common. HSV and VZV are double-stranded DNA viruses of the herpes group. Primary infection of VZV results in chickenpox (varicella). Reactivation of virus dormant in the sensory ganglion results in shingles (herpes zoster) of the innervated dermatome. Involvement of the ophthalmic branch of the trigeminal nerve (cranial nerve V1) occurs in

* Sydney Eye Hospital, Sydney, Australia
University of Sydney, Sydney, Australia
Westmead Children's Hospital, New South Wales, Australia

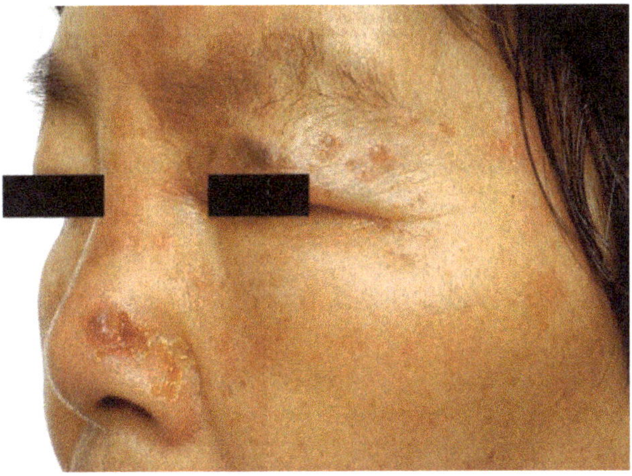

Figure 6.1. Nasociliary nerve involvement in herpes zoster ophthalmicus.

25% of shingles cases and results in herpes zoster ophthalmicus (HZO, Figure 6.1). VZV infection may be more severe in the immunosuppressed.[3]

Clinical features of HZO include a viral prodrome, preherpetic neuralgia (mild intermittent tingling to severe constant electric pain), rash (papules, vesicles, pustules, scabs) predominantly within the one dermatome (cranial nerve V1), and Hutchinson's sign (cutaneous involvement of the tip of the nose, indicating nasociliary nerve involvement and increased likelihood of ocular involvement, Figure 6.1) which may be disseminated (involving multiple dermatomes) in immunocompromised patients.[3,4] The most common ocular manifestation of HSV infection is a self-limiting blepharoconjunctivitis, characterized by periorbital vesicular rash, follicular conjunctivitis, and preauricular lymphadenopathy. Following this, the virus ascends the sensory nerve axon and, similar to VZV, resides in the trigeminal ganglion from where viral reactivation, replication, and retrograde migration may occur.

Corneal involvement can include: epithelial, stromal nummular keratitis with anterior stromal granular deposits; necrotizing keratitis with stromal infiltrates, thinning, and even perforation. Disciform endotheliitis, Descemet's folds, anterior uveitis and keratic precipitates (KPs – an inflammatory cellular deposit seen on the corneal endothelium) can also occur (Table 6.1, Figure 6.2). Neurotrophic changes can occur with corneal nerve damage causing persistent epithelial defects, thinning, and even perforation. The neurotrophic cornea is vulnerable to bacterial and

Table 6.1. SUN classification criteria for varicella zoster virus anterior uveitis.

Criteria: 1, 2 and 3

1. Evidence of anterior uveitis
   a. anterior chamber cells
   b. if anterior vitreous cells are present, severity is less than anterior chamber inflammation
   c. no evidence of retinitis

AND

2. Unilateral uveitis (unless there is a positive aqueous PCR for varicella zoster virus)

AND

3. Evidence of varicella zoster virus infection in the eye
   a. aqueous humor PCR positive for varicella zoster virus **OR**
   b. sectoral iris atrophy in a patient ≥60 years of age **OR**
   c. concurrent or recent dermatomal herpes zoster

Exclusions:

1. Positive serology for syphilis using a treponemal test
2. Evidence of sarcoidosis (either bilateral hilar adenopathy on chest imaging or tissue biopsy demonstrating noncaseating granulomata)
3. Aqueous specimen PCR positive for cytomegalovirus or herpes simplex virus

PCR = polymerase chain reaction. Adapted from The Standardization of Uveitis Nomenclature (SUN) Working Group. Classification criteria for varicella zoster virus anterior uveitis. Am J Ophthalmol 2021;228:165–73.[5]

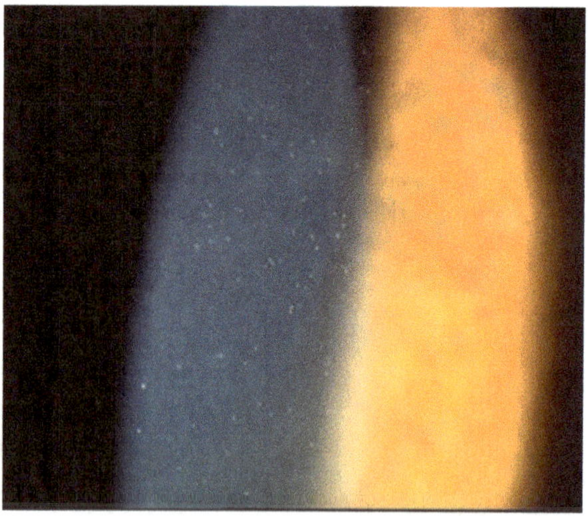

Figure 6.2. Anterior uveitis with keratic precipitates (KPs) on the endothelium.

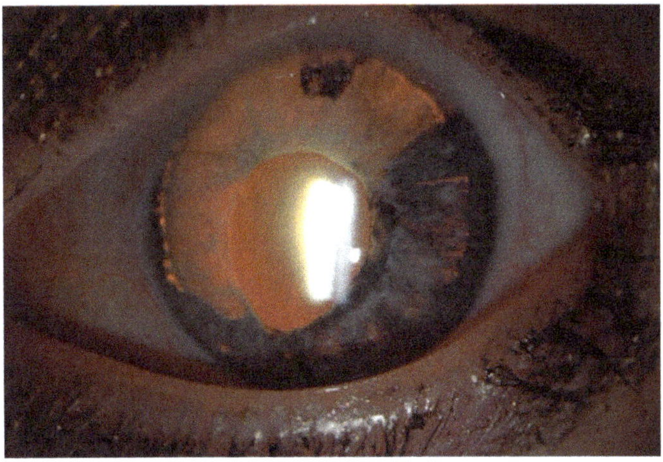

Figure 6.3. Iris transillumination defects in herpes zoster anterior uveitis.

Table 6.2. Directed treatment for anterior segment HSV and VZV infections.

Condition	Treatment	Duration
VZV keratouveitis	Valacyclovir 1 g orally q8h OR Famciclovir 500 mg orally q8h OR Acyclovir 800 mg orally 5 times daily	7 to 14 days
HSV keratouveitis	Valacyclovir 1 g orally q12h OR Famciclovir 500 mg orally q12h OR Acyclovir 800 mg orally 3 times daily	7 to 10 days

fungal keratitis. Mucus plaques with linear grey elevations, loosely adherent to underlying diseased epithelium/stroma can occur later on and be chronic.

Signs of HSV uveitis and herpes zoster sine herpete include elevated intraocular pressure, iris retroillumination defects (Figure 6.3) and KPs. Laboratory investigations include nucleic acid testing by VZV or HSV PCR.

Determining which layer of the eye is affected will dictate further localized treatment. Treatment options can include topical lubricants, topical acyclovir gel 5× per day and systemic antiviral +/- topical steroids, as indicated for anterior chamber inflammation (Table 6.2).[6] Treatments for post-herpetic neuralgia are often very important for the patient's recovery and include amitriptyline and gabapentin.

Table 6.3. SUN classification criteria for cytomegalovirus anterior uveitis.

Criteria: 1 and 2
1. Evidence of anterior uveitis
a. anterior chamber cells
b. if anterior vitreous cells are present, anterior chamber inflammation should be present
c. no evidence of retinitis
AND
2. Evidence of cytomegalovirus infection in the eye
a. Positive PCR for cytomegalovirus on aqueous specimen
Exclusions:
1. Positive serology for syphilis using a treponemal test
2. Evidence of sarcoidosis (either bilateral hilar adenopathy on chest imaging or tissue biopsy demonstrating noncaseating granulomata)
3. Aqueous specimen PCR positive for herpes simplex virus or varicella zoster virus

PCR = polymerase chain reaction. Adapted from The Standardization of Uveitis Nomenclature (SUN) Working Group. Classification criteria for cytomegalovirus anterior uveitis. Am J Ophthalmol 2021;228:89–95.[8]

6.1.2 Cytomegalovirus Anterior Uveitis

Cytomegalovirus (CMV) anterior uveitis is the most common ocular manifestation of CMV disease in immunocompetent individuals.[7] It is thought to be due to a local reactivation of latent CMV and is usually unilateral. The acute form may present as a Posner-Schlossman syndrome, a recurrent hypertensive anterior uveitis with few KPs. There are geographic differences in the chronic form of CMV anterior uveitis. Asian patients commonly present as Fuchs' uveitis syndrome with diffuse stellate KPs, while European patients present with a chronic hypertensive anterior uveitis with fewer KPs that are brown in color and located inferiorly. Characteristic features of CMV anterior uveitis include mild anterior chamber inflammation, elevated intraocular pressure, and stromal iris atrophy (Table 6.3). Synechia, macular edema and retinitis are typically absent. CMV disease may also be associated with the development of corneal endotheliitis with a reduced endothelial cell count.

6.1.3 Herpetic Viral Uveitis Acute Retinal Necrosis

Acute retinal necrosis (ARN) is primarily caused by VZV, HSV-1 or HSV-2 infection (Table 6.4). It may occur in the both the immunocompromised as well as healthy individuals of any age (Figure 6.4). Clinical findings

Table 6.4. SUN classification criteria for acute retinal necrosis.

Criteria: 1 and 2 or 3
1. Necrotizing retinitis involving the peripheral retina
AND (2 OR 3)
2. Evidence of infection with either HSV or VZV
a. Positive PCR for either HSV or VZV from either an aqueous or vitreous specimen
OR
3. Characteristic clinical picture
a. Circumferential or confluent retinitis **AND**
b. Retinal vascular sheathing and/or occlusion **AND**
c. More than minimal vitritis[a]
Exclusions:
1. Positive serology for syphilis using a treponemal test
2. Intraocular specimen PCR-positive for cytomegalovirus or *Toxoplasma gondii* (unless there is immunocompromise, morphologic evidence for >1 infection, the characteristic clinical picture of acute retinal necrosis, and the intraocular fluid specimen has a positive PCR for either HSV or VZV)

HSV = herpes simplex virus; PCR = polymerase chain reaction; VZV = varicella zoster virus.

[a]Vitritis criterion not required in immunocompromised patients.

Adapted from The Standardization of Uveitis Nomenclature (SUN) Working Group. Classification criteria for acute retinal necrosis syndrome. Am J Ophthalmol 2021;228:237–44.[9]

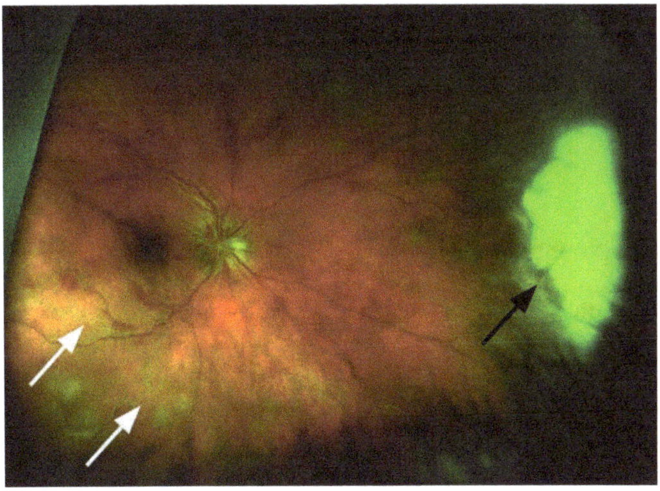

Figure 6.4. Widefield color fundus image of the left eye of a patient with acute retinal necrosis. Note the extensive retinal necrosis (black arrow), vitritis, hemorrhages and vasculitis (white arrows).

Table 6.5. Antiviral therapy for herpetic retinitis.

Systemic therapy	IV Acyclovir dose 5–10 mg/kg/d **OR** PO Valacyclovir 2 g q8h (VZV)/Valacyclovir 1 g q8h (HSV)[a] **AND** PO corticosteroid 1 mg/kg
Adjuvant intravitreal therapy	Foscarnet 2.4 mg/0.1 mL

[a]This dose is well documented and utilized routinely on the basis that this is as efficient as intravenous acyclovir 10 mg/kg tds without exposing patients to the side-effects associated with higher doses of valacyclovir.[10]

include either unilateral or bilateral decrease in visual acuity, floaters and discomfort. It is predominantly a peripheral disease comprising occlusive arteritis, full-thickness peripheral necrotizing retinitis (well demarcated, spread circumferentially), marked vitritis and anterior chamber activity. Complications include retinal detachment (up to 75%; rhegmatogenous or tractional) and ischemic optic neuropathy. Without prompt treatment second eye involvement occurs in around 30% and may occur simultaneously or up to several years later. With extended treatment the risk to the second eye reduces by 80%.

Patients with clinically suspected herpetic retinitis should be treated by a combination of systemic antivirals and systemic corticosteroids together with intravitreal foscarnet 2.4 mg/0.1 mL as adjunctive treatment (Table 6.5).[6] Retinal detachment repair is challenging due to the necrotic retina and number of breaks; vitrectomy with silicone oil injection is usually needed. Prophylactic barrier laser is controversial in these patients and its efficacy is varied.

6.1.4 *Progressive Outer Retinal Necrosis*

Progressive outer retinal necrosis (PORN) is a very rare devastating necrotizing retinitis caused by VZV or HSV infection in immunocompromised patients, such as advanced HIV infection (usually with CD4+ T-cell counts <50/L) or following solid organ transplantation. Clinical findings include bilateral, painless, rapid decrease in visual acuity. Retinal examination reveals rapidly coalescing white areas of outer retinal necrosis (often central as well as peripheral) but with minimal vasculitis, retinitis, vitritis or anterior uveitis (Figure 6.5). Treatment is double intravitreal antiviral and double systemic antiviral in addition to treatment for the underlying immunocompromised condition.[11]

Table 6.6. SUN classification criteria for cytomegalovirus retinitis.

Criteria: 1 and 2 and 3 or 4
1. Necrotizing retinitis with indistinct borders due to numerous small (<50 μm) satellites
AND
2. Immune compromise, either
a. Systemic (e.g., AIDS, organ transplant, chemotherapy) **OR**
b. Ocular (e.g., intraocular corticosteroids or chemotherapy)
AND (3 or 4)
3. Characteristic clinical picture (a or b or c and d)
a. Wedge-shaped area of retinitis **OR**
b. Hemorrhagic appearance of the retinitis **OR**
c. Granular appearance of the retinitis **AND**
d. Absent to mild vitritis
OR
4. Evidence of intraocular infection with cytomegalovirus
a. Positive PCR for cytomegalovirus from either the aqueous or vitreous specimen
Exclusions:
1. Positive serology for syphilis using a treponemal test
2. Intraocular specimen PCR-positive for infection by herpes simplex virus, varicella zoster virus, or *Toxoplasma gondii* (unless there is immune compromise, morphologic evidence for >1 infection, the characteristic picture of cytomegalovirus retinitis, and the intraocular fluid specimen also has a positive PCR result for cytomegalovirus)

PCR = polymerase chain reaction. Adapted from The Standardization of Uveitis Nomenclature (SUN) Working Group. Classification criteria for cytomegalovirus retinitis. Am J Ophthalmol 2021;228: 245–54.[13]

6.1.5 *CMV Retinitis*

In the 'pre-highly active antiretroviral therapy (HAART) era', CMV retinitis affected up to 40% of people with AIDS, but usually only when CD4+ T-cell counts were <50/L. Since the advent of combination antiretroviral therapy (ART), there has been a dramatic reduction in the incidence of CMV retinitis. We now see CMV retinitis in people who are immunocompromised in other ways, such as from chemotherapy.[12] Due to the absence of inflammation, the disease may be asymptomatic until late, and may present with decreased visual acuity (if macular involvement) and/or field loss or scotoma. Vitritis is usually mild/absent. CMV retinitis may be either 1) hemorrhagic (associated with necrosis), with loss of fundal details ('pizza pie' appearance, Figure 6.6), 2) granular, which is relatively indolent with minimal hemorrhages and vascular sheathing (Figure

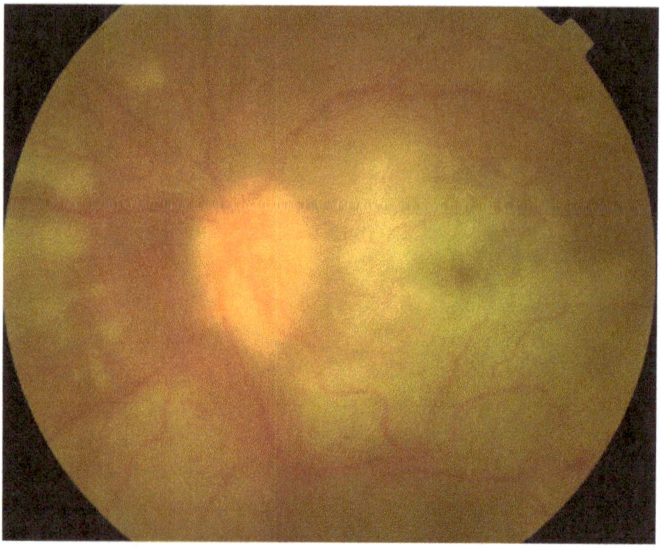

Figure 6.5. Color fundus photo of the left eye showing progressive outer retinal necrosis. Note the extensive necrotizing retinitis involving the posterior pole and lack of vitritis.

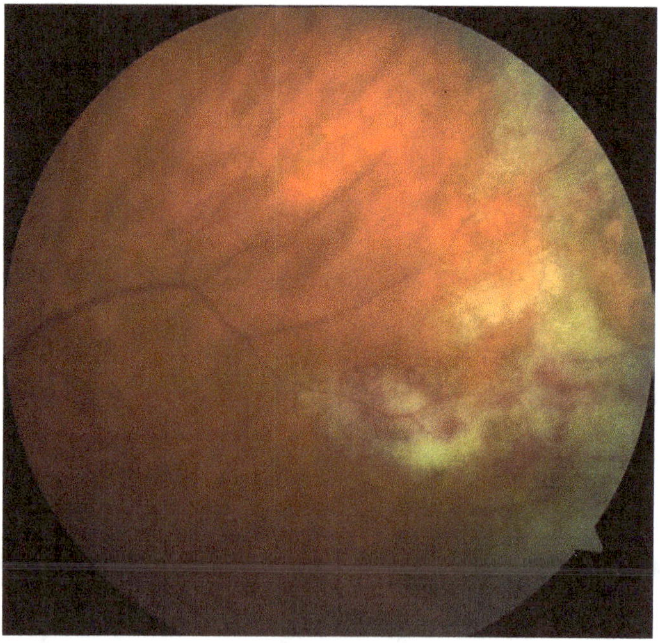

Figure 6.6. Color fundus image of a patient with CMV retinitis with CD4+ T-cell count of 30/L. Note the extensive retinitis, retinal hemorrhages and lack of vitritis.

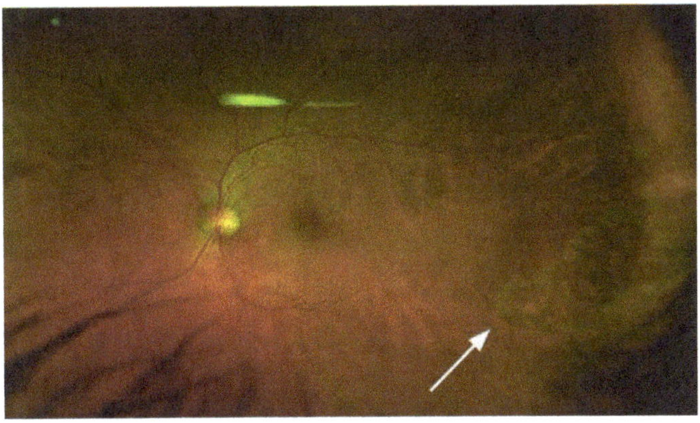

Figure 6.7. Widefield color fundus image of CMV retinitis in an elderly patient with HIV (arrow).

Table 6.7. Antiviral therapy for CMV retinitis.

Condition	Treatment
Systemic therapy	PO Valgancyclovir 900 mg q12h loading then 450 mg BD **OR** IV Ganciclovir 5 mg/kg q12h **OR** IV Foscarnet 90 mg/kg q12h **OR** IV Cidofovir 5 mg/kg weekly
Adjuvant intravitreal therapy	Ganciclovir 4 mg/0.1 mL, 1–4 doses

6.7), 3) perivascular, seen as 'frosted branch angiitis' which spreads along the course of the retinal vessels (Table 6.6, Figure 6.8). As it may be asymptomatic, regular screening should be performed in those at risk. Complications include retinal detachment (up to 30% of patients), retinal atrophy, and optic nerve disease (5%).[3]

CMV retinitis is usually treated with systemic antivirals (Table 6.7). Intravitreal foscarnet or ganciclovir is often used as well when the macula and optic discs are involved. HAART is an essential component of overall management if indicated; however, timing of ART should be discussed between an HIV physician and ophthalmologist. Anti-CMV maintenance therapy is continued until the CD4+ T-cell count is >100–150/L for 3–6 months. If stopped prior to this time the patient is at increased risk of immune reconstitution uveitis. Lifelong maintenance treatment is recommended for all patients without immune recovery.

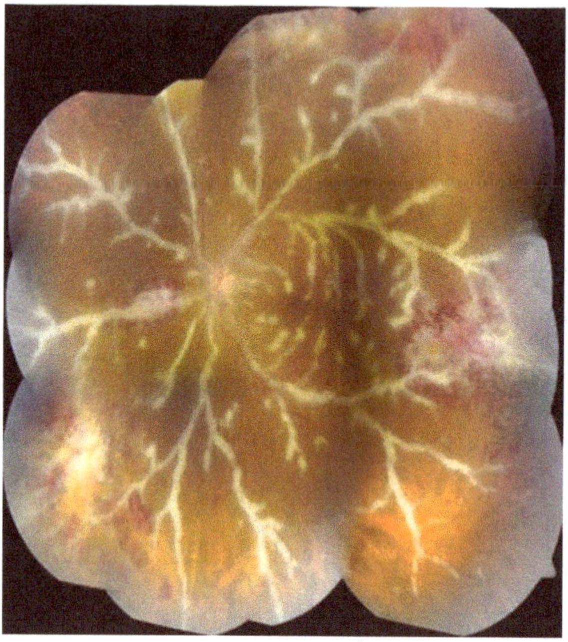

Figure 6.8. Frosted branch angiitis in CMV retinitis.

6.2 Toxoplasma Retinochoroiditis

Ocular infections by *Toxoplasma gondii* are still very common in the general immunocompetent population as well as the immunosuppressed. However, in immunosuppressed subjects it is often multifocal (even bilateral), associated with moderate/severe anterior uveitis and vitritis, and is commonly associated with neuro-toxoplasmosis. In contrast to immunocompetent individuals, it always requires treatment. Corticosteroids, if used, should be used extremely cautiously, and only in conjunction with antimicrobial agents.

Ocular toxoplasmosis occurs either as a primary infection or a reactivation along an old scar. Primary toxoplasmosis appears as a white, fluffy circumscribed area of retinitis when active (Figures 6.9 and 6.10) and becomes pigmented as it heals to form an atrophic scar. More commonly, reactivation of ocular toxoplasmosis happens along the borders of an old scar, resulting in its extension following healing (Figure 6.11). Ocular toxoplasmosis may include anterior uveitis (often with high intraocular pressure and KPs), vitritis (may have 'vitreous precipitates' on the posterior

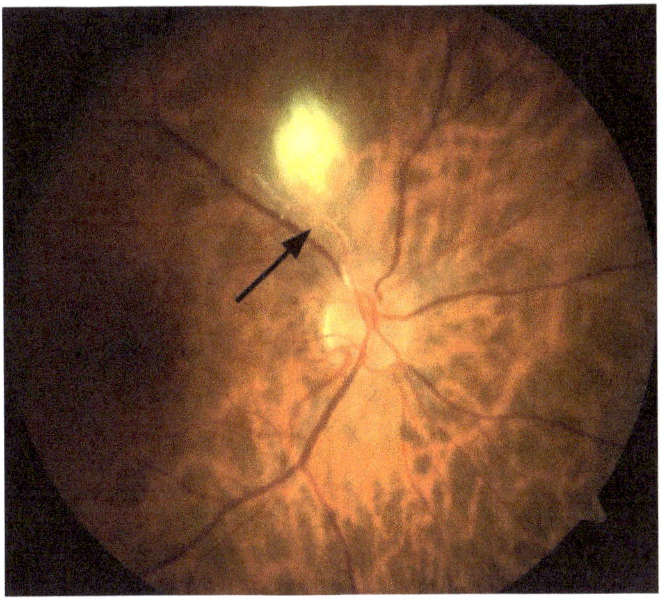

Figure 6.9. Fundal image showing focus of toxoplasma retinochoroiditis and associated retinal vasculitis (arrow).

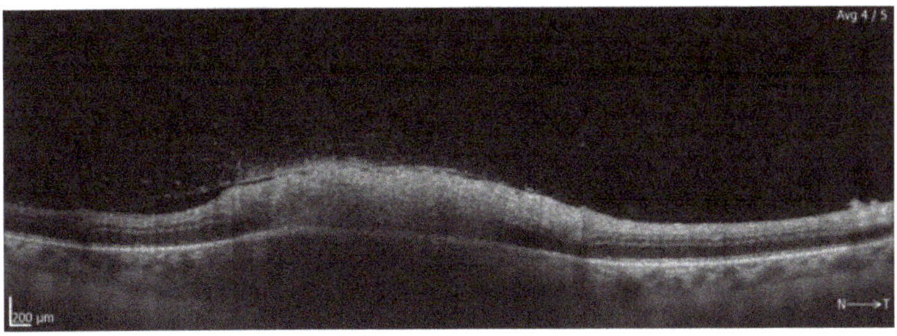

Figure 6.10. OCT through a toxoplasma retinochoroiditis lesion highlighting full thickness retinitis.

surface of a posterior vitreous detachment), retinitis and retinal vasculitis (most commonly periphlebitis but may develop arteritis, see Chapter 2, Figure 2.29). Other presentations include: scleritis, punctate outer retinitis (with quiet vitreous), large lesions, endophthalmitis-like, neuroretinitis, serous retinal detachments, and pigmentary retinopathy. Immunocompromised individuals may have life-threatening diseases, including encephalitis, intracerebral cysts, hepatitis and myocarditis.

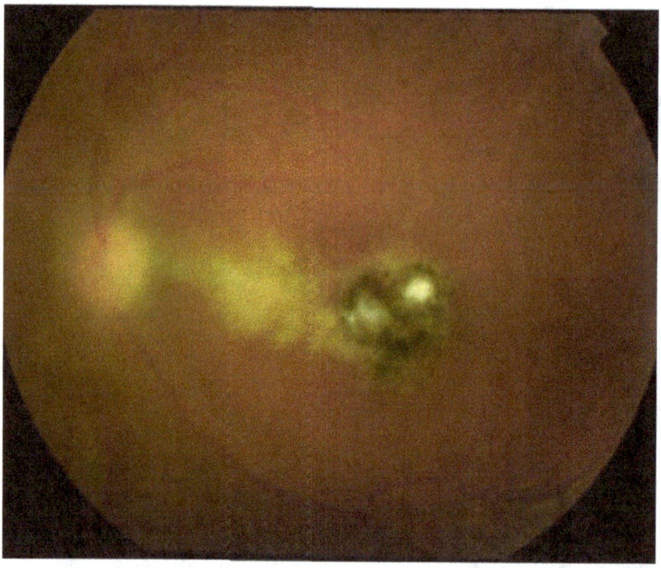

Figure 6.11. Reactivation of ocular toxoplasmosis along the nasal border of an old hyper-pigmented scar.

Toxoplasma retinochoroiditis is essentially a clinical diagnosis (Table 6.8). Positive serological tests must be interpreted with caution as a high proportion of the adult population has anti-toxoplasma IgG antibodies from previous exposure. Although IgM antibodies are suggestive of recently acquired infection, there may be IgM cross-reactivity and persistence. Negative serology in undiluted serum makes the diagnosis unlikely. Detection of toxoplasma DNA by PCR in intraocular fluids can be very useful diagnostically.

Systemic treatment varies depending on severity of HIV-associated immunosuppression. The mainstay of treatment is pyrimethamine with sulfadiazine and folinic acid. Trimethoprim/sulfamethoxazole, clindamycin or atovaquone are alternate treatment options (Table 6.9). Steroids should be used very cautiously in immunosuppressed individuals. In patients with recurrent reactivations or if the location of the scar threatens visual function (e.g., adjacent to the optic nerve, fovea or large blood vessels), extended prophylactic treatment should be considered. A commonly used regime includes trimethoprim/sulfamethoxazole 3 times a week, resulting in a decrease in reactivation.

A comparison between the clinical presentation of retinitis in acute retinal necrosis, CMV retinitis and toxoplasmosis is given in Table 6.10.

Table 6.8. SUN classification criteria for toxoplasmosis retinitis.

Criteria: Focal or paucifocal necrotizing retinitis* AND (1 or 2)

1. Evidence of infection with *Toxoplasma gondii*
   a) Positive PCR for *Toxoplasma gondii* from either the aqueous or vitreous specimen
   OR
   b) Positive serum IGM antibodies against *Toxoplasma gondii*

OR

2. Characteristic clinical ocular features
   a) Hyperpigmented and/or atrophic chorioretinal scar **AND** (b or c)
   b) Round or oval retinitis lesions **OR**
   c) Recurrent acute (episodic) course

Exclusions:

1. Both negative IgG AND IgM antibodies against *Toxoplasma gondii* (unless there is positive PCR for *Toxoplasma gondii* from aqueous or vitreous specimen)
2. Positive serology for syphilis using a treponemal test
3. Intraocular specimen PCR-positive for herpes simplex virus, varicella zoster or cytomegalovirus (unless there is immune compromise, morphologic evidence for >1 infection, the picture of toxoplasmic retinitis and the intraocular fluid specimen also has a positive PCR for *Toxoplasma gondii*)

**Active retinitis lesions in immunocompetent patients. Immunocompromised patients may have a multifocal or diffuse necrotizing retinitis. Number of scars may be >5.*

Adapted from Standardization of Uveitis Nomenclature Working Group. Classification criteria for toxoplasmic retinitis. Am J Ophthalmol 2021;228:134–41.[14]

Table 6.9. Antibiotic treatment protocols for toxoplasmic retinitis.

"Classic" protocol	PO Pyrimethamine 25 mg bid PO Sulfadiazine 1 gr qds PO Folinic acid 5 mg 2–7 times a week
Alternate protocols	PO Trimethoprim/sulfamethoxazole 960 g bid **OR** PO Clindamycin 300 mg bid **OR** PO atovaquone 1,500 mg bid
Prophylactic treatment	PO Trimethoprim/sulfamethoxazole 960 gr 3 times a week

6.3 Syphilis

Syphilis is well known for being the great masquerader. It must be included in all differentials and may be unilateral or bilateral, unifocal or multifocal, and cause inflammation throughout the eye (Table 6.11). Anterior uveitis

Table 6.10. Comparison of clinical presentation of retinitis in acute retinal necrosis (ARN), cytomegalovirus (CMV) retinitis and toxoplasmosis retinochroiditis.[6]

	ARN	CMV	Toxoplasmosis
Presentation	Painful visual loss in days <15 yr HSV2 Adults HSV1 & VZV	Painless	Painless
Immune status	Immunocompetent or compromised	CD4 <200 (Usually <50)	Immunocompetent or compromised
Early signs	Retinitis: – Sharp border – Homogeneous – Multifocal to confluent – Posterior pole involved late – Minimal hemorrhage Granulomatous anterior uveitis Vitritis Disc edema Periarteritis	Retinitis: – Fuzzy borders – Hemorrhage ++, necrosis – Slow but relentless brushfire extension along vessels – Involves optic disc Mild or no vitritis	Retinitis: – Solitary chorioretinal lesion, may be adjacent to old pigmented scar Granulomatous or non-granulomatous anterior uveitis Vitritis & detached hyaloid covered by inflammatory precipitates Vasculitis Papillitis
Late signs	Full-thickness retinal necrosis and rhegmatogenous retinal detachment	Diffuse atrophic Glial proliferation Hyperplastic RPE	Pigmented scar 50% recurrence in 3 years 3 attacks per lifetime

Table 6.11. Ophthalmic complications of syphilis.[15]

Anterior segment	Conjunctival chancre Pupillary conjunctivitis Episcleritis Scleritis Interstitial keratitis Anterior uveitis
Posterior segment	Multi-/unifocal choroiditis/chorioretinitis Neuroretinitis Retinal vasculitis

(*Continued*)

Table 6.11. (*Continued*)

Neuro-ophthalmic	Argyll Robertson pupils Papilloedema Retrobulbar neuritis Optic peri-neuritis Ocular motility disorders Visual field defects

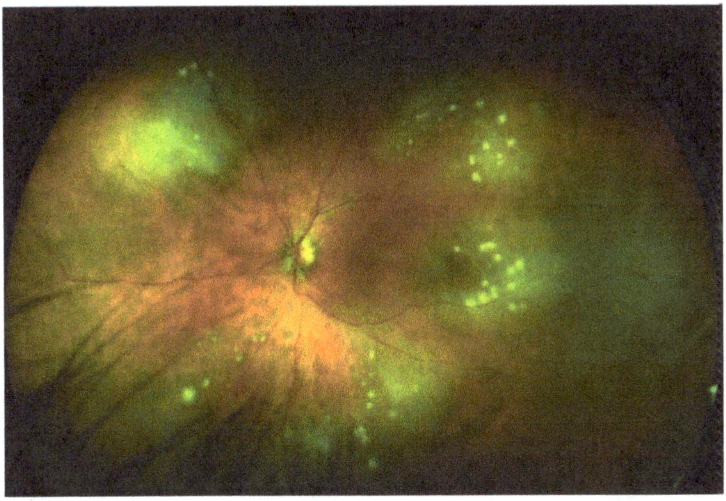

Figure 6.12. Color image of acute syphilitic posterior placoid chorioretinitis. Note the multi focal lesions throughout the retinal periphery.

associated with syphilis may be granulomatous or non-granulomatous. Posterior segment involvement can include retinitis, chorioretinitis, yellow plaque-like lesions at the level of the retinal pigment epithelium (RPE, Figures 6.12, 6.13, 6.14) with overlying vitritis and serous retinal detachment and optic peri-neuritis (Figure 6.15). Resolution of the lesions results in a pigmentary retinopathy.

Serum should be tested for antibodies to *Treponema pallidum* as evidence of current or previous infection and for 'non-treponemal antibodies' to assess disease stage or treatment response (see Chapter 4 for specific tests).

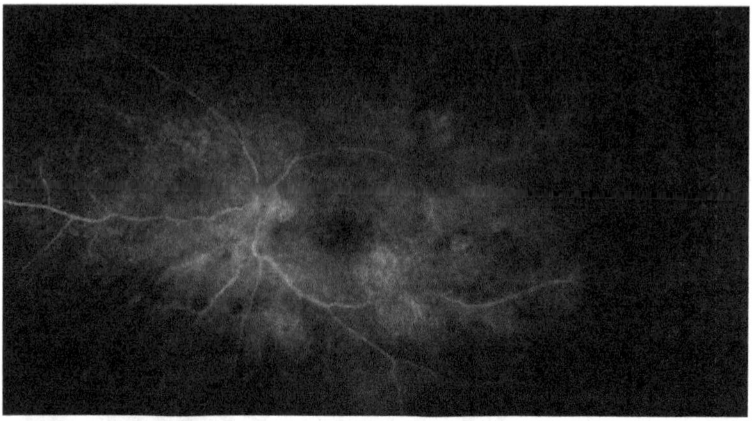

Figure 6.13. Fluorescein angiography of acute syphilitic posterior placoid chorioretinitis. Note the blocked fluorescence over the lesions and surrounding leakage.

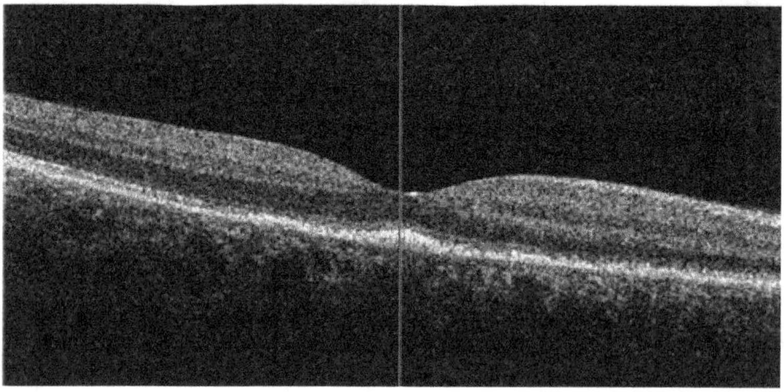

Figure 6.14. OCT image of acute syphilitic posterior placoid chorioretinitis. Note the hyperreflective nodularity of the choroid-retinal pigment epithelium complex.

Management of syphilitic eye disease should be undertaken in conjunction with an infectious disease or sexual health physician as treatment requires high-dose penicillin, with an extended regimen for late latent and tertiary syphilis. Spirochete death may transiently worsen inflammation (Jarisch-Herxheimer or J-H reaction). Systemic steroids are also used to treat the paradoxical J-H reaction and the intraocular and/or optic nerve inflammatory response.

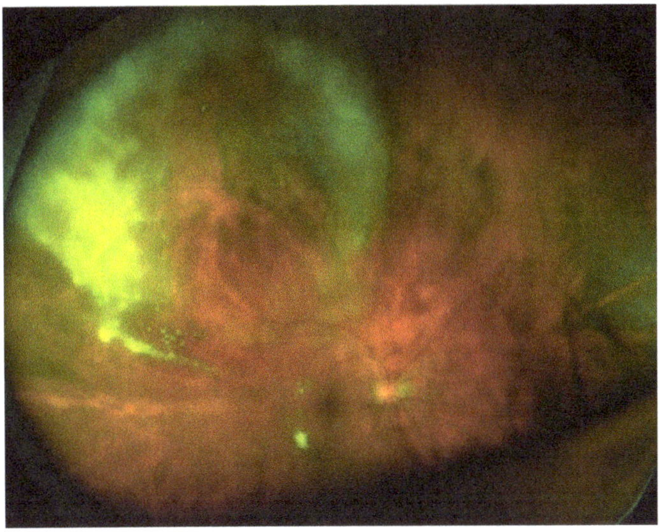

Figure 6.15. Syphilis uveitis. Note the extensive vitritis.

6.4 Tuberculosis

Latent tuberculosis (TB) is much more common in developed countries than active TB and causes infections in healthy people. The ocular manifestations of TB can be protean and depend on the exact pattern of systemic *Mycobacterium tuberculosis* infection (Table 6.12). Investigations for systemic TB should be performed through an interferon-gamma release assay (IGRA) or purified protein derivative (PPD) skin test (Mantoux), combined with chest X-ray, though ocular TB may occur without evidence of active, infectious extra-ocular disease (i.e., sputum cultures, chest X-ray). While PCR testing and culture of aqueous or vitreous fluid may be attempted, they are of low yield and the diagnosis is usually made on clinical grounds (Table 6.13).

Treatment is with a standard four-drug regimen +/- localized treatment of disease complications. Visual acuity should be checked before starting treatment with ethambutol and the patient is advised to report any disturbance of visual acuity, color vision or visual fields. With the development of multidrug-resistant strains, disease relapses are reported with

Table 6.12. Ocular manifestations of ocular tuberculosis.

Anterior segment	Episcleritis Scleritis Interstitial keratitis Anterior uveitis
Posterior segment	Vitritis Occlusive retinal vasculitis (Figure 6.16) – Periphlebitis – Ischemia – Neovascularization – Hemorrhage Macula edema Choroidal granulomata – Usually multifocal around the posterior pole Serpiginous choroidopathy (Figure 6.17)
Neuro-ophthalmic	Papilloedema Optic peri-neuritis Optic neuropathy

Table 6.13. SUN classification criteria for tubercular uveitis.

Criteria: 1 and 2

1. Evidence of a tubercular uveitis compatible uveitic syndrome
   a. anterior uveitis with iris nodules
   b. serpiginous-like tubercular choroiditis
   c. choroidal nodule (i.e., tuberculoma)
   d. in individuals with active systemic tuberculosis, multifocal choroiditis
   e. occlusive retinal vasculitis

AND

2. Evidence of infection with *Mycobacterium tuberculosis*, either
   a. histologically or microbiologically confirmed infection with *M. tuberculosis*[a] **OR**
   b. positive IGRA[b] **OR**
   c. positive tuberculin skin test[c]

Exclusions

1. Positive serology for syphilis using a treponemal test
2. Positive biopsy for sarcoidosis (and therefore an absence of histologic or microbiologic confirmation of infection with *M. tuberculosis*)

(*Continued*)

Table 6.13. (*Continued*)

3. Uveitic syndrome compatible with either sarcoidosis-associated uveitis or tubercular uveitis and bilateral hilar adenopathy on chest imaging without histologic or microbiologic confirmation of the diagnosis of infection with *M. tuberculosis*[d]

IGRA = interferon-gamma release assay.

[a]For example, biopsy, fluorochrome stain, culture, or polymerase chain reaction-based assay.

[b]For example, QuantiFERON gold or T-spot.

[c]For example, purified protein derivative skin test; a positive result should be >10 mm in duration. However, a positive skin test and a negative IGRA should be taken as evidence of atypical mycobacterial infection and not tuberculosis.

[d]In patients with a uveitic syndrome compatible either with sarcoidosis-associated uveitis or with tubercular uveitis, bilateral hilar adenopathy, and evidence of latent tuberculosis (e.g., positive tuberculin skin test or IGRA), the classification requires histologic or microbiologic confirmation of the diagnosis (i.e., classification cannot be made without such confirmation).

Adapted from The Standardization of Uveitis Nomenclature (SUN) Working Group. Classification criteria for tubercular uveitis. Am J Ophthalmol 2021;228:142–51.[16]

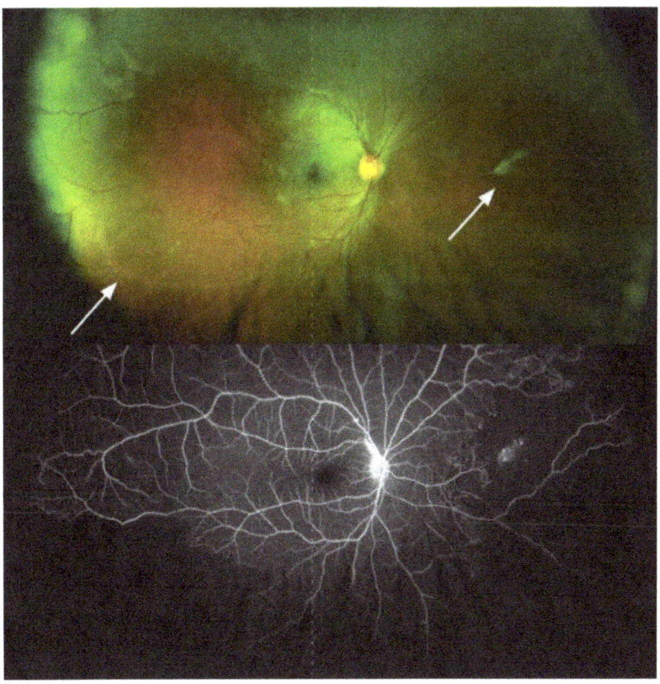

Figure 6.16. Occlusive vasculitis in a tuberculosis patient. In the color image (top) note the hemorrhages and occluded vessels ('ghost vessels', arrows). In fluorescein angiography (bottom) there are large corresponding areas of retinal ischemia.

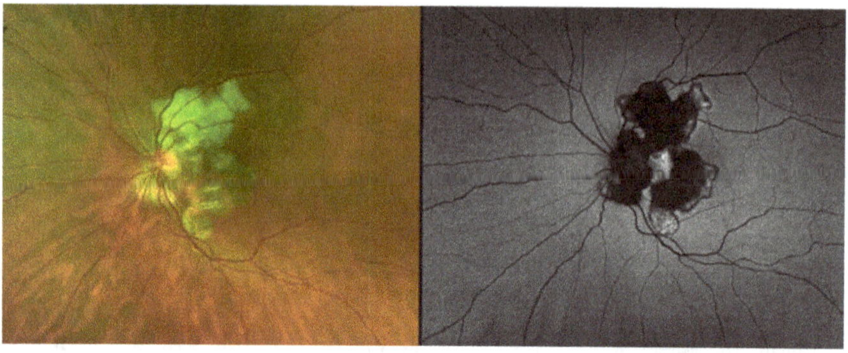

Figure 6.17. Serpiginous choroiditis. Color image (left) and fundus autofluorescence (right).

some patients having 3 or more events during their lifetime. Patients with a diagnosis of latent TB (a positive IGRA or PPD test without evidence of active disease), who are scheduled to receive extensive immunosuppression (particularly anti-tumor necrosis factor-α agents), must receive prophylactic anti-TB treatment before immunosuppression can be initiated.

6.5 Endogenous Endophthalmitis and Post-injection/Surgery Endophthalmitis

Risk factors for endogenous endophthalmitis include:

A) Immunocompromise — organ transplant, cancer, diabetes mellitus, liver failure, alcoholism
B) Sepsis — endocarditis, genitourinary, pneumonia
C) Specific risk factors for fungal endophthalmitis — intravenous drug use (IVDU), long-term indwelling catheter, ICU patient, any immunocompromise

Risk factors for post-operative or post-intravitreal injection endophthalmitis include having these procedures done, complicated surgery, history of reduced vision in acutely ill patient or immunocompromised host, and no history of intraocular surgery.

Organisms include:

- *Staphylococcus* or *Streptococcus* species
- Intravenous drug users: *Bacillus cereus, Candida albicans*
- Endocarditis: *Streptococcus viridians*
- Meningitis: *Streptococcus pneumonia, Haemophilus influenzae*
- Urinary tract injection: *Klebsiella pneumonia, Escherichia coli, Proteus sp.*
- Wounds: *Staphylococcus aureus, Streptococcus pyogenes*

For examination of decrease in visual acuity, pain, lid & conjunctival edema, corneal edema: if bacterial infection — anterior chamber activity, vitritis, retinal infiltrate, flame-shaped hemorrhage ± white center (Roth spots), panuveitis with choroidal lesions (Figure 6.18); if fungal infection — multifocal, yellow-white fluffy retinal lesions, spread into vitreous ('cotton balls', Figure 6.19).

Investigations and Treatment: Thorough history and examination is indicated. Once endophthalmitis is suspected a vitreous tap and injection are required. The vitreous sample must be sent for gram stain, microbacterial culture and fungal cultures. Normally antibiotics +/– antifungal agents are

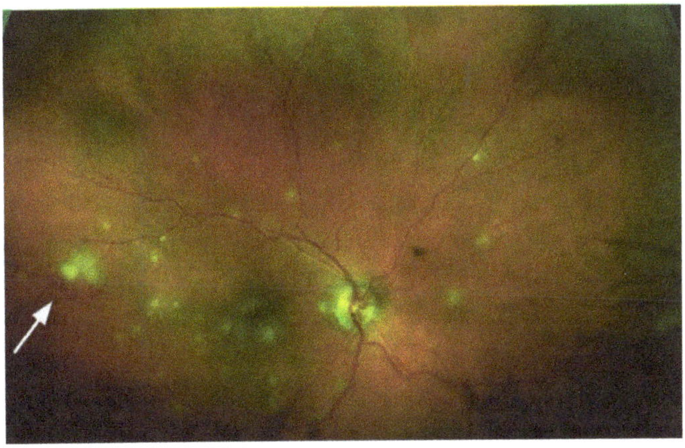

Figure 6.18. Widefield color photo of endogenous endophthalmitis associated with *Streptococcus mitis* infection. Note the multiple choroidal lesions and choroidal abscess (arrow).

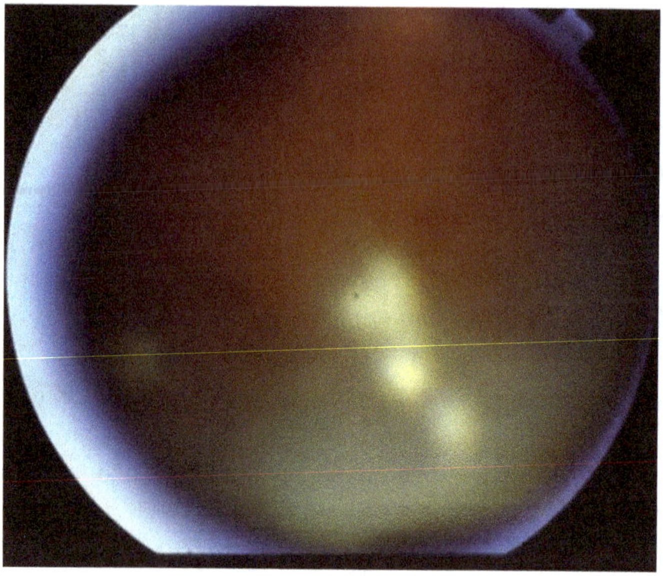

Figure 6.19. Fundus color image of *Candida* infection.

injected 0.1 mL of each at the same time. Systemic investigations including blood cultures, chest CT, brain MRI, and cardiac ECHO are also indicated for endogenous endophthalmitis as well as systemic antibiotics.

6.6 Bartonellosis

Bartonellosis is most commonly caused by *Bartonella henselae*, of which the major reservoir are cats. The infection is transmitted through breaks in the skin by contaminated cat claws. The most common ocular involvement is granulomatous conjunctivitis with regional lymphadenopathy and fever (Parinaud oculoglandular syndrome, Figure 6.20), though neuroretinitis is considered the recognizable manifestation (Figure 6.21).[17] Other clinical findings include vasculitis, retinitis, retinal vascular occlusion and vitritis. Diagnosis is based on suggestive clinical findings and a positive blood serology. During the first 2 weeks of infection positive IgM titters are commonly noted. Although self-limiting, treatment is recommended in vision-threatening diseases and includes a combination of antibiotics (typically doxycycline or rifampicin) and systemic corticosteroids.[18]

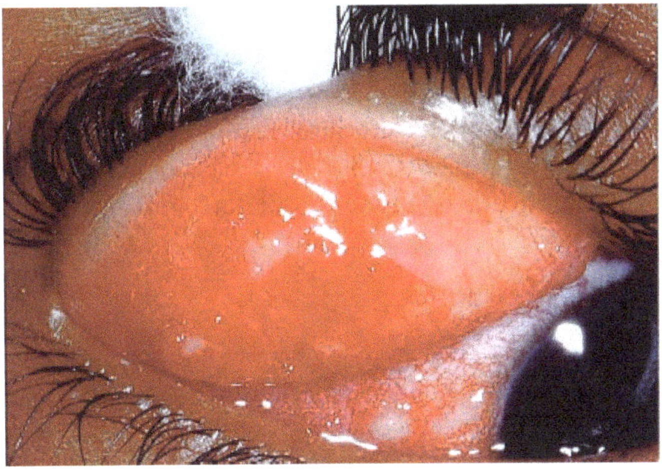

Figure 6.20. Granulomatous conjunctivitis in Parinaud oculoglandular syndrome.

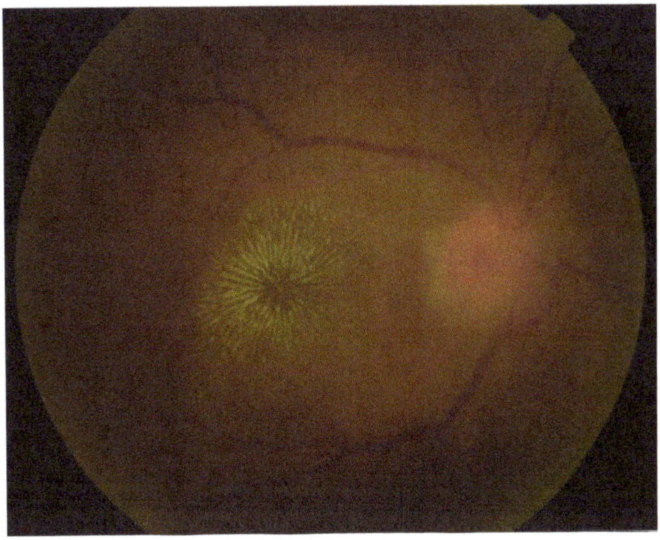

Figure 6.21. Neuroretinitis due to *Bartonella henselae.* Note the classic macular star formation and optic nerve hyperemia.

6.7 Lyme Disease

Lyme disease is caused by *Borrelia burgdorferi*, a spirochete transmitted by black-legged ticks. The animal reservoirs include rodents, deer, birds, cats or dogs, and patients typically recall recent contact. Ocular involvement in Lyme disease is uncommon, but clinical findings range from conjunctivitis, granulomatous anterior uveitis, vitritis, neuroretinitis, vasculitis or cranial nerve (CN) palsies.[19] The most common CN involvement is the facial nerve (VII) and patients can present with bilateral facial paralysis. Diagnosis is based on a suggestive history, clinical findings and a positive serology test. Treatment is based on doxycycline or amoxycillin, rifampicin, with topical steroids for anterior uveitis.

6.8 Toxocara

This is caused by *Toxocara canis* (Helminth parasite, intestinal roundworm of dogs). Pathogenesis is the ingestion of soil/food contaminated by ova (in dog or cat feces). Ova develop into larva (microfilaria) in the intestine and then disseminate. When they die, a granulomatous inflammation is produced.

Presentation may be asymptomatic or may be associated with decrease in vision (floaters in chronic endopthalmitis), leukocoria or strabismus (in younger children of amblyopic age).[20] The stages include:

1) Chronic endophthalmitis (present with endophthalmitis)
2) Posterior granuloma (looks like retinoblastoma)
3) Peripheral granuloma (Figure 6.22)

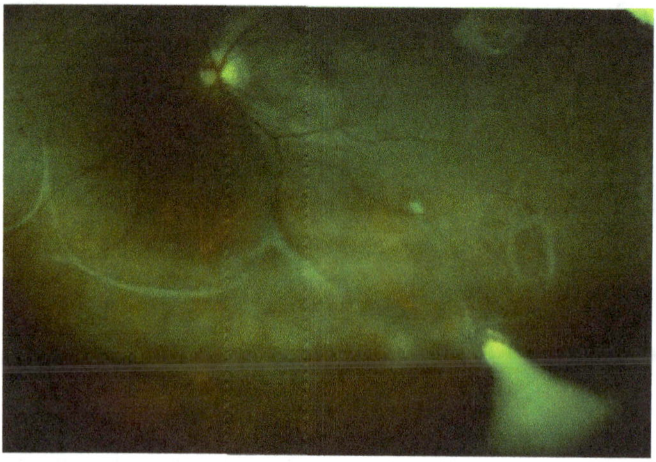

Figure 6.22. Toxocara infection with peripheral granuloma.

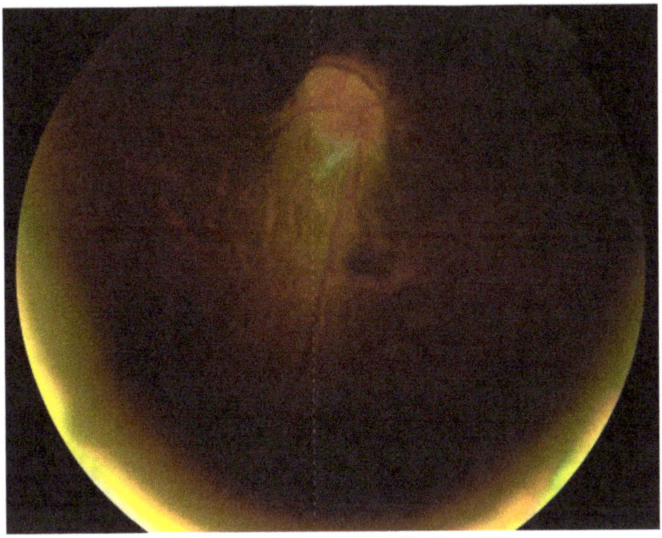

Figure 6.23. Dragged macula due to toxocara infection.

Complications can include hemorrhage, hard exudate posterior synechia, cataract, glaucoma, total retinal detachment, dragged macula (Figure 6.23), and phthisis.

Any titer for toxocara serology is significant (but not necessarily diagnostic) — IgM indicates recent acquired infection (<6 months). Exclude retinoblastoma, toxocara PCR, and eosinophilia.

Management includes:

1. Systemic and topical steroids
2. Mydriatics
3. Control of intraocular pressure
4. Argon laser for mobile larva

Thiobendazole is used for systemic but NOT ocular toxocariasis (death of the nematode results in increased inflammation).

6.9 Diffuse Unilateral Subacute Neuroretinitis

Diffuse unilateral subacute neuroretinitis (DUSN) is strictly unilateral and biphasic with the first phase, which is often associated with a decrease in vision and mild vitritis, multiple post-equatorial evanescent white dots,

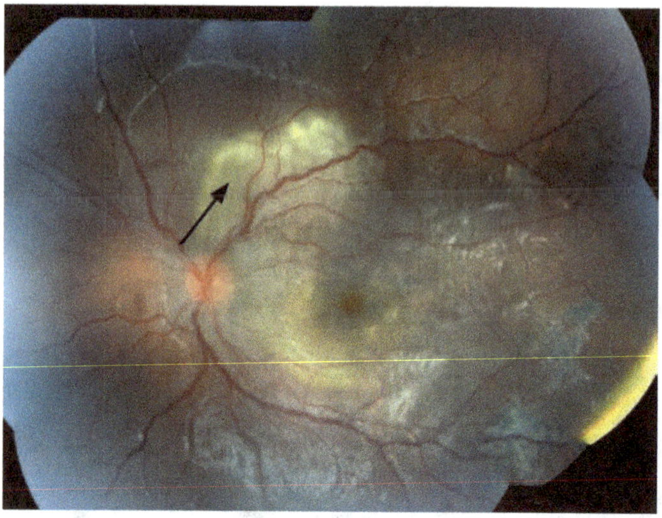

Figure 6.24. Color montage fundus image of right eye highlighting DUSN (arrow).

vasculitis, papillitis and motile nematode.[21] It is often confused with unilateral 'white dot syndromes' (Figure 6.24).

Late signs may include unilateral wipe-out (optic atrophy, arteriolar attenuation, pigmentary disruption). Can be confused with unilateral RP. Laser of the nematode may be performed if the worm can be visualised.

6.10 Other Rarer Infections

6.10.1 *Pneumocystis Jirovecii (Carinii)* Choroiditis

This cause of uveitis is now uncommon, as a result of the use of ART. The choroiditis is typically bilateral, comprising yellow choroidal patches of ¼- to 2-disc diameters in size around the posterior pole, with minimal vitritis.[22] It is often asymptomatic. Treatment is with trimethoprim/sulfamethoxazole, clindamycin/primaquine or pentamidine.

6.10.2 *Cryptococcus* Choroiditis

This rare condition is usually associated with cryptococcal meningitis and may be associated with an optic neuropathy or papilloedema.[22] It is characterized by multifocal off-white choroidal lesions, occasionally with

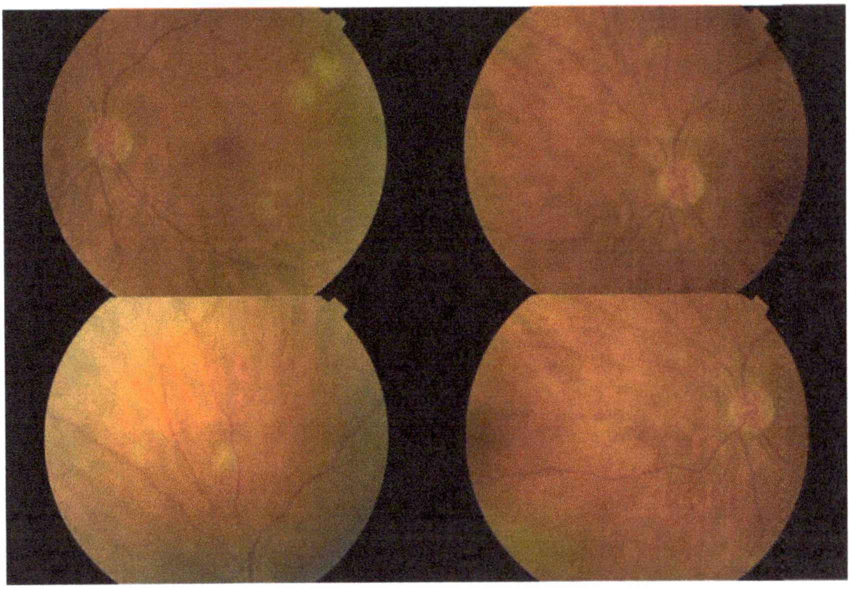

Figure 6.25. Cryptococcus choroiditis in a patient with HIV. Note the extensive choroidal lesions throughout the retina.

a retinitis or endophthalmitis (Figure 6.25). Treatment is as for cryptococcal meningitis with induction therapy using an antifungal agent, such as amphotericin B, followed by consolidation with fluconazole.

6.10.3 *Microsporidiosis*

Microsporidia are protozoan obligate intracellular parasites, of which four genera may cause the human disease microsporidiosis. This is usually seen in the immunocompromised (notably in AIDS) where it may present as chronic diarrhea respiratory infection, or keratoconjunctivitis.[23] Microsporidial keratouveitis presents with bilateral irritation and photophobia, punctate keratopathy, often with follicular conjunctivitis and/or anterior uveitis.

Teaching Points

- 25% of shingles cases involve cranial nerve V1 causing herpes zoster ophthalmicus.

- The diagnosis of ARN is caused by VZV, HSV-1 or HSV-2. Without timely treatment 30% will develop second eye involvement.
- CMV retinitis occurs in the immunosuppressed, e.g., AIDS, chemotherapy, etc., so may be asymptomatic until late due to the absence of inflammation.
- Toxoplasma retinochoroiditis in immunocompromised patients can lead to encephalitis, intracerebral cysts, hepatitis and myocarditis.
- Due to the wide variety of presentations that syphilis has, it should be included in all infectious uveitis differentials. Patients must be under the care of infectious disease or sexual health physicians as well.
- Before starting a patient on anti-tumor necrosis factor-α agents it is vital to check TB status, and if they have latent TB, give prophylactic TB treatment beforehand.
- Fungal endophthalmitis risk factors include intravenous drug use, long-term indwelling catheter, ICU patient and any immunocompromise.

References

1. Lin P. Infectious uveitis. *Curr Ophthalmol Rep* 2015;3(3):170–83.
2. Acharya NR, Tham VM, Esterberg E, *et al.* Incidence and prevalence of uveitis: results from the Pacific Ocular Inflammation Study. *JAMA Ophthalmol* 2013;131(11):1405–12.
3. Singalavanija T, Ausayakhun S, Tangmonkongvoragul C. Anterior segment and external ocular disorders associated with HIV infections in the era of HAART in Chiang Mai University Hospital, a prospective descriptive cross sectional study. *PLoS One* 2018;13(2):e0193161.
4. Bowling B. Kanski's Clinical Ophthalmology: A Systematic Approach (8th edition). United Kingdom: Saunders Ltd, 2015.
5. Standardization of Uveitis Nomenclature Working G. Classification criteria for varicella zoster virus anterior uveitis. *Am J Ophthalmol* 2021;228:165–73.
6. Zagora S, Pinto A, McCluskey P. Ocular disease in patients with HIV infection. ASHM 2019. Retrieved from https://hivmanagement.ashm.org.au/ocular-disease-in-patients-with-hiv-infection/.
7. Chan NS, Chee SP, Caspers L, Bodaghi B. Clinical features of CMV-associated anterior uveitis. *Ocul Immunol Inflamm* 2018;26(1):107–15.
8. Standardization of Uveitis Nomenclature Working G. Classification criteria for cytomegalovirus anterior uveitis. *Am J Ophthalmol* 2021;228:89–95.
9. Standardization of Uveitis Nomenclature Working G. Classification criteria for acute retinal necrosis syndrome. *Am J Ophthalmol* 2021;228:237–44.

10. Beutner KR. Valacyclovir: a review of its antiviral activity, pharmacokinetic properties, and clinical efficacy. *Antiviral Res* 1995;28(4):281–90.
11. Lo PF, Lim R, Antonakis SN, Almeida GC. Progressive outer retinal necrosis: manifestation of human immunodeficiency virus infection. *BMJ Case Rep* 2015;2015:bcr2014207344.
12. Ho M, Invernizzi A, Zagora S, *et al.* Presenting features, treatment and clinical outcomes of cytomegalovirus retinitis: Non-HIV patients vs HIV patients. *Ocul Immunol Inflamm* 2020;28(4):651–8.
13. Standardization of Uveitis Nomenclature Working G. Classification criteria for cytomegalovirus retinitis. *Am J Ophthalmol* 2021;228:245–54.
14. Standardization of Uveitis Nomenclature Working G. Classification criteria for toxoplasmic retinitis. *Am J Ophthalmol* 2021;228:134–41.
15. Denniston AKO, PL M. Oxford Handbook of Ophthalmology (3rd edition). United Kingdom: Oxford University Press, 2014.
16. Standardization of Uveitis Nomenclature Working G. Classification criteria for tubercular uveitis. *Am J Ophthalmol* 2021;228:142–51.
17. Niederer RL, Al-Ani HH. Bartonella neuroretinitis. *N Engl J Med* 2021; 384(10):952.
18. Bhatti MT, Lee MS. Should patients with bartonella neuroretinitis receive treatment? *J Neuroophthalmol* 2014;34(4):412–6.
19. Mikkila HO, Seppala IJ, Viljanen MK, *et al.* The expanding clinical spectrum of ocular lyme borreliosis. *Ophthalmology* 2000;107(3):581–7.
20. Woodhall D, Starr MC, Montgomery SP, *et al.* Ocular toxocariasis: epidemiologic, anatomic, and therapeutic variations based on a survey of ophthalmic subspecialists. *Ophthalmology* 2012;119(6):1211–7.
21. Curragh DS, Ramsey A, Christie S, McLoone E. Case report: a case of diffuse unilateral subacute neuroretinitis (DUSN) in a child. *BMC Ophthalmol* 2018;18(Suppl 1):218.
22. Cunningham ET, Jr. Uveitis in HIV positive patients. *Br J Ophthalmol* 2000;84(3):233–5.
23. Mohanty A, Mitra S, Mallick A, *et al.* Sequelae of microsporidial keratoconjunctivitis and its management. *Indian J Ophthalmol* 2021;69(6):1537–43.

https://doi.org/10.1142/9789811251474_0007

Chapter 7

Masquerade Syndromes

Yi-Hsing Chen,[*,†,‡] *Yih-Shiou Hwang*[†,‡]

7.1 Introduction

The term "uveitis masquerade syndrome (UMS)" is characterized by intraocular inflammation or pseudo-inflammation from non-inflammatory causes including malignancy and non-neoplastic proliferative conditions. UMS differs from other types of uveitis in that it may be refractory unilateral or bilateral asymmetrical ocular inflammation or pseudo-inflammation (e.g., pigment, blood, or malignant cells); particularly presenting in patients over the age of 60 but can occur in those much younger as well; history of systemic malignancy; the absence of other inflammatory signs such as ocular pain, keratic precipitates and synechia; and initial response and eventual resistance to corticosteroids.[1] The prevalence of UMS was reported as 5% in all uveitis from a tertiary centre.[1] Early diagnosis of the masquerading underlying disease, especially when malignant, may allow earlier intervention and better prognosis.

7.2 Retinal Detachment

Retinal detachment can occur as part of an inflammatory condition such as Vogt-Koyanagi-Harada disease (VKH) or sympathetic ophthalmia where it is exudative.[2–4] In patients with necrotizing retinitis such as cytomegalovirus, acute retinal necrosis, toxoplasmosis, etc., rhegmatogenous retinal detachment can occur due to the retinal necrosis. Patients with large retinal detachments, particularly giant tears, may have an accompanying

* UCL Institute of Ophthalmology, University College London, London, UK
† Department of Ophthalmology, Chang Gung Memorial Hospital, Taoyuan, Taiwan
‡ College of Medicine, Chang Gung University, Taoyuan, Taiwan

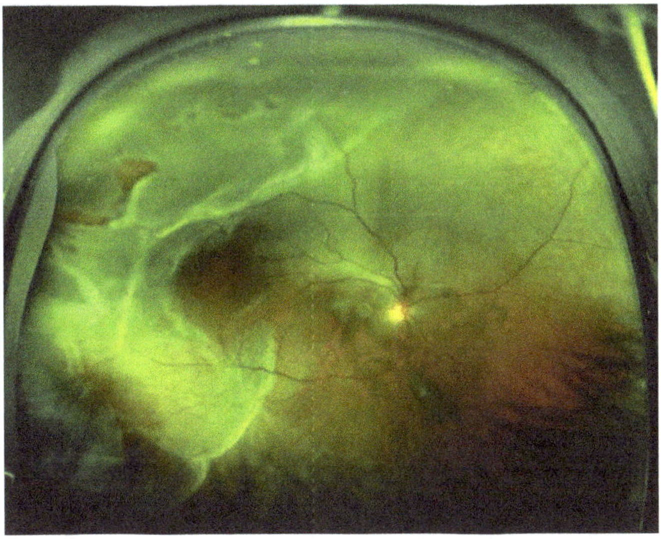

Figure 7.1. Giant retinal tear.

uveitis but this is secondary to the retinal detachment (Figure 7.1).[5] Careful investigation and dilated fundus examination are necessary to avoid misdiagnosis.

7.3 Retinitis Pigmentosa (RP)

Retinal pigmentary changes with coarse "bone spicule" clumps in the retinal pigment epithelium (RPE) are the typical presentation of RP (Figure 7.2). However, in younger patients with sectoral or asymmetric type of RP, these pigment changes may not be obvious, which can result in the

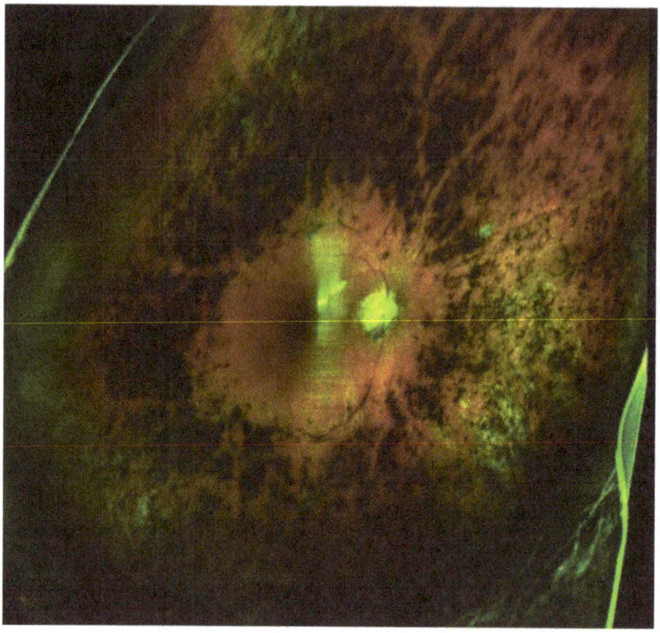

Figure 7.2. Retinitis pigmentosa with extensive bone spicules, attenuated blood vessels and a pale optic disc.

diagnosis being missed (Figure 7.3). Retinal pigmentary changes can also occur in the context of past ocular inflammation, for example, syphilis, toxoplasmosis, cytomegalovirus, rubella, measles or diffuse unilateral subacute neuroretinitis (DUSN), long-standing retinal vasculitis and toxic retinopathy.[6–9] Rarely, vasculitis, pars planitis, anterior uveitis, intermediate uveitis and macular edema have been reported in RP patients[8,10,11] and in other retinal dystrophies.

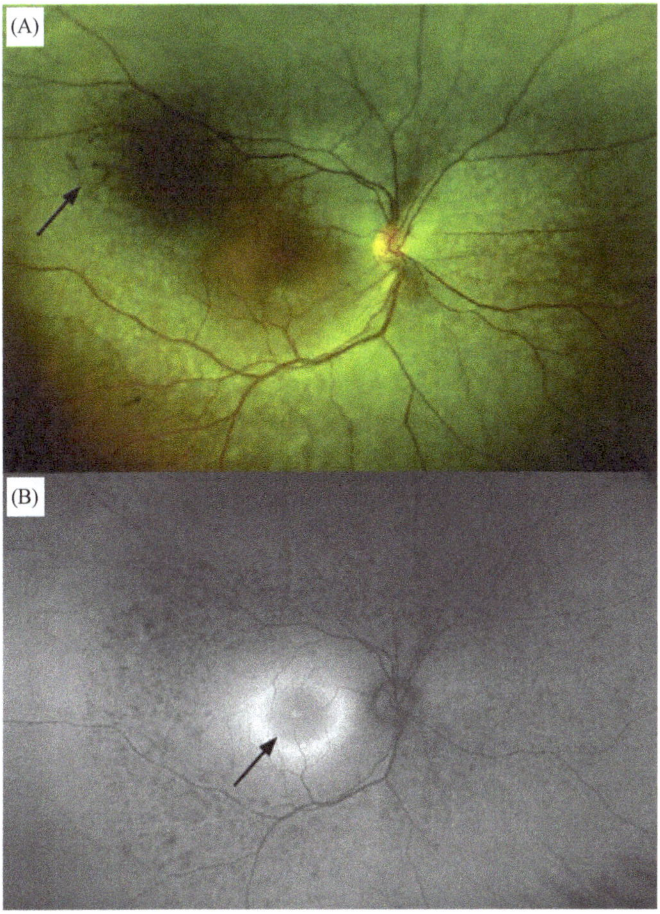

Figure 7.3. (A) A patient with early retinitis pigmentosa. Note the normal blood vessels and few bone spicules (arrow). (B) Fundus autofluorescence demonstrating the typical paracentral hypoautofluorescence (arrow).

7.4 Endogenous Endophthalmitis

Endogenous endophthalmitis results when there is ocular seeding from a bloodstream infection. It is typically found in patients who are immunosuppressed, diabetic, intravenous drug users or those who have chronic indwelling central venous catheters.[12] Endogenous endophthalmitis is suspected when clinical findings include anterior chamber inflammation,

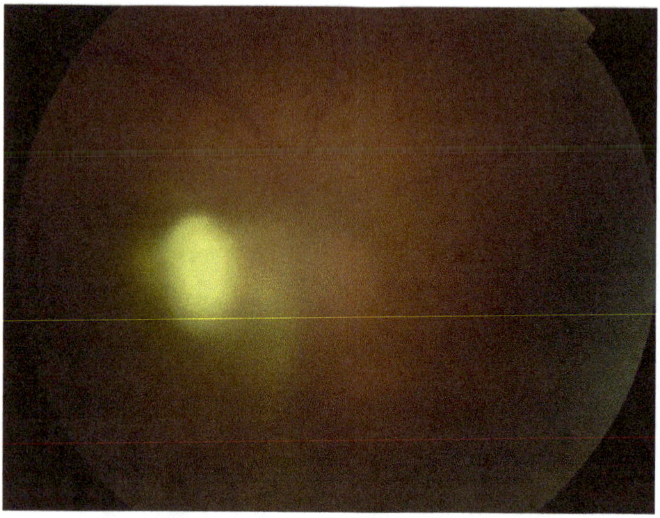

Figure 7.4. ***Candida albicans*** **endogenous endophthalmitis.**

hypopyon or fibrin in the anterior chamber, elevated intraocular pressure, vitritis and retinal hemorrhages and infiltrates (Figure 7.4).[13,14] The diagnosis is supported by positive blood cultures for either bacteremia or fungemia.[15] The gold standard for the diagnosis of endogenous endophthalmitis is obtaining a positive culture from intraocular fluids (primarily vitreous).[12] Specimens should be sent for gram staining and cultures. Polymerase chain reaction (PCR) is increasingly being used in the diagnosis of endophthalmitis.[16] A systemic evaluation is needed to locate the primary course of infection.

7.5 Chronic Endophthalmitis

When microbial organisms are introduced into the eye during surgery or penetrating trauma, the onset of inflammation is typically acute with symptoms and signs developing within a few days. However, organisms of low virulence may cause intraocular inflammation weeks or months after the event, presenting as insidious, low grade intraocular inflammation, commonly mistaken as immune-mediated uveitis.[17,18] Symptoms of chronic endophthalmitis differ from acute endophthalmitis and patients may only report a grumbling inflammation with minor discomfort and preserved visual acuity.[18,19] Signs suggestive of chronic endophthalmitis include granulomatous keratic precipitates, hypopyon, whitish nodules at the site of the corneal wound or overlying the intraocular lens, posterior capsule plaque or vitritis (Figures 7.5 and 7.6).[17]

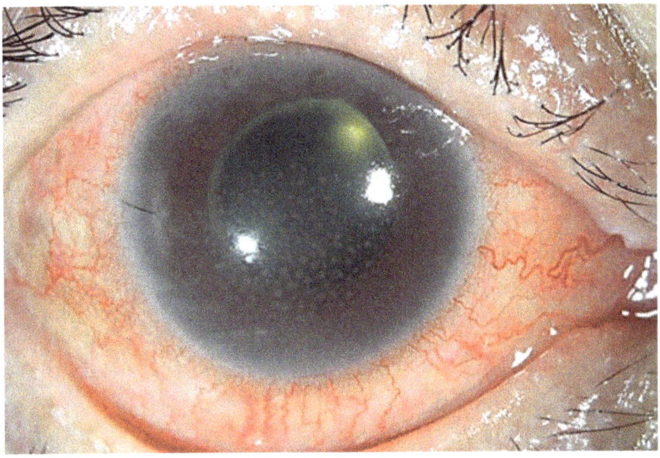

Figure 7.5. Chronic post-operative endophthalmitis with granulomatous keratic precipitates.

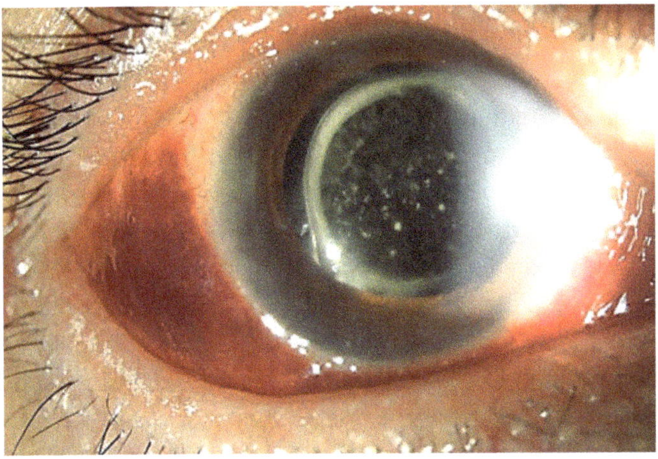

Figure 7.6. Chronic endophthalmitis following cataract surgery with posterior capsule plaque.

The diagnosis should be suspected in cases of prolonged inflammation following ocular surgery or trauma; when the inflammation relapses after weaning from topical corticosteroids; presence of a posterior capsule plaque (Figure 7.5) or the appearance of a hypopyon following laser capsulotomy.[20] Initial investigations, including ocular fluid sampling, may be negative and the inflammation could initially respond to topical corticosteroid treatment. Vitreous cultures may be negative in up to 50% of chronic endophthalmitis cases, due to slow growth of the organisms or their need for special conditions (anaerobic cultures or requiring high CO_2 concentrations).[21,22] Use of PCR increases the rates of detecting the causative organism and should be considered in suspected cases.[23] Cases of post-operative chronic endophthalmitis are typically caused by a single pathogen, with *Propionibacterium acnes* and coagulase-negative bacteria the most common causes.[24] Treatment options vary, depending on the severity of inflammation, identified pathogen and response to treatment. Treatment with antibiotics is an acceptable initial approach, combining intravitreal, topical and systemic drugs.[25] In many cases, surgical clearing of the intraocular contents is needed, including removal of the lens and capsular bag.[21] This combined approach improves clinical response and can prevent recurrences.

7.6 Drug-Induced Uveitis

Many systemic, intraocular or local medications as well as vaccines are associated with uveitis incidence (Table 7.1). Many drugs in the bisphosphonate class can induce uveitis, most commonly anterior uveitis (AU).[26–28] Onset of inflammation is usually within several days of drug exposure and responds rapidly to drug cessation and corticosteroids. Antimicrobial drugs including rifabutin and moxifloxacin are associated with uveitis.[29,30] Rifabutin-associated uveitis often presents with a hypopyon AU, similar to HLA-B27-associated uveitis, though many patients are HLA-B27 negative.[31] The emerging use of biologic therapies results in ever more intraocular inflammation being reported. Drug classes related to uveitis include anticancer immunotherapies, for example: immune checkpoint inhibitors (ICI), mitogen-activated protein (MEK) inhibitors or BRAF inhibitors.[31] Even drugs used to treat uveitis, such as tumor necrosis factor-α (TNF-α) inhibitors, particularly etanercept, have been reported to cause uveitis.[32]

Table 7.1. Drugs associated with uveitis.

Drug class	Drug name
Bisphosphonates	Alendronate
	Zoledronic acid
	Pamidronate
	Residronate
	Etidronate
Antimicrobials	Cidofovir
	Rifabutin
	Moxifloxacin
	Sulfonamides
Anti-TNF-α agents	Etanercept
	Infliximab
	Adalimumab
Anticancer immunotherapies	Vemurafenib
	Dabrafenib
	Trametinib
	Ipilimumab
	Pembrolizumab
	Nivolumab
Vaccines	Bacille Calmette-Guérin (BCG)
	Hepatitis B
	Influenza
	Human papillomavirus (HPV)
	Varicella
	Measles mumps rubella (MMR)

Among vaccines there are also reports relating to the occurrence of uveitis following vaccination, usually within 30 days.[33] Most cases are of AU with a good visual outcome, but several cases of Vogt-Koyanagi-Harada-like disease or multiple evanescent white dot syndrome (MEWDS) have also been reported.[34,35] The vaccines most associated with uveitis include those for hepatitis B, human papillomavirus, influenza virus and the Bacille Calmette-Guérin tuberculosis vaccine.

7.7 Primary Vitreoretinal Lymphoma/Primary Intraocular Lymphoma

Lymphoproliferative malignancies can present as intraocular inflammation. Intraocular lymphomas can be categorized into three main groups: primary vitreoretinal lymphoma (PVRL), primary uveal lymphoma and secondary intraocular lymphoma. PVRL is predominately diffuse large B-cell lymphoma and rarely T-cell lymphoma. Typical findings include vitritis, anterior chamber cells, and subretinal yellow infiltrates (Figure 7.7).[36] Vitreous cells appear as veils (Figure 7.8). It is characterized by hyperreflective subretinal infiltrates, hyperreflective infiltration in outer retinal layers, RPE undulation, clumps of vitreous cells, and sub-RPE deposits on optical coherence tomography (OCT) scans.[36–38] Of these, the hyperreflective subretinal infiltrates are unique to PVRL (Figure 7.9).[38]

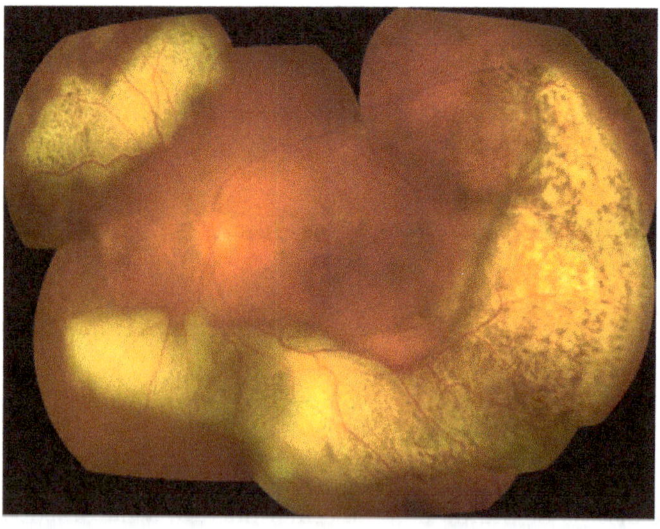

Figure 7.7. Yellow subretinal infiltrates in a patient with primary vitreoretinal lymphoma.

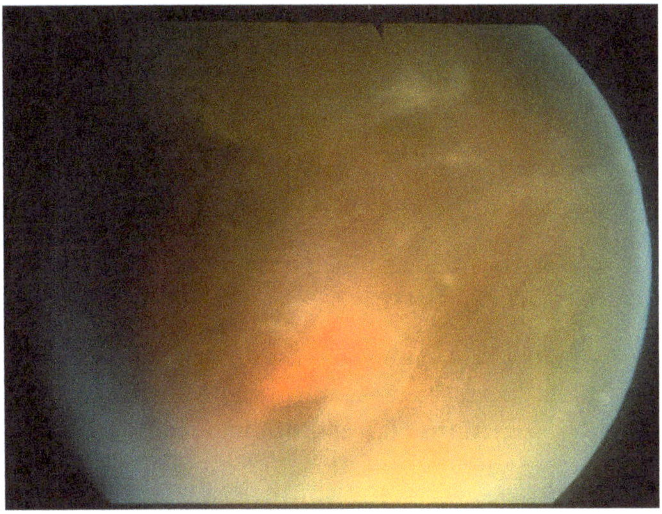

Figure 7.8. Vitreous veils in primary vitreoretinal lymphoma.

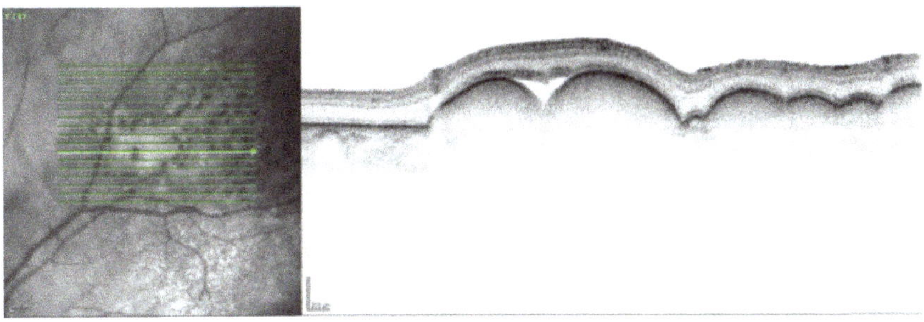

Figure 7.9. Ocular coherence tomography in a patient with primary vitreoretinal lymphoma, demonstrating subretinal infiltrates.

Vitreous biopsy and histological diagnostic techniques remain the gold standard for diagnosis. The cytokine level of IL-10 to IL-6 ratio greater than 1 in the vitreous is highly suggestive of PVRL; however, it cannot be used as a sole biomarker. Cytology by Giemsa staining for a large atypical lymphoid cell with large nuclei, prominent nucleoli, and scanty basophilic cytoplasm in a vitreous specimen is diagnostic.[39] Diagnosis is challenging because of the vulnerability and rarity of the atypical lymphoma cells, the influence of prior corticosteroid treatment on the morphology of cells, and mechanical damage during vitrectomy and sample processing. Monoclonal rearrangements of immunoglobulin heavy chain (IgH) and T-cell receptor genes detected by PCR provide higher test efficacy than cytology for B- and T-cell lymphoma.[40]

7.8 Chorioretinal Tumors

Chorioretinal tumors may mimic uveitis, for example, peripheral uveal melanoma including iris melanomas and melanoma of the ciliary body and retinoblastoma.[41,42] Anterior chamber cells can be the first clinical signs of chorioretinal tumors but this is rare (Figure 7.10). These cells are a mixture of tumor cells, pigment cells, and inflammatory macrophages, rather than the dominant $CD4^+$ T-cells in the immune-mediated uveitis.[41,43] Systemic investigation to exclude metastatic disease from the liver, lungs, and central nervous system is necessary when the diagnosis is suspected.

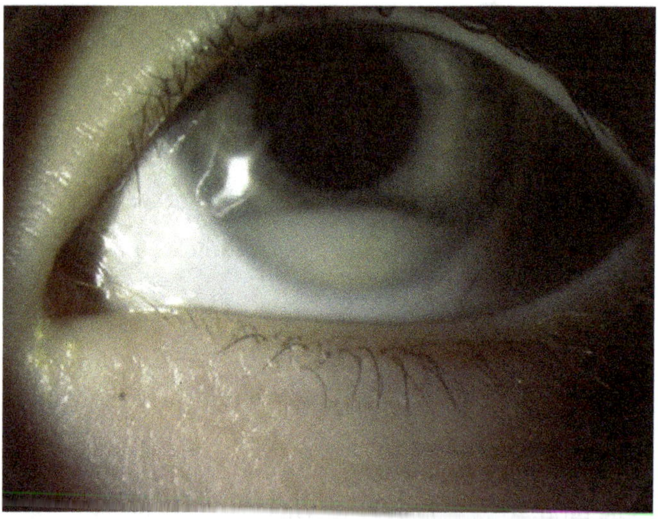

Figure 7.10. Endophytic retinoblastoma presenting with hypopyon in a three-year-old patient.

7.9 Metastatic Tumors

Metastatic disease can present as clinically diffuse choroidal infiltrates, optic nerve head infiltration (Figure 7.11) and diffuse serous retinal detachment (SRD), choroidal folds and thickening.[44] The metastatic cells may also respond to oral steroids.[45] The presentation of circumferential infiltrate, choroidal folds without SRD, and extrascleral nodules are suspicious for a lymphoproliferative process of the uvea (Figure 7.12).

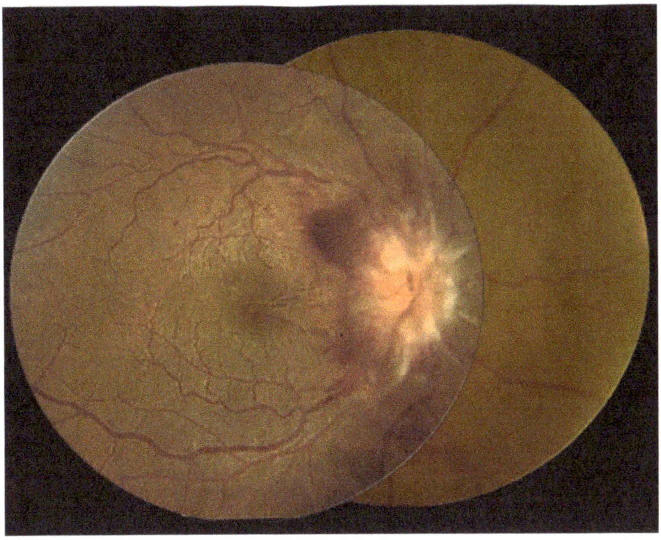

Figure 7.11. Optic nerve head infiltration of metastatic acute lymphoblastic leukemia.

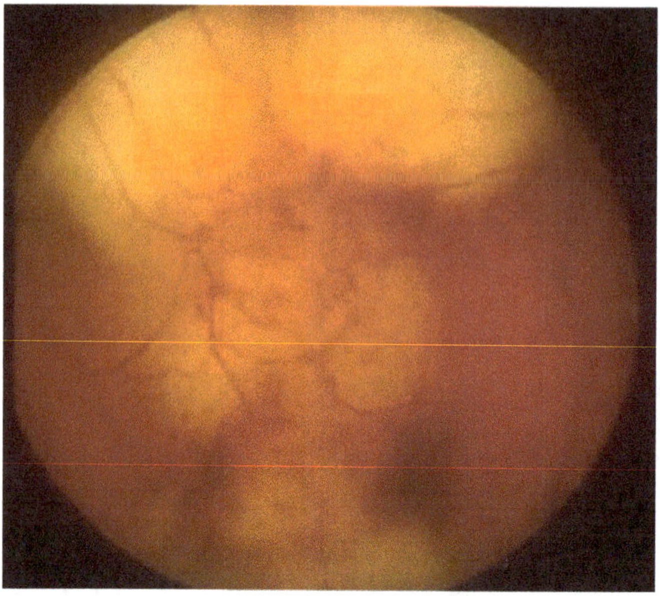

Figure 7.12. Choroidal lymphoma.

7.10 Intraocular Foreign Body

Though not typically regarded as a cause of masquerade, the clinical presentation of intraocular foreign body (IOFB) may be atypical, resulting in delay in diagnosis and management. In cases of small IOFBs they may be undetected and present as anterior, intermediate, or posterior uveitis especially if found in the angle, pars plana, and iris stroma.[46,47] In the early stage they may present as traumatic uveitis but have an occult foreign body. Common manifestations of chronic IOFBs also include cataract, diffuse pigmentary changes of the RPE, siderosis bulbi, iris heterochromia, dilated pupils, secondary glaucoma, iritis, and cystoid macular edema (Figure 7.13).[48] Meticulous clinical examination and a detailed clinical history are the cornerstones to reveal the unusual pathogenic mechanism. Ancillary tests such as ocular ultrasound, anterior chamber OCT, electroretinogram and computed tomography can confirm the clin-

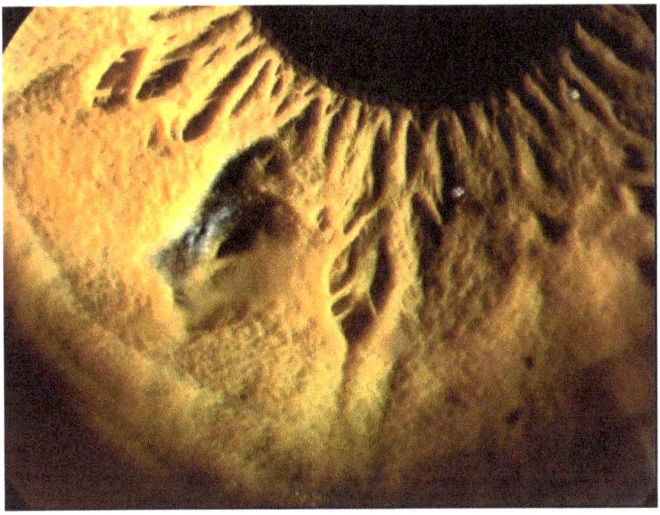

Figure 7.13. Intraocular foreign body.

ical diagnosis. Magnetic resonance imaging must not be used if the IOFB could be metallic.

Teaching Points

- Masquerade syndromes have intraocular inflammation or pseudo-inflammation from non-inflammatory causes including malignancy and non-neoplastic proliferative conditions.
- Chronic endophthalmitis should be considered when there is a grumbling inflammation, minor discomfort, and preserved visual acuity.
- Drug-induced uveitis can be triggered by bisphosphonates, rifabutin, moxifloxacin, biologics and vaccines.
- Primary vitreoretinal lymphoma / primary intraocular lymphoma is challenging to diagnose as it imitates uveitis, white dot syndromes or other neoplasms clinically, and additionally it initially responds to corticosteroid treatment. Once there is a clinical suspicion then a vitreous biopsy (and/or chorioretinal biopsy) is required.

References

1. Rothova A, Ooijman F, Kerkhoff F, *et al.* Uveitis masquerade syndromes. *Ophthalmology* 2001;108(2):386–99.
2. Fukutsu K, Namba K, Iwata D, *et al.* Pseudo-inflammatory manifestations of choroidal lymphoma resembling Vogt-Koyanagi-Harada disease: case report based on multimodal imaging. *BMC Ophthalmol* 2020;20(1):94.
3. Kinast RM, Solomon SD, Cubillan LD, *et al.* Prevalence and causes of clinically detectable uveitic serous retinal detachment. *Eur J Ophthalmol* 2021;31(6):3093–8.
4. Yassin MA, Ata F, Mohamed SF, *et al.* Ophthalmologic manifestations as the initial presentation of chronic myeloid leukemia: A review. *Surv Ophthalmol* 2022;67(2):530–43.
5. Arroyo JG, Jaffe GJ. Spontaneous giant retinal pigment epithelial tear associated with panuveitis. *Retina* 1997;17(3):254–6.
6. Sevgi DD, Davoudi S, Comander J, Sobrin L. Retinal pigmentary changes in chronic uveitis mimicking retinitis pigmentosa. *Graefes Arch Clin Exp Ophthalmol* 2017;255(9):1801–10.
7. Lam RW, Remick RA. Pigmentary retinopathy associated with low-dose thioridazine treatment. *Can Med Assoc J* 1985;132(7):737.
8. Vela JI, Marcantonio I, Díaz-Cascajosa J, *et al.* Progression of retinal pigmentation mimicking unilateral retinitis pigmentosa after bilateral pars planitis: a case report. *BMC Ophthalmol* 2018;18(1):242.
9. Yeung TL, Li PS, Li KK. Presumed topiramate retinopathy: a case report. *J Med Case Rep* 2016;10:210.
10. Tripathy K, Chawla R, Venkatesh P, *et al.* Ultra-wide field fluorescein angiography in retinitis pigmentosa with intermediate uveitis. *J Ophthalmic Vis Res* 2016;11(2):237–9.
11. Dutta Majumder P, Menia N, Roy R, *et al.* Uveitis in patients with retinitis pigmentosa: 30 years' consecutive data. *Ocul Immunol Inflamm* 2018;26(8):1283–8.
12. Binder MI, Chua J, Kaiser PK, *et al.* Endogenous endophthalmitis: an 18-year review of culture-positive cases at a tertiary care center. *Medicine (Baltimore)* 2003;82(2):97–105.
13. Nishida T, Ishida K, Niwa Y, *et al.* An eleven-year retrospective study of endogenous bacterial endophthalmitis. *J Ophthalmol* 2015;2015:261310.
14. Samalia PD, Welch S, Polkinghorne PJ, Niederer RL. Endogenous endophthalmitis: A 21-year review of cases at a tertiary eye care centre. *Ocul Immunol Inflamm* 2021;in press.
15. Patel AV, Young LH. Endogenous Endophthalmitis. In: Durand ML, Miller JW, Young LH, eds. Endophthalmitis: Springer, 2016.

16. Okhravi N, Adamson P, Lightman S. Use of PCR in endophthalmitis. *Ocul Immunol Inflamm* 2000;8(3):189–200.
17. Niederer RL, Bar A, Gilbert R, *et al.* Chronic Endophthalmitis Masquerading as Uveitis. In: Durand ML, Miller JW, Young LH, eds. Endophthalmitis: Springer, 2016.
18. Shirodkar AR, Pathengay A, Flynn HW, Jr., *et al.* Delayed-versus acute-onset endophthalmitis after cataract surgery. *Am J Ophthalmol* 2012;153(3):391–8 e2.
19. Meisler DM, Mandelbaum S. Propionibacterium-associated endophthalmitis after extracapsular cataract extraction. Review of reported cases. *Ophthalmology* 1989;96(1):54–61.
20. Chaudhry M, Baisakhiya S, Bhatia MS. A rare complication of Nd-YAG capsulotomy: propionibacterium acnes endopthalmitis. *Nepal J Ophthalmol* 2011;3(1):80–2.
21. Clark WL, Kaiser PK, Flynn HW, Jr., *et al.* Treatment strategies and visual acuity outcomes in chronic postoperative Propionibacterium acnes endophthalmitis. *Ophthalmology* 1999;106(9):1665–70.
22. Narang S, Gupta A, Gupta V, *et al.* Fungal endophthalmitis following cataract surgery: clinical presentation, microbiological spectrum, and outcome. *Am J Ophthalmol* 2001;132(5):609–17.
23. Lohmann CP, Linde HJ, Reischl U. Improved detection of microorganisms by polymerase chain reaction in delayed endophthalmitis after cataract surgery. *Ophthalmology* 2000;107(6):1047–51.
24. Winward KE, Pflugfelder SC, Flynn HW, Jr., *et al.* Postoperative Propionibacterium endophthalmitis. Treatment strategies and long-term results. *Ophthalmology* 1993;100(4):447–51.
25. Zambrano W, Flynn HW, Jr., Pflugfelder SC, *et al.* Management options for Propionibacterium acnes endophthalmitis. *Ophthalmology* 1989;96(7):1100–5.
26. Belliveau MJ, Almeida DR, Urton TE. Acute anterior uveitis following zoledronic acid infusion for osteoporosis. *Can J Ophthalmol* 2012;47(5):e22–3.
27. Tan YL, Sims J, Chee SP. Bilateral uveitis secondary to bisphosphonate therapy. *Ophthalmologica* 2009;223(3):215–6.
28. Samalia P, Sims J, Niederer RL. Drug-induced ocular inflammation. *N Z Med J* 2020;133(1527):83–94.
29. Wefers Bettink-Remeijer M, Brouwers K, van Langenhove L, *et al.* Uveitis-like syndrome and iris transillumination after the use of oral moxifloxacin. *Eye (Lond)* 2009;23(12):2260–2.
30. Abdalla Elsayed MEA, Kozak I. Pharmacologically induced uveitis. *Surv Ophthalmol* 2021;66(5):781–801.

31. Moorthy RS, Moorthy MS, Cunningham ET, Jr. Drug-induced uveitis. *Curr Opin Ophthalmol* 2018;29(6):588–603.
32. Lim LL, Fraunfelder FW, Rosenbaum JT. Do tumor necrosis factor inhibitors cause uveitis? A registry-based study. *Arthritis Rheum* 2007;56(10):3248–52.
33. Benage M, Fraunfelder FW. Vaccine-associated uveitis. *Mo Med* 2016;113(1):48–52.
34. Cunningham ET, Jr., Moorthy RS. Vaccine-associated posterior uveitis. *Retin Cases Brief Rep* 2022;16(1):1–4.
35. Cunningham ET, Jr., Moorthy RS, Fraunfelder FW, Zierhut M. Vaccine-associated uveitis. *Ocul Immunol Inflamm* 2019;27(4):517–20.
36. Hearne E, Tomkins-Netzer O, Lightman S. Learning points in intraocular lymphoma. *Eye (Lond)* 2021;35(7):1815–7.
37. Deák GG, Goldstein DA, Zhou M, *et al.* Vertical hyperreflective lesions on optical coherence tomography in vitreoretinal lymphoma. *JAMA Ophthalmol* 2019;137(2):194–8.
38. Barry RJ, Tasiopoulou A, Murray PI, *et al.* Characteristic optical coherence tomography findings in patients with primary vitreoretinal lymphoma: a novel aid to early diagnosis. *Br J Ophthalmol* 2018;102(10):1362–6.
39. Kinoshita Y, Takasu K, Adachi Y, *et al.* Retrospective cytological study of intraocular lymphoma using vitreous and intraocular perfusion fluid. *Diagn Cytopathol* 2012;40(7):604–7.
40. Wang Y, Shen D, Wang VM, *et al.* Molecular biomarkers for the diagnosis of primary vitreoretinal lymphoma. *Int J Mol Sci* 2011;12(9):5684–97.
41. Feng L, Zhu J, Gao T, *et al.* Uveal melanoma in the peripheral choroid masquerading as chronic uveitis. *Optom Vis Sci* 2014;91(9):e222–5.
42. Garg V, Gupta A, Pruthi SK, Khare P. Retinoblastoma in an adult. *J Cytol* 2018;35(2):120–4.
43. Lentz KJ, Burns RP, Loeffler K, *et al.* Uveitis caused by cytotoxic immune response to cutaneous malignant melanoma in swine: destruction of uveal melanocytes during tumor regression. *Invest Ophthalmol Vis Sci* 1983;24(8):1063–9.
44. Bhandari R, Dacey M, Schwartz S, *et al.* Vogt-Koyanagi-Harada disease masquerading as a lymphoproliferative process of the uvea. *Br J Ophthalmol* 2013;97(11):1482–3.
45. Cheung MK, Martin DF, Chan CC, *et al.* Diagnosis of reactive lymphoid hyperplasia by chorioretinal biopsy. *Am J Ophthalmol* 1994;118(4):457–62.
46. Politis M, Rosin B, Amer R. Ocular siderosis subsequent to a missed pars plana metallic foreign body that masqueraded as refractory intermediate uveitis. *Ocul Immunol Inflamm* 2018;26(4):598–600.

47. Mahmoud A, Messaoud R, Abid F, *et al.* Anterior segment optical coherence tomography and retained vegetal intraocular foreign body masquerading as chronic anterior uveitis. *J Ophthalmic Inflamm Infect* 2017;7(1):13.
48. Kannan NB, Adenuga OO, Rajan RP, Ramasamy K. Management of ocular siderosis: visual outcome and electroretinographic changes. *J Ophthalmol* 2016;2016:7272465.

https://doi.org/10.1142/9789811251474_0008

Chapter 8

Complications of Uveitis

Jay Meyer,[*,†] *Sonya Bennett,*[*] *Daniel Gosling,*[*]
Haya Al-Ani,[*] *Sarah Welch,*[*] *Rachael Niederer*[*,†]

Complications are common in patients with uveitis, particularly with chronic disease, delayed diagnosis or posterior uveitis. They may be associated with sequelae of inflammation, or iatrogenic, in particular secondary to the effect of corticosteroids. Careful control of inflammation, tapering steroid dose appropriately, and initiation of second-line immunosuppressive therapy properly are critical to reducing the incidence of complications.

8.1 Corneal Complications

8.1.1 *Endothelial Damage*

There is evidence that anterior chamber inflammation can adversely affect the endothelium. This endothelial damage is likely multifactorial and may be related to the duration of uveitis, elevation of intraocular pressure (IOP), inflammatory cytokines, and deposition of keratic precipitates on the endothelium.[1,2] Viral causes of uveitis may also directly affect the endothelium, resulting in endotheliitis with associated corneal edema.[3] Corneal decompensation in eyes with uveitis is a rare but significant complication.[4] As uveitic eyes frequently require surgery for other complications such as cataracts or glaucoma, there may be a higher risk of post-operative decompensation if the endothelium is already compromised prior to surgery.

[*] Department of Ophthalmology, Auckland District Health Board, Auckland, New Zealand
[†] University of Auckland, Auckland, New Zealand

8.1.2 Band Keratopathy

Band keratopathy (BK) is a frequent complication of chronic anterior uveitis and is characterised by calcium deposition at the level of Bowman's membrane. Clinically, this appears as a gray or white opacification with irregular borders in the superficial cornea, and typically develops over months or years. The BK initially develops in the nasal and temporal peripheral cornea (Figure 8.1) and may advance centrally to extend throughout the interpalpebral zone (Figure 8.2). In the initial stages, patients are often

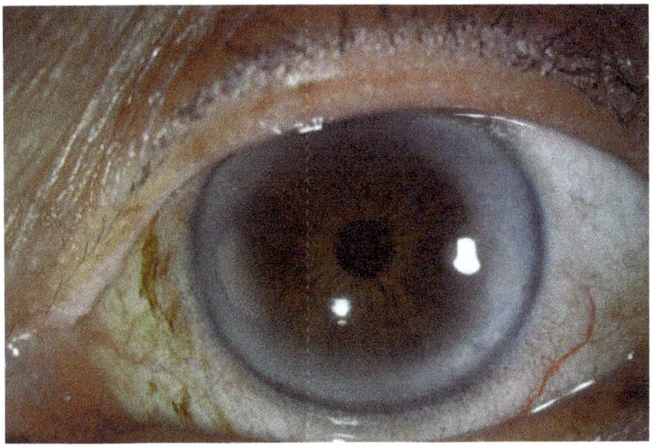

Figure 8.1. Early band keratopathy involving the nasal and temporal cornea.

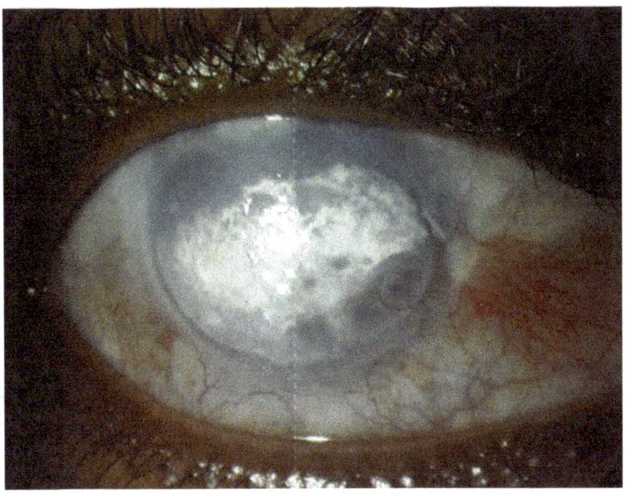

Figure 8.2. Band keratopathy involving the central cornea.

asymptomatic and treatment is rarely required. However, advanced BK can disrupt the epithelium and cause foreign body sensation, predispose to infection, or affect the central visual acuity.

The primary indications for BK removal include ocular discomfort, decreased visual acuity, or a poor view for clinical monitoring or surgical intervention. In eyes with significant neurotrophic keratopathy and/or ocular surface disease, there is a risk of precipitating a corneal melt and even perforation with treatment, and this must be taken in consideration when planning surgery and consenting patients.[5] Techniques to remove BK include mechanical debridement, chelation, and phototherapeutic keratectomy. A surgical technique of chelation is outlined in Chapter 10. Following treatment, there is a significant risk of recurrence over time, with up to 60% recurrence rate in eyes with uveitis.[6]

8.2 Cataract

Cataract is a common complication of uveitis and the leading cause of vision loss (Figure 8.3). It occurs in 50–78% of eyes, more commonly in chronic anterior uveitis and intermediate uveitis.[7–9] It is a result of both the primary inflammatory disease process and its subsequent treatment with corticosteroids. The predilection of uveitis to affect the working-age

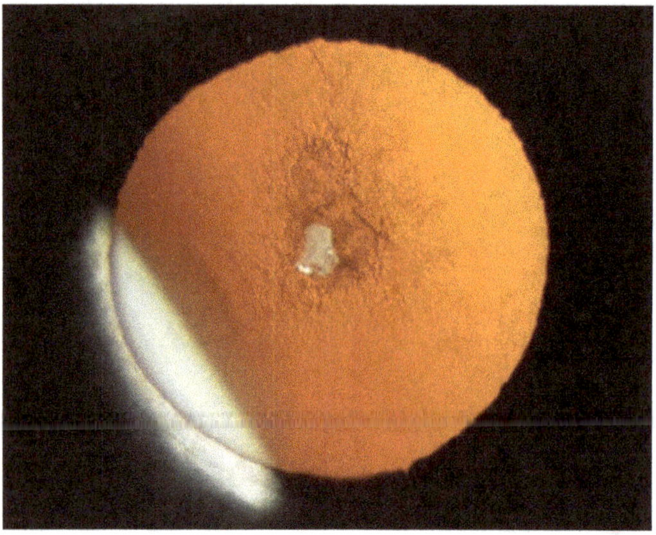

Figure 8.3. Posterior subcapsular lens opacification in a patient with uveitis.

population results in younger patients with more advanced cataract and higher rates of ocular co-morbidity compared to the non-uveitic population.[10]

Cataract surgery in uveitic eyes is indicated in 1) phacoantigenic uveitis, 2) visually significant cataract in quiet eyes with good visual prognosis, 3) impaired posterior segment examination due to cataract, and 4) cataract extraction to allow for visualization in posterior segment surgery.[8] Before surgery can be considered the eye must be quiescent for at least 3 months with or without treatment. Use of peri-operative systemic or intravitreal steroids must be considered to prevent disease relapse following surgery.[10,11] Surgery is often complex, requiring additional intra-operative procedures to manage structural abnormalities (Figure 8.4), such as posterior synechiae peel or iris hooks; this complexity is reflected in the higher complication rates compared to non-uveitic eyes (see Chapter 11).[12]

Post-operative cystoid macular edema occurs more frequently with uveitic cataract surgery, with reported rates ranging from 12–59%.[13,14] Pre-operative inflammation control and prophylactic steroid use are essential in reducing the risk of poor visual outcome.[15,16] It is also important to consider recurrence of inflammation; it is encouraging that published studies have demonstrated that with adequate treatment the risk of uveitis

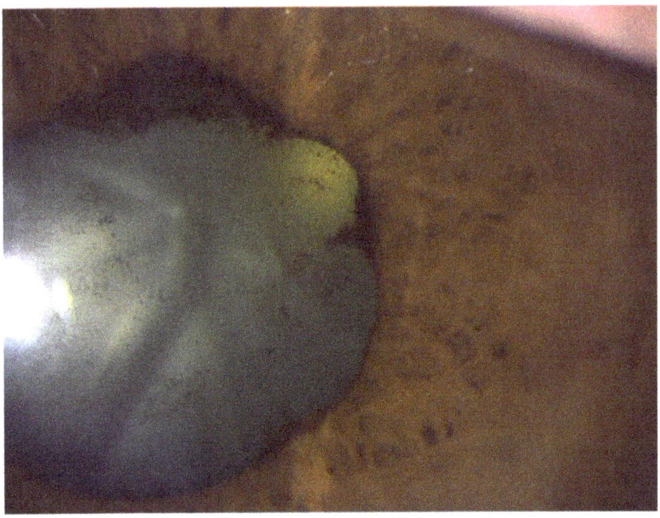

Figure 8.4. Posterior synechiae and cataract in a patient with HLA-B27-associated uveitis.

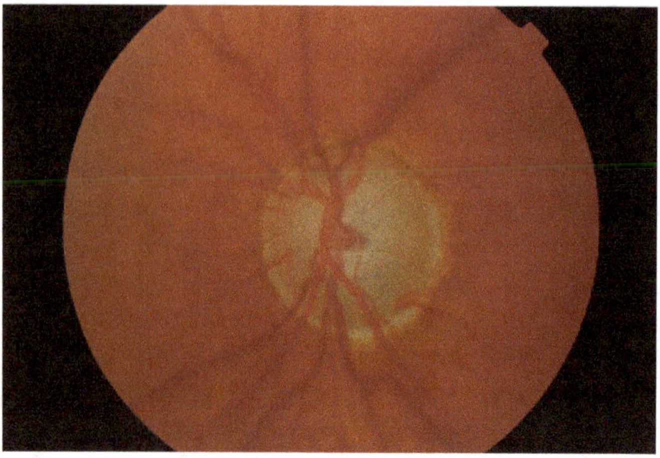

Figure 8.5. Extensive optic nerve cupping in uveitic glaucoma.

relapse does not increase following cataract surgery, with lower rates of recurrence compared to the pre-operative period.[14]

8.3 Uveitic Glaucoma

Uveitic glaucoma is a characteristic glaucomatous optic neuropathy (GON), featuring optic disc cupping and loss of visual function, and associated with raised IOP as a sequelae of intraocular inflammation (Figure 8.5). Surveys of uveitis cohorts show annual incidence of 14% ocular hypertension (OHT),[17] and a 77% 10-year conversion rate from OHT to manifest glaucoma.[18] Rates of glaucoma are higher in chronic uveitis and anterior segment involvement.[17,18] Patients with uveitic glaucoma are at high risk of blindness, therefore aggressive treatment and careful monitoring are required. The etiologies of raised IOP in uveitis are many, and often multifactorial. These mechanisms can be divided into those with an open or closed iridocorneal angle.

8.3.1 Open Angle — Altered Aqueous Outflow

In uveitis, increased permeability of the blood-aqueous barrier alters aqueous outflow dynamics. Viscosity increases and cells and inflammatory debris accumulate in trabecular meshwork (TM). In acute uveitis, effective treatment can lead to normalization of the IOP. However, in chronic or recurrent disease, baseline IOP can become permanently elevated by pathological changes of outflow. These patients are at high risk of GON.

8.3.2 Open Angle — *Steroid Response*

Raised IOP as a response to topical or systemic corticosteroid use, occurring in up to a third of patients (steroid responders), is a well-recognized but poorly understood phenomenon. Swelling of TM cells and increased extracellular matrix degradation products likely play a role.[19] Increased corticosteroid use in uveitis is a strong risk factor for developing OHT.[17] This may be due to steroid response, or simply association with severity of uveitis.

Onset of OHT can vary but is usually within a few weeks of starting treatment. Offset is variable. Adequate treatment of inflammation is the first priority, and should not be avoided for fear of inducing OHT. IOP should then be treated secondarily.

8.3.3 Open Angle — *Trabeculitis*

Inflammation can occur directly in the TM cells causing edema and loss of permeability. Trabeculitis is differentiated by a very high IOP, with relatively minor anterior chamber activity. It responds rapidly to topical corticosteroid, and there is an association with infectious etiologies,[20] but is most often idiopathic. Anterior chamber tap for viral PCRs (HSV, VZV, CMV) can be helpful to establish a cause. Later subjects may develop iris atrophy (Figure 8.6). Prophylactic antivirals may benefit IOP control in these cases. Recurrent episodes of symptomatic raised IOP due to trabeculitis, whether idiopathic or infective, are termed Posner-Schlossman syndrome.

8.3.4 Closed Angle — *Seclusio Pupillae*

The formation of posterior synechia at the pupil margin restricts flow of aqueous between the posterior and anterior chambers. If 360 degrees of adhesions form (seclusio pupillae, Figure 8.7), then iris bombé occurs with angle closure crisis (Figure 8.8).

Iridotomy is necessary to resolve the problem, but laser iridotomy can be problematic, due to inflammation and risk of damage to endothelium. Surgical iridotomy is often required.[21]

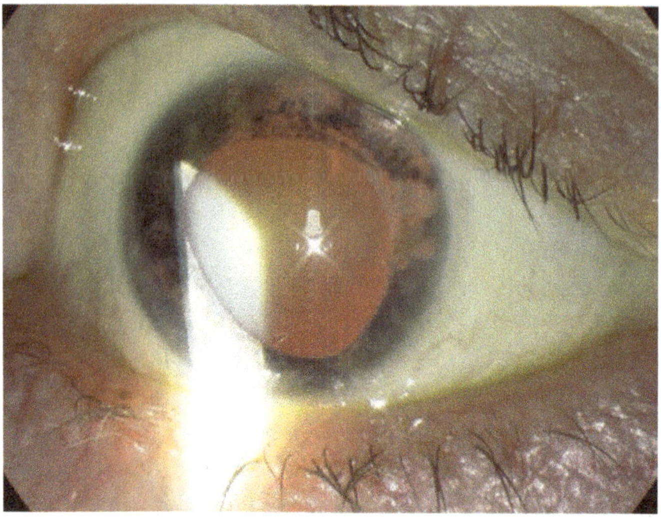

Figure 8.6. Iris atrophy in herpes simplex virus anterior uveitis.

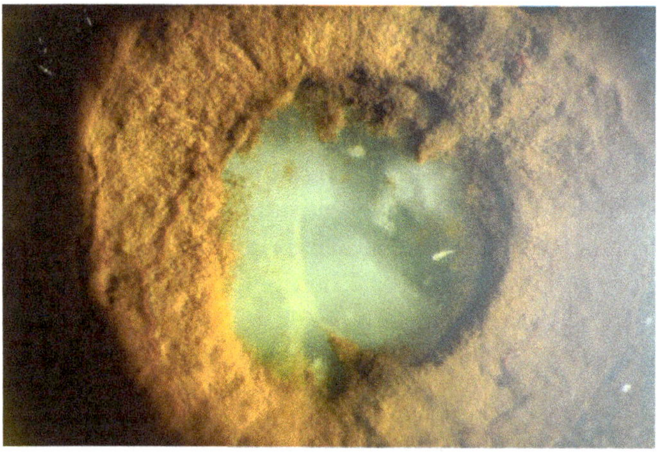

Figure 8.7. Extensive posterior synechia in a patient with sarcoidosis uveitis.

8.3.5 Closed Angle — Synechial Angle Closure

Peripheral anterior synechiae (PAS) can be diagnosed on gonioscopy, occluding the trabecular meshwork. Chronic or recurrent uveitis can lead to increasing areas of PAS and once a threshold is met (often between 180

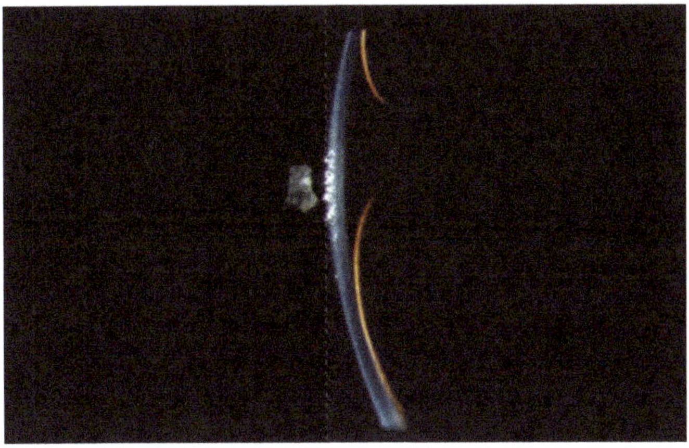

Figure 8.8. Angle closure due to posterior synechiae and iris bombé.

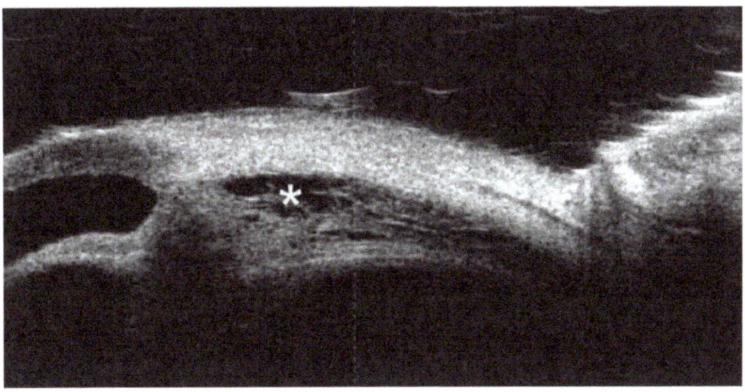

Figure 8.9. Ultrasound biomicroscopy (UBM) demonstrating ciliary body detachment in panuveitis. Note the fluid between the ciliary body and sclera (asterisk).

and 270 degrees of occlusion), outflow facility is reduced and IOP rises. Glaucoma tube surgery is then indicated.

8.3.6 *Closed Angle — Choroidal Effusion*

Rarely, inflammation and ischemia of the ciliary body cause swelling and forward rotation, precipitating closure of the drainage angle. This can be diagnosed by recognizing a shallow anterior chamber, myopic shift and ciliary body swelling on ultrasound biomicroscopy (Figure 8.9).

8.4 Retinal Detachment

Retinal detachment is common in eyes with uveitis, with up to 1–3% of eyes developing a rhegmatogenous retinal detachment or a serous detachment.[22–24] Any form of retinal detachment which involves the posterior segment occurs more commonly in uveitis. The diagnosis of retinal detachment can be challenging when there is fulminant vitritis or other media opacity and in many cases a B-scan can be helpful. Once the diagnosis of retinal detachment is made, it is important to distinguish what type of detachment it is as this will determine the ideal management.

8.4.1 *Serous Retinal Detachment*

The hallmarks of serous retinal detachment are shifting subretinal fluid and absence of a retinal break. In the context of uveitis, when a difficult view of the retina is common, then ascertaining whether the fluid is shifting or not is probably the best method of confirming the detachment is serous. One way to check this is to look at the patient while sitting upright, when the detachment will be inferior as the fluid moves with gravity and then lay the patient down and view the retina with the indirect ophthalmoscope to see the detachment at the posterior pole. If the retina is not visible due to media opacity then perform this maneuver with the B-scan.

Some uveitic conditions are nearly always associated with serous retinal detachment, such as Vogt-Koyanagi-Harada (VKH). In this entity, the serous detachments more commonly present as multiple small areas, but in some severe cases the areas may coalesce and large detachments may occur (Figure 8.10). The presence of signs in both eyes can help make the diagnosis and differentiate from a rhegmatogenous detachment.[25]

In nearly all cases, the treatment of serous retinal detachment associated with uveitis is to treat the underlying cause rather than proceed to surgery. The mechanism of the detachment is the production of excessive sub-retinal fluid overwhelming the retinal pigment epithelium (RPE) pump, and stopping the production of excess fluid by treating the infection or inflammation allows the RPE pump to slowly restore the normal anatomy. In most cases, once the underlying cause of the uveitis is adequately treated then the serous detachment resolves. Visual recovery usually depends on the extent of damage to the retina by the infection or inflammation and vision loss from serous detachments alone is less common.

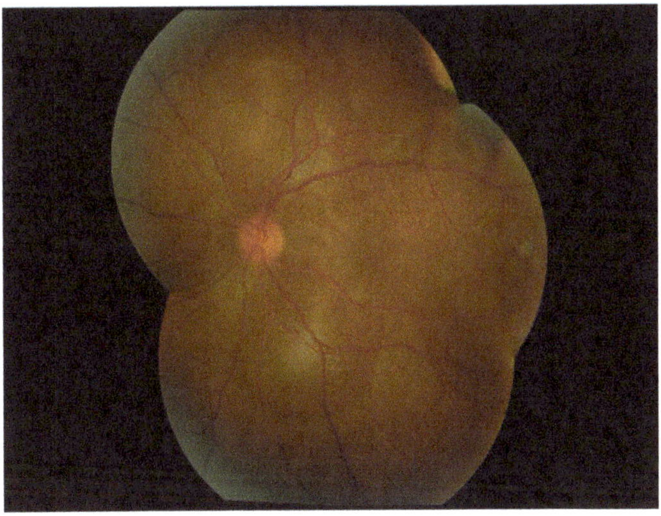

Figure 8.10. Serous retinal detachment due to Vogt-Koyanagi-Harada syndrome.

8.4.2 Rhegmatogenous Retinal Detachment

Rhegmatogenous retinal detachment (RRD) is less common than serous detachment in uveitis but can be visually devastating — in some series of uveitic RRD, up to 50% of eyes have moderate to severe visual loss. RRD is over a hundred times more common in eyes with uveitis compared to the general population due to the damage uveitis processes cause to the retina.[26–28] Retinal breaks may occur in thinned, atrophic retina associated with chronic inflammation particularly in the periphery, or in the case of severe infectious retinitis, in entities like ARN (acute retinal necrosis) or PORN (progressive outer retinal necrosis), large necrotic breaks may occur adjacent to areas of active necrosis (Figures 8.11 and 8.12). Peripheral breaks may be very small and difficult to identify making it hard to differentiate from serous detachments. The location and behavior of the subretinal fluid as well as the behaviors of the overlying retina can aid in achieving the correct diagnosis.

RRD in infectious retinitis like ARN or PORN often progresses very quickly with multiple breaks and can be technically challenging to repair. In most cases, the use of silicon oil as a tamponade is required. In ARN, laser retinopexy (barrier laser) around areas of necrosis used to be recommended to try to prevent retinal detachments but this remains controversial and there is no compelling evidence that laser prevents retinal

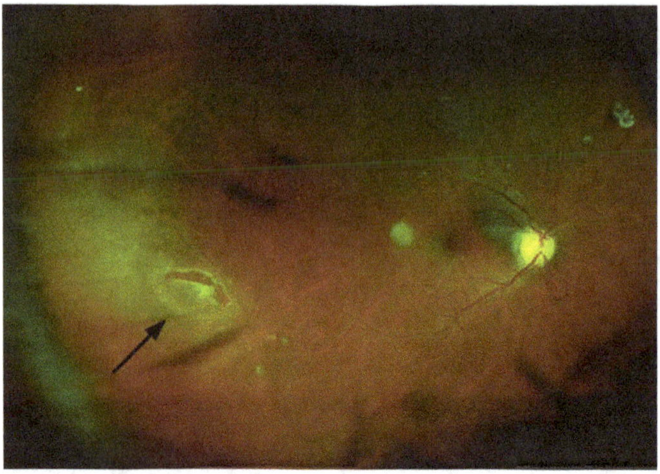

Figure 8.11. Retinal tear in patient with intermediate uveitis (arrow).

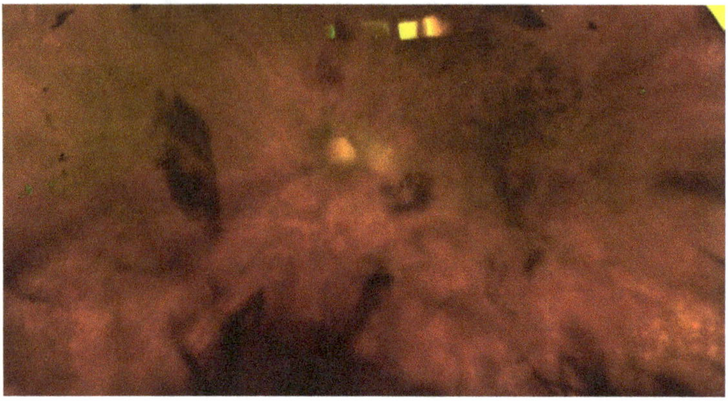

Figure 8.12. Inferior retinal detachment following acute retinal necrosis. Note dense vitritis and extensive retinal hemorrhages.

detachments. In cases of CMV retinitis, laser retinopexy may even increase the risk of breaks at the site of laser treatment.

Proliferative vitreoretinopathy (PVR) is common in eyes with uveitis and RRD and contributes to the technically challenging surgery associated with these detachments as well as the poor visual outcomes. PVR makes re-detachments more common and also requires the use of oil as a tamponade in many cases. In most cases, the retina can be re-attached despite these challenges but the vision is often compromised and sometimes long-term oil tamponade is required.

Some chronic RRDs present with significant anterior segment inflammation as well as vitritis mimicking a retinal detachment that has occurred in the presence of uveitis. These cases can be difficult to reach the correct diagnosis (see Chapter 7). A history, review of systems and careful examination of the other eye may be helpful. Choroidal effusions and relative hypotony in the affected eye are common findings. A short course of steroids (once an infectious etiology has been ruled out) will typically demonstrate a more limited response than expected for a serous retinal detachment and in some cases a diagnostic vitrectomy can reveal the underlying pathology.

In most cases of RRD associated with uveitis then a vitrectomy is the treatment of choice as it provides an opportunity to perform diagnostic biopsy as needed, as well as removing visually significant vitritis and potentially reducing the inflammatory load.

8.4.3 *Tractional Retinal Detachment*

Tractional retinal detachment (TRD) is less common in uveitis than the other forms of retinal detachment. It may arise in the presence of PVR with recurrent retinal detachments sometimes causing a combined RRD and TRD. TRD may also arise as a consequence of peripheral neovascularization response to severe ischemia in vasculitic conditions (Figure 8.13).

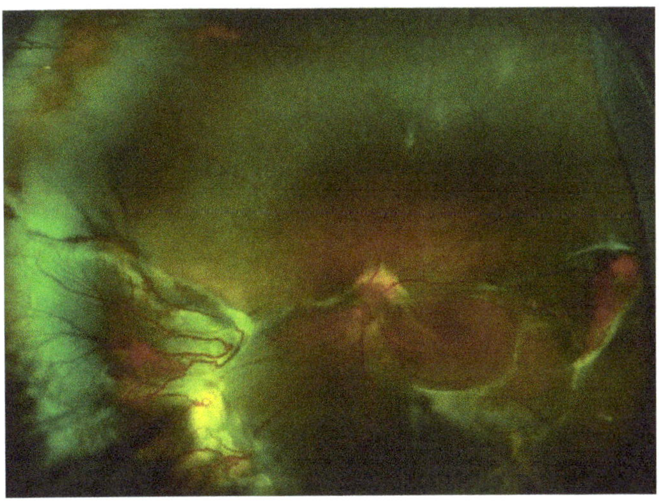

Figure 8.13. Tractional retinal detachment in tuberculosis panuveitis.

Rarely, severe chronic posterior uveitis that is poorly controlled may form fibrotic bands causing TRD. Surgery is indicated for those cases that are progressive or threatening the macula, but in many cases observation is sufficient.

8.5 Epiretinal Membrane

Epiretinal membranes (ERM) are common in uveitis, with some studies finding they occur in 40–50% of uveitic eyes. As expected, they are more likely to occur in eyes with posterior segment involvement of the uveitic process, but they occur in all forms of uveitis more commonly than in eyes without uveitis. Like idiopathic ERM, not all affect vision, but they can cause visual disturbances such as micropsia, metamorphopsia and reduced visual acuity. The best way to diagnose and monitor an ERM is with OCT, which may reveal ERM that are not visible on clinical exam or fundal photography (Figure 8.14). Careful review of the OCT examining the foveal contour is the best way to determine if the membrane is visually significant or not. A membrane which spares the center and does not distort or thicken the fovea is unlikely to cause visual symptoms even if it causes obvious retinal distortion in other areas of the macula. Increasing thickness of the fovea on OCT is correlated with reduction of visual acuity. Any treatment for the ERM should only be considered if there is significant visual disturbance.

Cystoid macula edema (CME) is common in uveitis for many reasons and may often be present associated with ERM (Figure 8.15). Eyes with both CME and ERM are more likely to have reduced vision. In these cases, it is often difficult to know if the CME is due to traction associated with the ERM or due to inflammation associated with the uveitis. Practically,

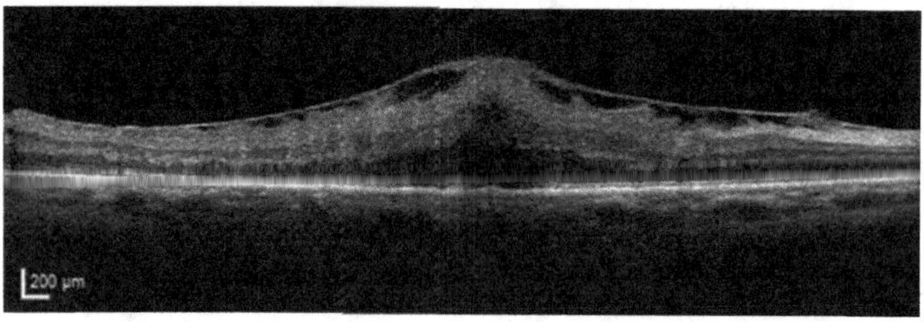

Figure 8.14. Epiretinal membrane in patient with uveitis.

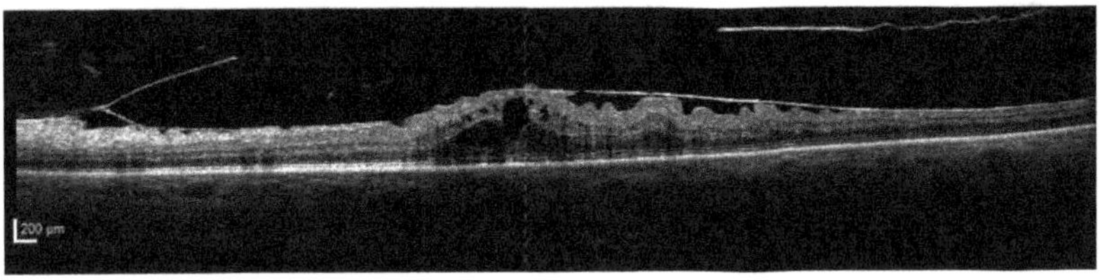

Figure 8.15. Epiretinal membrane and cystoid macular edema.

it is worth trying to modify the inflammation as much as possible to see if the CME settles with medical treatment alone. If it does, and the vision improves, then surgery for the ERM is not recommended. If the CME does not settle with medical treatment alone then surgery can be considered. Vitrectomy and ERM peel can improve vision by removing media opacity as well as restoring normal architecture at the macula, but persistent CME after surgery is not uncommon and long-term topical, periocular or intra-ocular steroids may be required to control this. Many surgeons use intra-vitreal steroid at the time of surgery to help control post-operative CME.

8.6 Choroidal Neovascular Membrane

Choroidal neovascularization (CNV) is a significant complication of uveitis, accounting for up to 6% of patients developing moderate or severe vision loss.[9] Uveitis is a leading cause of CNV following age-related macular degeneration and pathological myopia. It can occur as an early or late complication in both infectious and non-infectious uveitis, with a prevalence of 0.11–2% and most commonly in posterior or panuveitis.[29]

CNV is typical of the 'white dot syndromes', which are defined by multiple white-yellow inflammatory lesions at the outer retina, RPE, and choroid. In non-infectious uveitis, the most common conditions with CNV are punctate inner choroiditis and multifocal choroiditis[30,31] (Figure 8.16) but it is also seen in serpiginous choroiditis, Vogt-Koyanagi-Harada syndrome, birdshot chorioretinitis, toxoplasmosis, and sympathetic ophthalmia (Figure 8.17).[32–34]

Ocular conditions with chorioretinal scarring have a risk of choroidal blood vessels invading the retina, particularly in cases of choroidal inflammation. Disruption of Bruch's membrane due to inflammatory injury causes choroidal blood vessels to breach through the break resulting in

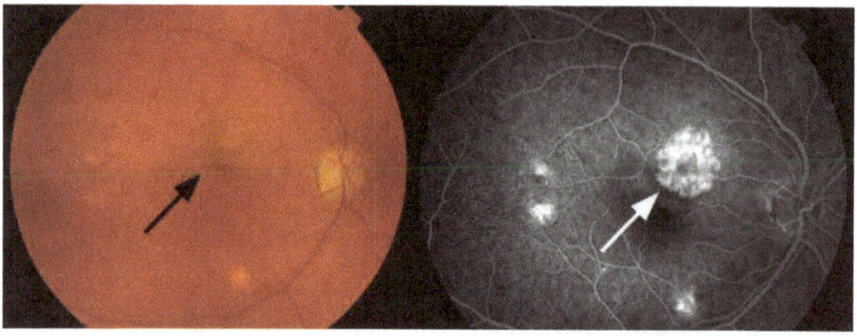

Figure 8.16. Choroidal neovascular membrane due to punctate inner choroiditis (black arrow) and on fluorescein angiography (white arrow).

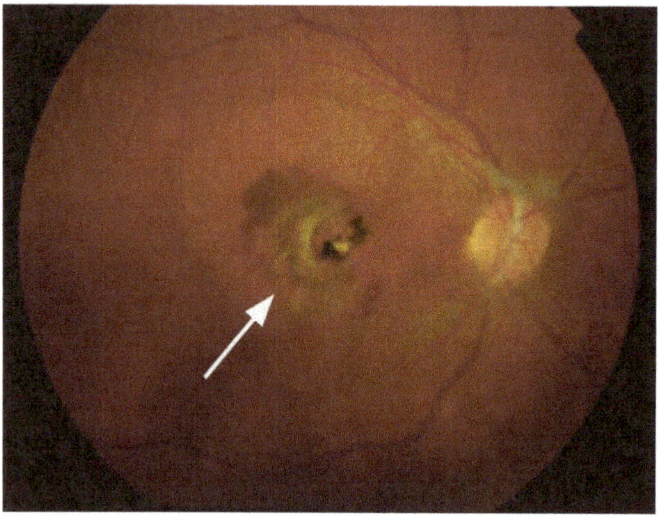

Figure 8.17. Choroidal neovascular membrane in a patient with previous toxoplasmosis panuveitis (arrow).

CNV formation,[35] with the subsequent inflammatory process causing retinal scarring and permanent vision loss.[9]

CNV usually presents as blurred vision, scotomas or metamorphopsia. The presence of CNV at presentation is associated with more than four times higher odds of severe vision loss (≤6/60) than those without CNV.[29] As it tends to occur in younger patients (<50 years) with good RPE function, clinical examination or OCT imaging may not show intraretinal or subretinal fluid but fluorescein angiography will show significant vessel leak.[36] Dual therapy is required to manage the leakage from CNV as well as the active inflammation triggering its formation, i.e., intravitreal anti-VEGF therapy and oral steroids, respectively. Concomitant immunosuppression (e.g., methotrexate or mycophenolate moftil) is an important consideration to reduce recurrence rates and formation of new inflammatory lesions.[37,38]

8.7 Cystoid Macular Edema

Cystoid macular edema (CME) is a common complication of uveitis, occurring in 8.3% of all cases, including 5.1% of anterior uveitis[39] and 40.7% of intermediate uveitis.[40] Risk factors include non-infectious uveitis (higher risk than infectious), chronic disease, intermediate uveitis, older age, presence of epiretinal membrane, and recent cataract surgery. Diagnosis is typically via OCT and/or FFA (Figures 8.18 and 8.19).

The POINT study examined treatment of uveitic CME in intermediate, posterior or panuveitis with either periocular triamcinolone acetonide, intravitreal triamcinolone acetonide, or intravitreal dexamethasone implant (ozurdex). At 8 weeks, the intravitreal route was superior, with no significant difference observed between intravitreal triamcinolone and dexamethasone implant. Interestingly, there was also no difference observed in the frequency of IOP rise (≥24 mmHg) between the two intravitreal groups.[41] Retisert (0.59 mg fluocinolone acetonide intravitreal implant) may be used to treat uveitic CME with high efficacy. The MUST trial demonstrated a significant reduction in CME, but there was a high

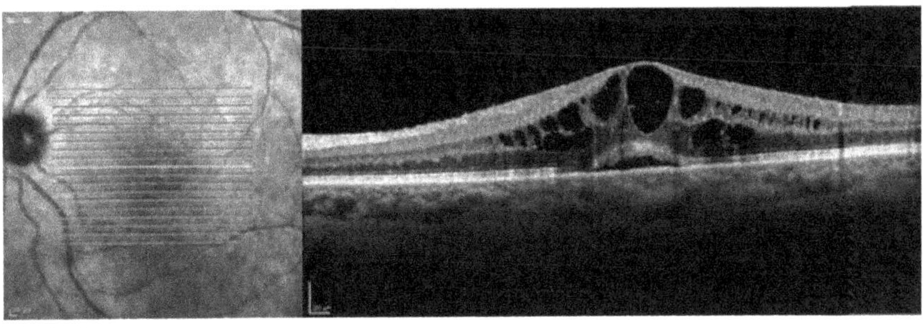

Figure 8.18. Ocular coherence tomography of cystoid macular edema in a patient with intermediate uveitis.

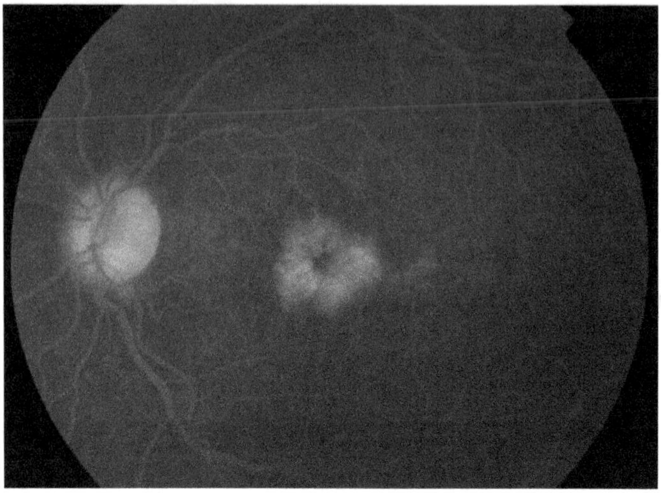

Figure 8.19. Fundus fluorescein angiography of cystoid macular edema in a patient with intermediate uveitis. Note the petaloid foveal pattern.

rate of ocular complications, in particular IOP rise, glaucoma (frequently necessitating surgery), and cataract. During the follow-up period an IOP rise of greater than 10 mmHg from baseline was noted in 67% of patients, and 40% of patients required glaucoma surgery.[42] Other intravitreal agents such as methotrexate or ranibizumab have also been reported to be used in uveitic CME, but efficacy is variable.

Systemic therapy may also be utilized in the management of uveitic CME, particularly in subjects with bilateral disease, recurrent involvement, or in steroid responders. It may also be of value in children who would require anesthetic to administer local therapy. Systemic treatment may include oral corticosteroid, immunomodulatory therapy, anti-TNF therapy or other biologics. A recent study shows that tocilizumab may have an advantage over anti-TNF therapy in the treatment of uveitic CME.[43]

In the MUST trial 7-year results, the cumulative proportion of eyes with CME resolving at any point was 94%. Subjects with epiretinal membrane on OCT were less likely to have resolution of CME. Recurrence was observed in 43%.[44] Subjects with uveitic CME will require long-term monitoring for recurrence, other complications of uveitis, and complications of local steroid treatment, in particular delayed IOP rise.

Teaching Points

- Complications of uveitis can be split into two main categories: sequelae of inflammation and iatrogenic.
- Following band keratopathy removal there is a significant risk of recurrence over time, with up to 60% recurrence rate in eyes with uveitis.
- Very common sequelae of inflammation are cataract, epiretinal membrane, and cystoid macula edema.
- Post-operative cystoid macular edema occurs in up to 60% of eyes following uveitic cataract surgery.
- Iatrogenic complications are usually the secondary effect of the corticosteroids used to treat uveitis. The most common are a raised IOP and cataract.
- Raised IOP as a response to topical or systemic corticosteroid use occurs in up to a third of patients, usually within a few weeks of starting treatment.

References

1. Alfawaz AM, Holland GN, Yu F, Margolis MS, Giaconi JA, Aldave AJ. Corneal endothelium in patients with anterior uveitis. *Ophthalmology* 2016;123(8):1637–45.
2. Trinh L, Brignole-Baudouin F, Labbé A, Raphaël M, Bourges JL, Baudouin C. The corneal endothelium in an endotoxin-induced uveitis model: Correlation between in vivo confocal microscopy and immunohistochemistry. *Mol Vis* 2008;14:1149–56.
3. Suzuki T, Ohashi Y. Corneal endotheliitis. *Semin Ophthalmol* 2008;23(4):235–40.
4. Wong SW, Carley F, Jones NP. Corneal decompensation in uveitis patients: Incidence, etiology, and outcome. *Ocul Immunol Inflamm* 2021;29(4):771–5.
5. Trollip JC, Meyer JJ, McGhee CNJ, Liu K, Danesh-Meyer HV, Niederer RL. Ethylenediaminetetraacetic acid chelation in herpes zoster ophthalmicus is associated with a high rate of corneal melt and perforation. *Cornea* 2021;40(3):277–81.
6. Najjar DM, Cohen EJ, Rapuano CJ, Laibson PR. EDTA chelation for calcific band keratopathy: Results and long-term follow-up. *Am J Ophthalmol* 2004;137(6):1056–64.

7. Okhravi N, Lightman S, Towler HM. Assessment of visual outcome after cataract surgery in patients with uveitis. *Ophthalmology* 1999;106(4):710–22.
8. Foster CS, Fong LP, Singh G. Cataract surgery and intraocular lens implantation in patients with uveitis. *Ophthalmology* 1989;96(3):281–8.
9. Tomkins-Netzer O, Talat L, Bar A, *et al.* Long-term clinical outcome and causes of vision loss in patients with uveitis. *Ophthalmology* 2014;121(12):2387–92.
10. Elgohary MA, McCluskey PJ, Towler HM, *et al.* Outcome of phacoemulsification in patients with uveitis. *Br J Ophthalmol* 2007;91(7):916–21.
11. Belair ML, Kim SJ, Thorne JE, *et al.* Incidence of cystoid macular edema after cataract surgery in patients with and without uveitis using optical coherence tomography. *Am J Ophthalmol* 2009;148(1):128–35 e2.
12. Moshirfar M, Somani AN, Motlagh MN, Ronquillo YC. Management of cataract in the setting of uveitis: A review of the current literature. *Curr Opin Ophthalmol* 2020;31(1):3–9.
13. Ganesh SK, Babu K, Biswas J. Phacoemulsification with intraocular lens implantation in cases of pars planitis. *J Cataract Refract Surg* 2004;30(10): 2072–6.
14. Sharief L, Lightman S, Baltinas J, Tomkins-Netzer O. Long-term effect of cataract phacoemulsification on the inflammation control and clinical outcome in uveitis patients. *Clin Exp Ophthalmol* 2018;46(9):1048–1054.
15. Mehta S, Linton MM, Kempen JH. Outcomes of cataract surgery in patients with uveitis: A systematic review and meta-analysis. *Am J Ophthalmol* 2014;158(4):676–92 e7.
16. Dada T, Dhawan M, Garg S, Nair S, Mandal S. Safety and efficacy of intraoperative intravitreal injection of triamcinolone acetonide injection after phacoemulsification in cases of uveitic cataract. *J Cataract Refract Surg* 2007;33(9):1613–8.
17. Daniel E, Pistilli M, Kothari S, *et al.* Risk of Ocular hypertension in adults with noninfectious uveitis. *Ophthalmology* 2017;124(8):1196–1208.
18. Ma T, Sims JL, Bennett S, Chew S, Niederer RL. High rate of conversion from ocular hypertension to glaucoma in subjects with uveitis. *Br J Ophthalmol* 2021;in press. doi:10.1136/bjophthalmol-2021–318809.
19. Tawara A, Tou N, Kubota T, Harada Y, Yokota K. Immunohistochemical evaluation of the extracellular matrix in trabecular meshwork in steroid-induced glaucoma. *Graefes Arch Clin Exp Ophthalmol* 2008;246(7):1021–8.
20. Choi JA, Kim JE, Noh SJ, Kyoung Kim E, Park CK, Paik SY. Enhanced cytomegalovirus infection in human trabecular meshwork cells and its implication in glaucoma pathogenesis. *Sci Rep* 2017;7:43349.
21. Betts TD, Sims JL, Bennett SL, Niederer RL. Outcome of peripheral iridotomy in subjects with uveitis. *Br J Ophthalmol* 2020;104(1):8–10.

22. Kerkhoff FT, Lamberts QJ, van den Biesen PR, Rothova A. Rhegmatogenous retinal detachment and uveitis. *Ophthalmology* 2003;110(2):427–31.
23. Simmons-Rear A, Yeh S, Chan-Kai BT, *et al.* Characterization of serous retinal detachments in uveitis patients with optical coherence tomography. *J Ophthalmic Inflamm Infect* 2012;2(4):191–7.
24. Young-Zvandasara T, Brunner D, Welch S, *et al.* Rhegmatogenous retinal detachment presentation and surgery in uveitic eyes. *Br J Ophthalmol* 2021;in press. doi:10.1136/bjophthalmol-2021–319268.
25. O'Keefe GA, Rao NA. Vogt-Koyanagi-Harada disease. *Surv Ophthalmol* 2017;62(1):1–25.
26. Slingsby TJ, Pecen PE, Palestine AG. Outcomes and complications associated with noninfectious uveitis in patients presenting with rhegmatogenous retinal detachment. *Ophthalmol Retina* 2020;4(8):823–8.
27. Nicholson BP, Zhou M, Rostamizadeh M, *et al.* Epidemiology of epiretinal membrane in a large cohort of patients with uveitis. *Ophthalmology* 2014;121(12):2393–8.
28. Fardeau C, Champion E, Massamba N, LeHoang P. Uveitic macular edema. *Eye (Lond)* 2016;30(10):1277–92.
29. Baxter SL, Pistilli M, Pujari SS, *et al.* Risk of choroidal neovascularization among the uveitides. *Am J Ophthalmol* 2013;156(3):468–77 e2.
30. Niederer RL, Gilbert R, Lightman S, Tomkins-Netzer O. Risk factors for developing choroidal neovascular membrane and visual loss in punctate inner choroidopathy. *Ophthalmology* 2018;125(2):288–94.
31. Thorne JE, Wittenberg S, Jabs DA, *et al.* Multifocal choroiditis with panuveitis incidence of ocular complications and of loss of visual acuity. *Ophthalmology* 2006;113(12):2310–6.
32. Nazari Khanamiri H, Rao NA. Serpiginous choroiditis and infectious multifocal serpiginoid choroiditis. *Surv Ophthalmol* 2013;58(3):203–32.
33. Moorthy RS, Chong LP, Smith RE, Rao NA. Subretinal neovascular membranes in Vogt-Koyanagi-Harada syndrome. *Am J Ophthalmol* 1993;116(2):164–70.
34. Wang JC, McKay KM, Sood AB, Lains I, Sobrin L, Miller JB. Comparison of choroidal neovascularization secondary to white dot syndromes and age-related macular degeneration by using optical coherence tomography angiography. *Clin Ophthalmol* 2019;13:95–105.
35. Olsen TW, Capone A, Jr., Sternberg P, Jr., Grossniklaus HE, Martin DF, Aaberg TM, Sr. Subfoveal choroidal neovascularization in punctate inner choroidopathy. Surgical management and pathologic findings. *Ophthalmology* 1996;103(12):2061–9.
36. Levison AL, Baynes KM, Lowder CY, Kaiser PK, Srivastava SK. Choroidal neovascularisation on optical coherence tomography angiography in

punctate inner choroidopathy and multifocal choroiditis. *Br J Ophthalmol* 2017;101(5):616–22.

37. Turkcuoglu P, Chang PY, Rentiya ZS, *et al.* Mycophenolate mofetil and fundus autofluorescence in the management of recurrent punctate inner choroidopathy. *Ocul Immunol Inflamm* 2011;19(4):286–92.
38. Wu W, Li S, Xu H, *et al.* Treatment of punctate inner choroidopathy with choroidal neovascularization using corticosteroid and intravitreal ranibizumab. *Biomed Res Int* 2018;2018:1585803.
39. Al-Ani HH, Sims JL, Tomkins-Netzer O, Lightman S, Niederer RL. Vision loss in anterior uveitis. *Br J Ophthalmol* 2020;104(12):1652–7.
40. Niederer RL, Sharief L, Bar A, Lightman S, Tomkins-Netzer O. Predictors of long-term visual outcome in intermediate uveitis. *Ophthalmology* 2017;124(3):393–8.
41. Thorne JE, Sugar EA, Holbrook JT, *et al.* Periocular triamcinolone vs. intravitreal triamcinolone vs. intravitreal dexamethasone implant for the treatment of uveitic macular edema: The PeriOcular vs. INTravitreal corticosteroids for uveitic macular edema (POINT) trial. *Ophthalmology* 2019;126(2):283–95.
42. Tomkins-Netzer O, Lightman S, Drye L, *et al.* Outcome of treatment of uveitic macular edema: The multicenter uveitis steroid treatment trial 2-year results. *Ophthalmology* 2015;122(11):2351–9.
43. Leclercq M, Andrillon A, Maalouf G, *et al.* Anti-tumor necrosis factor alpha versus tocilizumab in the treatment of refractory uveitic macular edema: A multicenter study from the French uveitis network. *Ophthalmology* 2021; in press. doi:10.1016/j.ophtha.2021.11.013.
44. Tomkins-Netzer O, Lightman S, Burke AE, *et al.* Seven-year outcomes of uveitic macular edema: The multicenter uveitis steroid treatment trial and follow-up study results. *Ophthalmology* 2021;128(5):719–728.

https://doi.org/10.1142/9789811251474_0009

Chapter 9

Medical Management of Uveitis

Asaf Bar,[*,†] Tal Koval,[*,†] Eli Neimark,[*,†] Ron Eremenko*[*,†]

Treatment of uveitis is primarily based on the use of pharmacological agents. The inflammatory process is destructive to ocular structures and can lead to irreversible vision loss. The main objective of treatment is to suppress the intraocular inflammation, preserve visual function and prevent relapses, and anti-inflammatory agents are used in most cases of infectious and non-infectious uveitis. Some diseases are self-limiting and may resolve on their own, with a favorable visual prognosis (e.g., acute posterior multifocal placoid pigment epitheliopathy and multiple evanescent white dot syndrome); the majority of these diseases do not need treatment.[1] Acute monophasic and recurring acute uveitis (such as spondylitis/HLA-B27-associated uveitis) usually only require treatment during active episodes. On the other hand, many chronic, non-infectious uveitides require long-standing therapy to control the inflammation.[1,2] In cases of infectious uveitis, treatment must address the pathogen and antimicrobial drugs used accordingly. Drugs can be delivered locally or systemically, and consideration must be taken to pharmacokinetics and penetration of the drugs across the ocular barriers and into the eye.[1] In-vitro efficacy is not a clear enough indication of a drug's pharmacological effect on the human eye.[3] Topical corticosteroids have variable penetration across the cornea, methylated corticosteroids cross the cornea easily, while fluorinated molecules have very poor penetration. Topical fluocinolone is considered a weak corticosteroid, used mainly for surface disease with little intraocular effect.[4] However, intravitreal fluocinolone implants are highly effective in

*Ophthalmology Department, E. Wolfson Medical Centre, Holon, Israel
†Sackler Faculty of Medicine, Tel Aviv, Israel

controlling intraocular inflammation but the high rate of complications must be considered, including raised intraocular pressure (IOP) and cataract.[5,6] Similarly, oral acyclovir is used for controlling corneal or anterior segment infection, but blood concentrations are not high enough for adequate blood-retinal barrier penetration and treating posterior disease. In cases of acute retinal necrosis, use of high-dose intravenous acyclovir or oral valacyclovir is indicated.[7]

9.1 Corticosteroids

Corticosteroids are the primary agents used in managing uveitis. They are used to treat active inflammation in the anterior chamber, vitreous, retina and to manage complications such as macular edema. Treatment choices for uveitis are based on drug potency (Table 9.1), anatomic location, disease course, and natural history.[2] The anatomic location, laterality, systemic associations and drug penetration dictate the choice of therapeutic agent for uveitis. Topical corticosteroids are used to treat anterior uveitides; regional corticosteroid injections or oral corticosteroids and immunosuppression are used to treat intermediate uveitides; and systemic corticosteroids and immunomodulatory drugs are used to treat posterior and panuveitides.[2,8]

Table 9.1. Relative potencies of corticosteroids are compared to the reference of hydrocortisone.

Corticosteroids	Systemic equivalent (mg)	Relative potency
Betamethasone	0.6	33
Dexamethasone	0.75	26
Methylprednisolone	4	5
Triamcinolone	4	5
Prednisolone	4	5
Prednisone	5	4
Hydrocortisone	20	1
Cortisone	25	0.8

Adapted from Cantrill HL, Palmberg PF, Zink HA, *et al.* Comparison of in vitro potency of corticosteroids with ability to raise intraocular pressure. *Am J Ophthalmol* 1975;79(6):1012–7.[9]

9.1.1 *Topical Corticosteroids*

Topical corticosteroids are beneficial in the treatment of anterior uveitis and episcleritis because they penetrate well only into the anterior segment of the eye. They are given at intervals ranging from once daily to hourly, depending on the severity of the inflammation. The most common options for topical steroid therapy are prednisolone acetate suspension 1%, dexamethasone suspension 0.1%, difluprednate emulsion 0.05%, loteprednol etabonate suspension 0.5%, and fluorometholone suspension 0.1%.[10] The intraocular efficacy of topical corticosteroids mostly depends on their intraocular permeability through the cornea. Lipophile derivatives such as dexamethasone and prednisolone acetate penetrate better into the anterior chamber than hydrophilic derivatives.[11] Loteprednol and fluorometholone have a slightly weaker anti-inflammatory effect, but they induce less elevation of IOP and might be beneficial treating steroid responders. In addition to their therapeutic effects, topical corticosteroids can result in a number of adverse effects, including cataract formation, increased susceptibility to microbial infection, delayed wound healing, and increased IOP.[4]

9.1.2 *Regional Corticosteroids*

Regional corticosteroid injections may be delivered via a periocular or intravitreal route. They are commonly used to treat active intraocular inflammation or macular edema in cases of unilateral or asymmetric inflammation. They are used either as the only treatment or as an adjuvant to systemic therapy in cases of chronic or resistant disease.[12–16] Their effect is noted within days to weeks, though recovery of visual acuity may lag for weeks or months.[17] Corticosteroid-induced rise of IOP/glaucoma and cataract are serious side effects that may result in considerable ocular morbidity.[18]

9.1.2.1 *Periocular Corticosteroids*

Periocular injections are administered into the subconjunctival space, the sub-tenon space or into the inferior orbital space along the orbital floor. The most frequently used drugs are triamcinolone acetonide 40 mg/mL

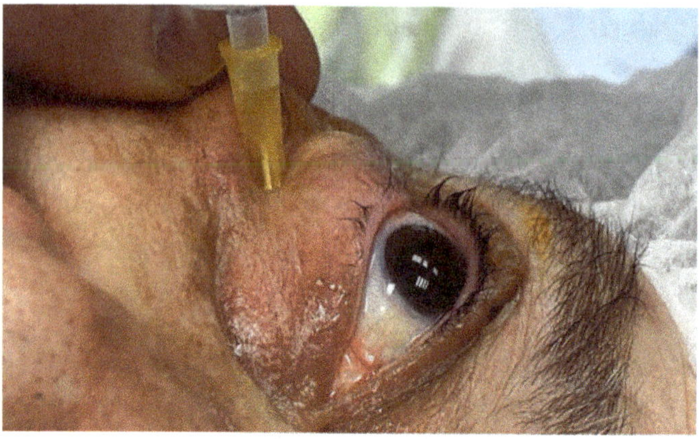

Figure 9.1. Orbital floor injection.

and methylprednisolone acetate 40–80 mg (Figure 9.1).[17] The advantage of regional administration is that it reduces systemic side effects while increasing medication delivery to the target tissue. While less effective than intravitreal injections, they are also less likely to result in increased IOP and cataract.

9.1.2.2 *Intravitreal Corticosteroids*

Intravitreal corticosteroid injections are used to treat vision-threatening inflammation or macular edema and can be used either for short-term treatment or, with intraocular implants, to achieve extended disease control and remission.[10]

Triamcinolone acetonide (40 mg/mL) is a water-insoluble corticosteroid that is administered intravitreally at a dose of 2–4 mg (0.05–0.1 mL).[10] It is highly effective in controlling intraocular inflammation and in non-vitrectomized eyes; measurable concentrations of a 4-mg intravitreal dosage are sustained for about 3 months.[19]

Dexamethasone is five times more potent and hydrophilic than triamcinolone acetonide, allowing for larger vitreous concentrations.[20] Because of the short half-life of dexamethasone in the vitreous cavity, a sustained-release intravitreal implant was developed (Figure 9.2). The Ozurdex (Allergan, Inc., Irvine, CA) dexamethasone intravitreal implant contains 0.7 mg preservative-free dexamethasone that delivers a sustained release of

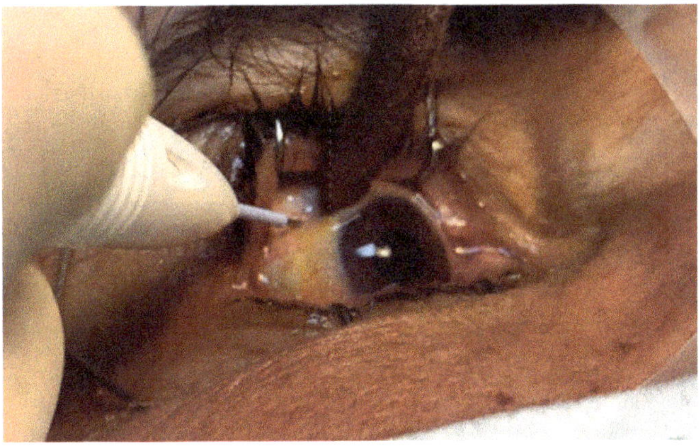

Figure 9.2. Intravitreal injection of a dexamethasone implant.

dexamethasone up to 6 months through a solid polymer delivery system.[21] Studies in non-infectious uveitis demonstrate a rapid response in both adults and children, resulting in resolution of macular edema lasting up to a median of 10 months.[12,22,23] Their use can result in reducing the burden of systemic corticosteroids.[24] The Ozurdex implant is inserted through a 22 g injector. During implantation conjunctival displacement should be performed and an arching scleral tunnel created, to prevent leakage at the site of injection.

Fluocinolone acetonide is a corticosteroid with low solubility in aqueous solution, allowing steroid release over a much longer time period.[25] This led to the study and development of sustained release fluocinolone acetonide intravitreal implants. Two implants are currently available, a surgically inserted implant (Retisert, Bausch & Lomb, Laval, Canada, 0.59 mg, Figure 9.3)[6] and an injectable implant (Iluvien, EyePoint Pharmaceuticals, Inc., Watertown, MA, 0.18 mg).[26] The implant creates a steady release of steroids at a rate of about 0.3–0.4 μg/day and can last up to about 3 years.[27,28] The implant was evaluated in a large prospective clinical trial, the Multicenter Uveitis Steroid Treatment (MUST), showing good efficacy of the implant in controlling uveitis. Over 24 months the implant group had a higher rate of glaucoma (hazard ratio 4.2) and cataract surgery (hazard ratio 3.33), compared to the systemic therapy group.[29]

The PeriOcular vs. INTravitreal corticosteroids for uveitic macular edema (POINT) trial examined periocular and intravitreal corticosteroid

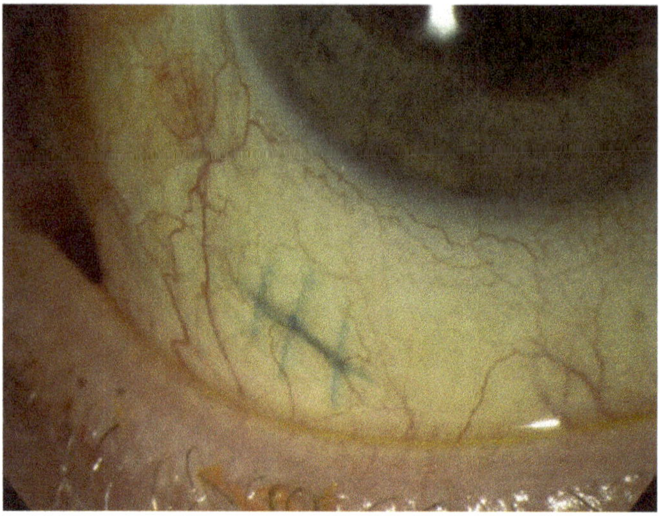

Figure 9.3. Sutures at insertion site of the Retisert implant.

therapy for uveitic macular edema. Researchers found that intravitreal corticosteroids (triamcinolone injections or dexamethasone implants) were significantly superior to periocular triamcinolone in achieving sustained macular edema resolution.[30] The groups treated intravitreally had a more rapid resolution of the macular edema and greater improvement in BCVA by more than 5 letters. However, there was an increased risk of IOP reaching 24 mmHg. According to the study, over 40% of patients in all groups required IOP-lowering medication.

9.1.3 *Systemic Corticosteroids*

Systemic corticosteroids are used for vision-threatening chronic uveitis when local corticosteroids are insufficient or contraindicated or when systemic disease also requires therapy. They are highly effective at controlling intraocular inflammation, lead to rapid stabilization and preserve vision. Many cases of uveitis that require oral glucocorticoids or other immunosuppressive medicines are chronic and treatment should strive to reach the lowest effective dose.

Dosage: A common initial dose of prednisone is 1 mg/kg/day up to a maximum of 60 mg/day.[3] Doses greater than 60 mg per day have been

Table 9.2. Suggested tapering schedules for prednisone.

Prednisone dose (mg/day)	Decrement (mg/day)	Taper interval	
		Rapid	**Standard**
60–30	10	2 days	Weekly
30–15	5	2 days	Weekly
15–7.5	2.5	2 days	Weekly
<7.5	2.5–1	2–7 days	Weekly to monthly

Adapted from Jabs DA, Rosenbaum JT, Foster CS, *et al.* Guidelines for the use of immunosuppressive drugs in patients with ocular inflammatory disorders: recommendations of an expert panel. *Am J Ophthalmol* 2000;130(4):492–513.[3]

linked to an increased risk of ischemic necrosis of the bone and should be avoided. Prednisone should be decreased after 2–4 weeks down to a dose of 7.5 mg/day. A systematic review of randomized trials of prednisone 7.5 mg/day in rheumatoid arthritis showed no increased risk of corticosteroid adverse effects over a few years.[31] To reduce the risk of relapse and withdrawal in patients receiving long-term treatment, tapering should be done gradually (Table 9.2).[3]

Adverse effects: Extended use of high dose may lead to increased body weight, high blood pressure, elevated blood glucose and low bone density.[3] Mood alteration may occur with both depression, suicidality and mania reported. Although daily doses ≤7.5 mg are considered safe, studies in rheumatoid arthritis demonstrate that large cumulative doses of prednisone increase the risk of cardiovascular disease and mortality.[32]

Monitoring and recommendations: Patients should be monitored monthly for weight, blood pressure and blood glucose levels. If treating for over a year, consider a bone density scan.

The MUST Trial and Follow-up Study was a randomized trial that compared treatment efficacy of non-infectious uveitis with either intraocular fluocinolone implants or systemic therapy with oral corticosteroids and immunosuppression.[29] The trial demonstrated comparable inflammatory control after 2 and 5 years follow-up,[33] but by 7 years there was an advantage to systemic treatment.[6] There was no increased risk of systemic adverse effects compared to intravitreal corticosteroid therapy, with the exception of increased antibiotic use for infections. The strict adherence to maintain prednisone doses of less than 7.5 mg/day was a major element in the relative safety noted in the trial.

9.2 Immunomodulatory Therapy

Most patients with non-infectious uveitis will respond well to glucocorticoids. However, in approximately 30% adequate inflammatory control is not achieved and the addition of second-line immunomodulatory therapy (IMT) is considered for a steroid-sparing effect. Indications for the use of IMT include inability to control the inflammation only with corticosteroids, disease relapse when the dose of oral glucocorticoids is lowered to ≤7.5 mg/day, corticosteroid-related adverse events, severe vision-threatening intraocular inflammation, or ocular or systemic disease known to have poor outcomes with glucocorticoid monotherapy (such as birdshot chorioretinitis or granulomatosis with polyangiitis).[34]

Before starting treatment with IMT, patients must undergo a systemic workup to verify there is no active ocular or systemic infection. Careful consideration should be given to risk of tuberculosis and hepatitis. It is also important to ensure syphilis has been excluded. A complete blood count (CBC) should be obtained to ascertain the patient is not immunosuppressed, and renal or hepatic functions should be determined as baseline values, depending on the route of metabolism of the

Table 9.3. Immunomodulatory drugs used for treating uveitis.

Drug	Metabolism	Tests prior to initiation	Monitoring
Azathioprine	Hepatic, renal	CBC, blood chemistry, LFT, syphilis serology, IGRA, PPD, check TMPT levels	CBC, blood chemistry, LFT
Methotrexate	Intestinal flora	CBC, blood chemistry, LFT, syphilis serology, IGRA, PPD, rule out pregnancy	CBC, blood chemistry, LFT
Mycophenolate mofetil	Hepatic	CBC, blood chemistry, LFT, syphilis serology, IGRA, PPD, rule out pregnancy	CBC, LFT
Cyclosporine A	Hepatic	CBC, blood chemistry, LFT, syphilis serology, IGRA, PPD, rule out pregnancy	CBC, renal function, LFT

Table 9.3. (*Continued*)

Drug	Metabolism	Tests prior to initiation	Monitoring
Tacrolimus	Hepatic	CBC, blood chemistry, LFT, syphilis serology, IGRA, PPD	CBC, blood chemistry, LFT, Tacrolimus levels
Sirolimus	Hepatic	CBC, blood chemistry, LFT, syphilis serology, IGRA, PPD, rule out pregnancy	CBC, LFT, Sirolimus levels
Cyclophosphamide	Hepatic	CBC, blood chemistry, LFT, syphilis serology, IGRA, PPD, rule out pregnancy	CBC, blood chemistry, urinalysis
Chlorambucil	Unknown	CBC, blood chemistry, LFT, syphilis serology, IGRA, PPD	CBC, LFT

CBC = complete blood count; IGRA = interferon-gamma release assay; LFT = liver function test; PPD = purified protein derivative; TMPT = Thiopurine methyltransferase

chosen drug (Table 9.3). Some drugs are contraindicated for pregnant or breastfeeding women. In case of systemic disease, cooperation with a rheumatologist or other treating physician is advised, to monitor systemic response and adverse effects.

9.2.1 *Antimetabolites*

9.2.1.1 *Azathioprine*

Mechanism of action: Azathioprine is a prodrug that is converted to 6-mercaptopurine in the liver. It is a purine nucleoside analogue that inhibits the proliferation of white blood cells. It is particularly effective for treating intermediate uveitis.

Dosage: It is administered orally as a daily dose of 1–3 mg/kg/day. Treatment effect is seen after 4–12 weeks.[35]

Adverse effects: Gastrointestinal upset, bone marrow suppression and hepatotoxicity. About one-fourth of patients discontinue the treatment because of the side effects (mostly reversible).

Monitoring and recommendations: Monitoring of CBC and blood chemistry every 4–6 weeks and liver function test (LFT) every 3 months. The use of azathioprine in children is uncommon because of data insufficiency.

9.2.1.2 *Methotrexate*

Mechanism of action: Methotrexate is a folic acid analogue that inhibits cellular replication, through purine metabolism inhibition. It is highly effective as an immunosuppressive agent, with a good safety profile and is widely used, even among children.[36–38]

Dosage: It is administered orally or subcutaneously on a weekly basis. The initial dose is 10–15 mg/week, which can be increased up to a maximum of 25 mg/week. Treatment effect is usually seen after 6–12 weeks but can take even up to 6 months. Folic acid is given within 24 hours after drug administration to reduce systemic side effects related to folate deficiency (anemia, weakness, nausea, stomach pains and hepatic dysfunction).[38]

Adverse effects: gastrointestinal discomfort, reversible hepatotoxicity, leukopenia, and pneumonitis.

Monitoring and recommendations: Patients require 1–2 monthly monitoring of CBC and LFT. In case of elevated liver enzymes, consider dose reduction or stopping treatment. After 5 years of treatment patients should undergo a liver fibroscan, even in the presence of normal LFTs. Alcohol consumption should be avoided while taking methotrexate. Methotrexate is highly teratogenic and female patients must be advised not to become pregnant while taking the drug.

9.2.1.3 *Mycophenolate Mofetil*

Mechanism of action: Mycophenolate mofetil (MMF) inhibits cellular replication by blocking purine synthesis. It has particular effect on highly replicating cells, inhibiting B- and T-cell proliferation.[38]

Dosage: It is administered orally twice daily at doses of 500–1,500 mg.[39]

Adverse effects: Diarrhea, bone marrow suppression and hepatotoxicity (mostly reversible).

Monitoring and recommendations: Patients require monthly monitoring of CBC and LFT. In case of elevated liver enzymes, dose reduction or stopping treatment should be considered. It is highly teratogenic and both female and male patients must be advised to avoid pregnancy while on the drug.[40]

The First-line Antimetabolites as Steroid-sparing Treatment (FAST) trial compared methotrexate and MMF for the treatment of non-infectious uveitis. Primary outcome was control of uveitis in both eyes with prednisone ≤7.5 mg/day and ≤2 drops of prednisolone acetate 1% a day, at 6 months follow-up. There was no significant difference between the methotrexate (66.7%) and MMF (57.1%) treatment success rates.[37]

9.2.2 Calcineurin Inhibitors

Calcineurin inhibitors are immunosuppressants that inhibit the phosphatase calcineurin signaling and restrict T-cell proliferation and IL-2 receptor expression.

9.2.2.1 *Cyclosporine A*

Dosage: It is administered once or twice a day orally at a daily dose of 3–5 mg/kg to reach the target serum level of 100–150 ng/mL.[41]

Adverse effects: Headaches, gingival hyperplasia, hypertension, nephrotoxicity, anemia and hirsutism. Systemic side effects can be severe and limit the effectiveness of this drug.

Monitoring and recommendations: Patients require monthly monitoring of CBC and renal function.

9.2.2.2 *Tacrolimus*

Tacrolimus is a calcineurin inhibitor that shows similar efficacy for long-term control of posterior segment intraocular inflammation as cyclosporine A, with a favorable safety profile.[42]

Dosage: It is administered orally with doses starting from 1–3 mg BID. Therapeutic effect is seen by 2–6 weeks from the first dose.[1]

Adverse effects: Nephrotoxicity, neurotoxicity, diabetes mellitus, hypertension and increased risk of systemic infections.

Monitoring and recommendations: Patients require monthly monitoring of CBC, hepatic and renal function.

9.2.2.3 *Sirolimus*

Sirolimus is another calcineurin inhibitor that shows promising efficacy in limited studies. It was shown to be effective in most patients with non-infectious uveitis and reduced the need for long term supplementary corticosteroid therapy.[43] More studies are needed to establish the efficacy and safety of the drug.

Dosage: Yet to be determined. However, intravitreal 440 μg and 1320 μg subconjunctival injections show promising results with increased safety.[44,45]

Adverse effects: No non-ocular adverse effects were noted. The most common ocular adverse effect is iridocyclitis.[44,45]

Monitoring and recommendations: Undetermined for ocular use. Patients who receive systemic treatment for other indications should be monitored every 4–6 weeks with CBC, hepatic and renal function.

9.2.3 *Alkylating Agents*

These are historically reported as treatment options for uveitis, but are currently rarely used. They have a limited role in the treatment of refractory, vision-threatening disease, such as necrotizing scleritis.

9.2.3.1 *Cyclophosphamide*

Mechanism of action: Cyclophosphamide forms irreversible DNA cross-links that lead to cell apoptosis. It is reserved for selected cases with severe vision-threatening intraocular inflammation.[46] Disease remission can be achieved in most patients who are able to tolerate the treatment.[47]

Dosage: The drug is administered intravenously at a starting dose of 500–1000 mg/m^2, followed by an oral maintenance dose of 1–2 mg/kg/day.

Adverse effects: Gastrointestinal toxicity, hepatotoxicity, bladder toxicity, hematologic toxicity, and an increased risk for opportunistic infections.

Monitoring and recommendations: Weekly monitoring of CBC, urea and electrolytes. There is an increased risk of secondary malignancies, particularly carcinoma of bladder.[48] It is highly teratogenic and toxic to both male and female fertility, leading to sterility. Patients should be instructed to retain sperm or eggs before beginning treatment.

9.2.3.2 Chloramb ucil

Chlorambucil is another alkylating immunosuppressive agent with a similar side effects profile. It was shown to be a reasonable treatment option for intractable sight-threatening uveitis with 68% positive clinical response, even after cessation of systemic prednisone.[49]

Mechanism of action: Alkylating and crosslinking of DNA, thus intervening with synthesis and transcription.

Dosage: The drug is given orally at a dose of 0.1–0.2 mg/kg/day. However, the dose can be increased to achieve a quicker remission.[50]

Adverse effects: Bone marrow suppression, gonadal dysfunction, and increased risk of subsequent development of malignancy.[49]

Monitoring and recommendations: CBC including platelet count and LFTs weekly.

9.3 Biologics

Biologic response modifiers ('biologics') are the next step in the ladder of treatment for specific types of non-infectious uveitis and are generally considered for patients whose disease is inadequately controlled by standard corticosteroids and second-line immunosuppressive drugs.[34]

The biologics used most often in the field of uveitis are the tumor necrosis factor (TNF)-α modifiers adalimumab (Humira) and infliximab (Remicade). For uveitis, most biologics are used as off-label drugs, with the exception of adalimumab. Other biologics which are more rarely used are lymphocyte inhibitors (e.g., rituximab and abatacept), interleukin inhibitors (e.g., anakinra, tocilizumab) and interferons. Patients must undergo screening before starting treatment with biologic drugs (Table 9.4).

9.3.1 *TNF-α Inhibitors*

Anti-TNF-α agents are most effective in Behçet's disease-related uveitis, HLA-B27-associated uveitis, and juvenile idiopathic arthritis-associated uveitis.[1]

Other TNF inhibitors such as etanercept and golimumab were not proven to be as effective for uveitis as adalimumab and infliximab, and de novo uveitis has been reported in subjects with ankylosing spondylitis following commencement of etanercept.

Table 9.4. Screening tests before starting treatment with biologic agents.[51]

	Investigations
Medical history	Exclusion of infections (HIV, HBV, HCV, syphilis, TB) Exclusion of malignancy Known demyelinating disease (including multiple sclerosis) Pregnancy
Blood tests	CBC ANA
Serology	HBsAg, HBsAb, HBcAb HAV-Ab HCV-Ab HIV
TB	CXR PPD/IGRA

TB = Tuberculosis, HIV = human immunodeficiency virus, HAV = hepatitis A virus, HBV = hepatitis B virus, HCV = hepatitis C virus, CBC = complete blood count, ANA = antinuclear antibody, CXR = chest roentgenogram, PPD = purified protein derivative, IGRA = interferon-gamma release assay.

9.3.1.1 *Infliximab*

Mechanism of action: Chimeric anti-TNF-α monoclonal antibody.

Dosage: Intravenously administered at a dose of 3–5 mg/kg loading at weeks 0, 2, and 6, then maintenance 3–10 mg/kg every 8 weeks. Escalation of the maintenance dose to weekly infusions is possible in persistent cases. The maximal dose in children is 20 mg/kg administered every 2 weeks.[52]

Adverse effects: See Table 9.5.

Monitoring and recommendations: CBC, LFT, urea and electrolytes — before each infusion. Patients should avoid live immunizations 6 months following treatments. See Table 9.5 for information regarding pregnancy and lactation.

9.3.1.2 *Adalimumab*

Mechanism of action: Fully human anti-TNF-α monoclonal antibody.

Table 9.5. Adverse effects related to TNF inhibitors.[39,53–55]

System	Adverse effects	Remarks
Local	Injection site reaction	May respond to oral antihistamine given at time of administration
Immune-related	Allergic reaction Hypersensitivity reactions Lupus-like syndrome	
Infectious disease concerns	Susceptibility to infections Reactivation of tuberculosis, histoplasmosis, hepatitis B, and fungal infection	
Neurologic	Demyelinating disease	
Malignancy	Non-melanoma skin cancer Reports on carcinoid tumor of gastrointestinal tract and glioblastoma multiforme	
Hematologic	Thromboembolic events	
Cardiac	Congestive heart failure	
Pregnancy	No risk of fetal malformations when administered during the first 2 trimesters of pregnancy (until week 30). Administration during the third trimester is related to newborn neutropenia.	TNF-α inhibitors should be administered only when clearly indicated.
Lactation	Compatible. Minimal transfer to the breast milk and feeding baby.	

Dosage: Subcutaneous injections. Adult patients: initial dose of 80 mg followed by 40 mg 2-week intervals, beginning 1 week after the initial dose. Pediatric patients: 40 mg every 1–2 weeks (if bodyweight <30 kg, 20 mg every 2 weeks).

Adverse effects: See Table 9.5.

Monitoring and recommendations: CBC, LFT, urea and electrolytes — monthly for 3 months; then 3-monthly. Patients should avoid live immunizations 6 months following treatments. See Table 9.5 for information regarding pregnancy and lactation.

Adalimumab is U.S. Food and Drug Administration approved for the treatment of non-infectious intermediate, posterior, and panuveitis.[1] It was investigated in two randomized, placebo-controlled clinical trials of adult patients with active[56] and inactive[57] non-infectious uveitis (VISUAL I & II) and was demonstrated to have about 50% reduction in the relapse rate following oral corticosteroid taper.[1] It also showed superiority in preventing recurrence and in reducing systemic side effects.[1] In children with JIA-associated uveitis, adalimumab was demonstrated to be an effective addition to methotrexate in two placebo-controlled, randomized trials.[58,59] An Expert Panel of the American Uveitis Society recommended infliximab or adalimumab as a first-line therapy for Behçet's disease and as a second-line therapy for JIA-associated uveitis.[60]

9.3.2 *Rituximab*

Indicated for the treatment of granulomatosis with polyangiitis. Effective in treating scleritis, ocular cicatricial pemphigoid and autoimmune retinopathy.[61–64] Also utilized in primary intraocular lymphoma.

Mechanism of action: Chimeric murine/human monoclonal IgG, kappa antibody directed against the CD20 antigen.

Dosage: Intravenous injections of 500 or 1,000 mg at week 0 and 2; may repeat 6–12 months thereafter.

Adverse effects: Infusion reactions, muscle spasm, headaches, renal toxicity, increased risk of infections, increased risk of cardiovascular event, delayed onset neutropenia, progressive multifocal leukoencephalopathy.

Monitoring and recommendations: LFT every 1–2 months, CBC at 2- and 4-month intervals during treatment. Rituximab should be discontinued 3 months prior to pregnancy due to risk of teratogenicity (risk of 2.2% fetal anomalies). Also risk of newborn lymphocytopenia. Not recommended during lactation.

9.3.3 *Other Biologic Agents*

In general, these have fewer data, typically consisting of small case series.[65–68]

- Interleukin (IL) inhibitors: e.g., anakinra (anti-IL-1 receptor), secukinmunab (anti-IL-17 receptor). Tocilizumab (anti-IL-6 receptor) is being trialed as treatment for patients with anti-TNF-α resistant disease.[69]

- Other lymphocyte inhibitors: e.g., daclizumab and abatacept.
- Interferons: Interferon α-2a and 2b, as well as Interferon 2β, are effective in treating uveitis related to Behçet's disease.[70]

Teaching Points

- Self-limiting uveitides may not require treatment, and include acute posterior placoid multifocal choroidopathy and multiple evanescent white dot syndrome.
- Regional injections of corticosteroids are generally considered in unilateral or asymmetrical disease. They can also be used as adjuvant treatment to systemic therapy in cases of chronic or resistant disease.
- Corticosteroids are the backbone of treatment in uveitis. Their common side effects of IOP/glaucoma and cataract should be constantly monitored. There are various methods of delivery including topical, periocular, intravitreal and systemic.
- Immunomodulatory therapy (IMT) is the next step after corticosteroids. Drugs include Azathioprine, Methotrexate, Mycophenolate mofetil, Cyclosporine A, Tacrolimus, Sirolimus, Cyclophosphamide and Chlorambucil. Before starting IMT, ensure the relevant tests are acquired prior to initiation and that monitoring is undertaken (Table 9.3).
- Biologics are the next step after IMT. TNF-α modifiers adalimumab (Humira) and infliximab (Remicade) are commonly used. Ensure screening tests are undertaken before initiating therapy (Table 9.4) and appropriate monitoring is performed. It is important to check for MS prior to commencing anti-TNF therapy in patients with intermediate uveitis.

References

1. Jabs DA. Immunosuppression for the uveitides. *Ophthalmology* 2018; 125(2):193–202.
2. Jabs DA, Nussenblatt RB, Rosenbaum JT. Standardization of uveitis nomenclature for reporting clinical data. Results of the First International Workshop. *Am J Ophthalmol* 2005;140(3):509–16.

3. Jabs DA, Rosenbaum JT, Foster CS, *et al.* Guidelines for the use of immunosuppressive drugs in patients with ocular inflammatory disorders: recommendations of an expert panel. *Am J Ophthalmol* 2000;130(4):492–513.
4. McGhee CN, Dean S, Danesh-Meyer H. Locally administered ocular corticosteroids: benefits and risks. *Drug Saf* 2002;25(1):33–55.
5. Kempen JH, Van Natta ML, Friedman DS, *et al.* Incidence and outcome of uveitic glaucoma in eyes with intermediate, posterior, or panuveitis followed up to 10 years after randomization to fluocinolone acetonide implant or systemic therapy. *Am J Ophthalmol* 2020;219:303–16.
6. Writing Committee for the Multicenter Uveitis Steroid Treatment T, Follow-up Study Research G, Kempen JH, *et al.* Association between long-lasting intravitreous fluocinolone acetonide implant vs systemic anti-inflammatory therapy and visual acuity at 7 years among patients with intermediate, posterior, or panuveitis. *JAMA* 2017;317(19):1993–2005.
7. Baltinas J, Lightman S, Tomkins-Netzer O. Comparing treatment of acute retinal necrosis with either oral Valacyclovir or intravenous Acyclovir. *Am J Ophthalmol* 2018;188:173–80.
8. Jabs DA. Treatment of ocular inflammation. *Ocul Immunol Inflamm* 2004;12(3):163–8.
9. Cantrill HL, Palmberg PF, Zink HA, *et al.* Comparison of in vitro potency of corticosteroids with ability to raise intraocular pressure. *Am J Ophthalmol* 1975;79(6):1012–7.
10. Valdes LM, Sobrin L. Uveitis therapy: the corticosteroid options. *Drugs* 2020;80(8):765–73.
11. McGhee CN. Pharmacokinetics of ophthalmic corticosteroids. *Br J Ophthalmol* 1992;76(11):681–4.
12. Tomkins-Netzer O, Taylor SR, Bar A, *et al.* Treatment with repeat dexamethasone implants results in long-term disease control in eyes with noninfectious uveitis. *Ophthalmology* 2014;121(8):1649–54.
13. Habot-Wilner Z, Sallam A, Roufas A, *et al.* Periocular corticosteroid injection in the management of uveitis in children. *Acta Ophthalmol* 2010;88(8):e299–304.
14. Habot-Wilner Z, Sallam A, Pacheco PA, *et al.* Intravitreal triamcinolone acetonide as adjunctive treatment with systemic therapy for uveitic macular edema. *Eur J Ophthalmol* 2011;21 Suppl 6:S56–61.
15. Tomkins-Netzer O, Lightman S, Burke AE, *et al.* Seven-year outcomes of uveitic macular edema: The Multicenter Uveitis Steroid Treatment trial and follow-up study results. *Ophthalmology* 2021;128(5):719–28.
16. Sallam A, Taylor SR, Habot-Wilner Z, *et al.* Repeat intravitreal triamcinolone acetonide injections in uveitic macular oedema. *Acta Ophthalmol* 2012;90(4):e323–5.

17. Ferrante P, Ramsey A, Bunce C, Lightman S. Clinical trial to compare efficacy and side-effects of injection of posterior sub-Tenon triamcinolone versus orbital floor methylprednisolone in the management of posterior uveitis. *Clin Experiment Ophthalmol* 2004;32(6):563–8.
18. Jea SY, Byon IS, Oum BS. Triamcinolone-induced intraocular pressure elevation: intravitreal injection for macular edema and posterior subtenon injection for uveitis. *Korean J Ophthalmol* 2006;20(2):99–103.
19. Beer PM, Bakri SJ, Singh RJ, *et al.* Intraocular concentration and pharmacokinetics of triamcinolone acetonide after a single intravitreal injection. *Ophthalmology* 2003;110:681–6.
20. London NJ, Chiang A, Haller JA. The dexamethasone drug delivery system: indications and evidence. *Adv Ther* 2011;28(5):351–66.
21. Lowder C, Belfort R, Jr., Lightman S, *et al.* Dexamethasone intravitreal implant for noninfectious intermediate or posterior uveitis. *Arch Ophthalmol* 2011;129(5):545–53.
22. Taylor SR, Tomkins-Netzer O, Joshi L, *et al.* Dexamethasone implant in pediatric uveitis. *Ophthalmology* 2012;119(11):2412.e2.
23. Tomkins-Netzer O, Talat L, Seguin-Greenstein S, *et al.* Outcome of treating pediatric uveitis with dexamethasone implants. *Am J Ophthalmol* 2016;161:110–5.e1–2.
24. McCartney M, McCluskey P, Zagora S. Intravitreal dexamethasone implants for non-infectious uveitis. *Clin Exp Ophthalmol* 2019;47(9):1156–63.
25. Jaffe GJ, Yang CH, Guo H, *et al.* Safety and pharmacokinetics of an intraocular fluocinolone acetonide sustained delivery device. *Invest Ophthalmol Vis Sci* 2000;41(11):3569–75.
26. Jaffe GJ, Lin P, Keenan RT, *et al.* Injectable fluocinolone acetonide long-acting implant for noninfectious intermediate uveitis, posterior uveitis, and panuveitis: two-year results. *Ophthalmology* 2016;123(9):1940–8.
27. Cai CX, Skalak C, Keenan RT, *et al.* Time to disease recurrence in noninfectious uveitis following long-acting injectable fluocinolone acetonide implant. *Graefes Arch Clin Exp Ophthalmol* 2020;258(5):1023–30.
28. Driot JY, Novack GD, Rittenhouse KD, *et al.* Ocular pharmacokinetics of fluocinolone acetonide after Retisert intravitreal implantation in rabbits over a 1-year period. *J Ocul Pharmacol Ther* 2004;20(3):269–75.
29. Multicenter Uveitis Steroid Treatment Trial Research G, Kempen JH, Altaweel MM, *et al.* Randomized comparison of systemic anti-inflammatory therapy versus fluocinolone acetonide implant for intermediate, posterior, and panuveitis: the multicenter uveitis steroid treatment trial. *Ophthalmology* 2011;118(10):1916–26.
30. Thorne JE, Sugar EA, Holbrook JT, *et al.* Periocular Triamcinolone vs. Intravitreal Triamcinolone vs. intravitreal dexamethasone implant for the

treatment of uveitic macular edema: The PeriOcular vs. INTravitreal corticosteroids for uveitic macular edema (POINT) trial. *Ophthalmology* 2019;126(2):283–95.

31. Suhler EB, Thorne JE, Mittal M, *et al.* Corticosteroid-related adverse events systematically increase with corticosteroid dose in noninfectious intermediate, posterior, or panuveitis: post hoc analyses from the VISUAL-1 and VISUAL-2 trials. *Ophthalmology* 2017;124(12):1799–807.
32. del Rincon I, Battafarano DF, Restrepo JF, *et al.* Glucocorticoid dose thresholds associated with all-cause and cardiovascular mortality in rheumatoid arthritis. *Arthritis Rheumatol* 2014;66(2):264–72.
33. Multicenter Uveitis Steroid Treatment Trial Research G, Kempen JH, Altaweel MM, *et al.* Benefits of systemic anti-inflammatory therapy versus fluocinolone acetonide intraocular implant for intermediate uveitis, posterior uveitis, and panuveitis: fifty-four-month results of the Multicenter Uveitis Steroid Treatment (MUST) trial and follow-up study. *Ophthalmology* 2015;122(10):1967–75.
34. Dick AD, Rosenbaum JT, Al-Dhibi HA, *et al.* Guidance on noncorticosteroid systemic immunomodulatory therapy in noninfectious uveitis: Fundamentals Of Care for UveitiS (FOCUS) initiative. *Ophthalmology* 2018;125(5): 757–73.
35. Pasadhika S, Kempen JH, Newcomb CW, *et al.* Azathioprine for ocular inflammatory diseases. *Am J Ophthalmol* 2009;148(4):500–9.e2.
36. Rathinam SR, Gonzales JA, Thundikandy R, *et al.* Effect of corticosteroid-sparing treatment with mycophenolate mofetil vs methotrexate on inflammation in patients with uveitis: a randomized clinical trial. *JAMA* 2019;322(10):936–45.
37. Rathinam SR, Babu M, Thundikandy R, *et al.* A randomized clinical trial comparing methotrexate and mycophenolate mofetil for noninfectious uveitis. *Ophthalmology* 2014;121(10):1863–70.
38. Simonini G, Cantarini L, Bresci C, *et al.* Current therapeutic approaches to autoimmune chronic uveitis in children. *Autoimmun Rev* 2010;9(10):674–83.
39. Pasadhika S, Rosenbaum JT. Update on the use of systemic biologic agents in the treatment of noninfectious uveitis. *Biologics* 2014;8:67–81.
40. Anderka MT, Lin AE, Abuelo DN, *et al.* Reviewing the evidence for mycophenolate mofetil as a new teratogen: case report and review of the literature. *Am J Med Genet A* 2009;149A(6):1241–8.
41. Nussenblatt RB, Palestine AG, Chan CC, *et al.* Randomized, double-masked study of cyclosporine compared to prednisolone in the treatment of endogenous uveitis. *Am J Ophthalmol* 1991;112(2):138–46.

42. Murphy CC, Greiner K, Plskova J, *et al.* Cyclosporine vs tacrolimus therapy for posterior and intermediate uveitis. *Arch Ophthalmol* 2005;123(5):634–41.
43. Shanmuganathan VA, Casely EM, Raj D, *et al.* The efficacy of sirolimus in the treatment of patients with refractory uveitis. *Br J Ophthalmol* 2005; 89(6):666–9.
44. Nguyen QD, Merrill PT, Clark WL, *et al.* Intravitreal sirolimus for noninfectious uveitis: a phase III Sirolimus study Assessing double-masKed Uveitis tReAtment (SAKURA). *Ophthalmology* 2016;123(11):2413–23.
45. Ibrahim MA, Sepah YJ, Watters A, *et al.* One-year outcomes of the SAVE study: Sirolimus as a therapeutic Approach for uVEitis. *Transl Vis Sci Technol* 2015;4(2):4.
46. Suelves AM, Arcinue CA, Gonzalez-Martin JM, *et al.* Analysis of a novel protocol of pulsed intravenous cyclophosphamide for recalcitrant or severe ocular inflammatory disease. *Ophthalmology* 2013;120(6):1201–9.
47. Pujari SS, Kempen JH, Newcomb CW, *et al.* Cyclophosphamide for ocular inflammatory diseases. *Ophthalmology* 2010;117(2):356–65.
48. Radis CD, Kahl LE, Baker GL, *et al.* Effects of cyclophosphamide on the development of malignancy and on long-term survival of patients with rheumatoid arthritis. A 20-year followup study. *Arthritis Rheum* 1995;38(8):1120–7.
49. Miserocchi E, Baltatzis S, Ekong A, *et al.* Efficacy and safety of chlorambucil in intractable noninfectious uveitis: the Massachusetts Eye and Ear Infirmary experience. *Ophthalmology* 2002;109(1):137–42.
50. Goldstein DA, Fontanilla FA, Kaul S, *et al.* Long-term follow-up of patients treated with short-term high-dose chlorambucil for sight-threatening ocular inflammation. *Ophthalmology* 2002;109(2):370–7.
51. Wakefield D, McCluskey P, Wildner G, *et al.* Inflammatory eye disease: Pre-treatment assessment of patients prior to commencing immunosuppressive and biologic therapy: Recommendations from an expert committee. *Autoimmun Rev* 2017;16(3):213–22.
52. Angeles-Han ST, Ringold S, Beukelman T, *et al.* 2019 American College of Rheumatology/Arthritis Foundation Guideline for the screening, monitoring, and treatment of juvenile idiopathic arthritis-associated uveitis. *Arthritis Care Res (Hoboken)* 2019;71(6):703–16.
53. Gamalero L, Simonini G, Ferrara G, *et al.* Evidence-based treatment for uveitis. *Isr Med Assoc J* 2019;21(7):475–9.
54. Wolfe F, Michaud K. Biologic treatment of rheumatoid arthritis and the risk of malignancy: analyses from a large US observational study. *Arthritis Rheum* 2007;56(9):2886–95.
55. Wolfe F, Michaud K. The effect of methotrexate and anti-tumor necrosis factor therapy on the risk of lymphoma in rheumatoid arthritis in 19,562

patients during 89,710 person-years of observation. *Arthritis Rheum* 2007;56(5):1433–9.

56. Jaffe GJ, Dick AD, Brezin AP, *et al.* Adalimumab in patients with active non-infectious uveitis. *N Engl J Med* 2016;375(10):932–43.
57. Nguyen QD, Merrill PT, Jaffe GJ, *et al.* Adalimumab for prevention of uveitic flare in patients with inactive non-infectious uveitis controlled by corticosteroids (VISUAL II): a multicentre, double-masked, randomised, placebo-controlled phase 3 trial. *Lancet* 2016;388(10050):1183–92.
58. Ramanan AV, Dick AD, Jones AP, *et al.* Adalimumab plus methotrexate for uveitis in juvenile idiopathic arthritis. *N Engl J Med* 2017;376(17):1637–46.
59. Quartier P, Baptiste A, Despert V, *et al.* ADJUVITE: a double-blind, randomised, placebo-controlled trial of adalimumab in early onset, chronic, juvenile idiopathic arthritis-associated anterior uveitis. *Ann Rheum Dis* 2018;77(7):1003–11.
60. Levy-Clarke G, Jabs DA, Read RW, *et al.* Expert panel recommendations for the use of anti-tumor necrosis factor biologic agents in patients with ocular inflammatory disorders. *Ophthalmology* 2014;121(3):785–96.e3.
61. Tomkins-Netzer O, Taylor SR, Lightman S. Can rituximab induce long-term disease remission in patients with intra-ocular non-infectious inflammation? *Ophthalmologica* 2013;230(3):109–15.
62. Miserocchi E, Pontikaki I, Modorati G, *et al.* Anti-CD 20 monoclonal antibody (rituximab) treatment for inflammatory ocular diseases. *Autoimmun Rev* 2011;11(1):35–9.
63. Cao JH, Oray M, Cocho L, Foster CS. Rituximab in the treatment of refractory noninfectious scleritis. *Am J Ophthalmol* 2016;164:22–8.
64. Ng CC, Sy A, Cunningham ET, Jr. Rituximab for non-infectious uveitis and scleritis. *J Ophthalmic Inflamm Infect* 2021;11(1):23.
65. Zulian F, Balzarin M, Falcini F, *et al.* Abatacept for severe anti-tumor necrosis factor alpha refractory juvenile idiopathic arthritis-related uveitis. *Arthritis Care Res (Hoboken)* 2010;62(6):821–5.
66. Mesquida M, Molins B, Llorenc V, *et al.* Long-term effects of tocilizumab therapy for refractory uveitis-related macular edema. *Ophthalmology* 2014;121(12):2380–6.
67. Brambilla A, Caputo R, Cimaz R, Simonini G. Canakinumab for childhood sight-threatening refractory uveitis: a case series. *J Rheumatol* 2016;43(7):1445–7.
68. Deuter CM, Koetter I, Guenaydin I, *et al.* Interferon alfa-2a: a new treatment option for long lasting refractory cystoid macular edema in uveitis? *A pilot study. Retina* 2006;26(7):786–91.

69. Ramanan AV, Dick AD, Guly C, *et al.* Tocilizumab in patients with anti-TNF refractory juvenile idiopathic arthritis-associated uveitis (APTITUDE): a multicentre, single-arm, phase 2 trial. *Lancet Rheumatol* 2020;2(3):e135-e41.
70. Lightman S, Taylor SR, Bunce C, *et al.* Pegylated interferon-alpha-2b reduces corticosteroid requirement in patients with Behcet's disease with upregulation of circulating regulatory T cells and reduction of Th17. *Ann Rheum Dis* 2015;74(6):1138–44.

https://doi.org/10.1142/9789811251474_0010

Chapter 10

Surgical Management of Complications of Uveitis

Sonya Bennett, Sarah Welch,* Jay Meyer,*,† Daniel Gosling,* Rachael Niederer*,†*

Complications are frequent in uveitis, occurring both acutely and as the long-term sequelae of chronic disease. Surgical intervention may be required to manage complications, optimize visual outcome, prevent further damage or to provide intraocular samples to aid the diagnosis. Where possible, surgery is best performed on a quiet eye, and careful attention should be paid to pre-operative, peri-operative and post-operative management of uveitis.

10.1 Surgical Management of Band Keratopathy

Surgical management of band keratopathy may be performed for ocular discomfort, decreased visual acuity, poor view for clinical monitoring or surgical intervention (Figure 10.1). Patient selection is important, as patients with significant ocular surface disease such as severe dry eye, neurotrophic keratopathy, or limbal stem cell deficiency risk a persistent epithelial defect after treatment and may not be good candidates for intervention.[1] Risks to discuss with patients prior to procedure include corneal melt, infection, incomplete removal, irregular astigmatism and recurrence.

* Department of Ophthalmology, Auckland District Health Board, Auckland, New Zealand
† Department of Ophthalmology, University of Auckland, Auckland, New Zealand

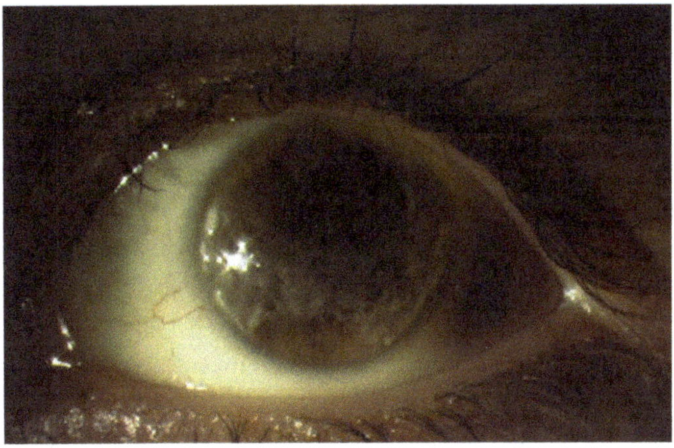

Figure 10.1. Band keratopathy.

Control of underlying inflammation is vital to decrease the risk of recurrence post-treatment.

Techniques for surgical removal or band keratopathy include manual debridement, chelation and phototherapeutic keratectomy (PTK). The goals of treatment include removal of corneal opacities and restoration of a smooth ocular surface.[2] Simple manual debridement alone may reduce plaque-like opacities, but is less effective for more diffuse opacification and may induce irregular astigmatism. PTK can be used and may produce a smooth corneal surface, but is costly, not readily available to all surgeons due to the use of an excimer laser, and can result in a refractive shift. Chelation is the most widely used procedure as it is cost-effective, can reduce focal or diffuse opacification, and does not involve ablation of tissue. Chelation is typically performed using compounded disodium ethylenediaminetetraacetic acid (Na_2 EDTA) according to the technique described below. Alternatively, chelation using dipotassium EDTA (K_2 EDTA) has been reported, with the advantage that it can be prepared in clinic using readily available blood collection tubes,[3] although care must be taken to use the correct tube size to avoid concentration errors. Chelation can be performed in a reclined slit-lamp examination chair, in a procedure room, or in the operating theatre.

10.1.1 *Na_2 EDTA Chelation Procedure*

Topical anesthetic is adequate for most patients although younger patients may require a local or general anesthetic. The eye is prepped with topical povidone–iodine 5% applied to the ocular surface and a lid speculum inserted. The epithelium overlying the band keratopathy is removed with a sponge or blade to allow penetration of the EDTA. If desired or required for large treatment areas, alcohol (20%) can be applied for 30–40 seconds using a sponge or surgical well to loosen the epithelium prior to debridement, followed by a saline rinse. Disodium EDTA (0.05 mol/L) drops are then applied directly or into a sponge or surgical well to contain the solution over the band keratopathy. At approximately 5-minute intervals, gentle mechanical debridement using a blunt or sharp instrument can be performed as needed to facilitate removal of loosened calcium plaques. Application of EDTA is continued until adequate dissipation of the calcium is achieved (typically 15–40 minutes). Often, it is not possible to remove the opacification completely. If a topical anesthetic has been used, a bandage contact lens can be placed. A topical antibiotic and corticosteroid are typically given post-operatively with dosing based on the underlying condition as well as post-operative healing and inflammation. For neurotrophic eyes or those with significant ocular surface disease, amniotic membrane placement at the conclusion of the procedure can be considered as well as preservative-free medications to facilitate epithelial healing. In eyes with underlying herpetic disease, a course of oral antiviral medication should also be considered during the peri-operative period. In patients with cataracts requiring surgery, chelation should be performed before biometric readings are obtained, as the procedure can affect keratometry.

10.2 Glaucoma Surgery

Surgical intervention in uveitic glaucoma is indicated when inadequate disease control occurs despite maximal tolerated medical therapy. One study showed a glaucoma surgery rate of 40% over 10 years.[4] It may be required for overall intraocular pressure (IOP) lowering, control of IOP spikes, to reduce reliance on topical drops, rescue in acute cases, or to resolve secondary angle closure.

In acute episodes of uveitis with transitory raised IOP, a healthy nerve may be resilient to short periods of ocular hypertension (OHT). However, clinicians should be very cautious in chronic or recurrent uveitis,[5] as there are high rates of conversion to glaucomatous optic neuropathy (GON) and associated blindness. Our approach is to offer surgical intervention for those with inadequate IOP control on maximal therapy, even without manifest GON. Patients with progressive GON on maximal therapy should also be offered surgery, regardless of IOP measurement. Careful monitoring of the optic nerve and visual field will identify surgical candidates. This monitoring should be more frequent than would be performed in primary glaucoma.

A quiescent period of at least 3 months before surgery is preferable. However, if urgent surgery is indicated, aggressive peri-operative management of the uveitis will be needed to achieve optimal outcomes.

10.2.1 *Trabeculectomy*

In most cases requiring filtration surgery, trabeculectomy with mitomycin-C (MMC) is appropriate as the primary procedure (Figure 10.2). Post-operative control of inflammation is essential to success.[6] Intra-operative MMC application is widely used (we routinely apply high concentration 0.5 mg/mL for 3 minutes), and intensive post-operative steroid treatment (Table 10.1). There is some evidence that uveitis may be less severe after trabeculectomy, due to filtration of aqueous.[7]

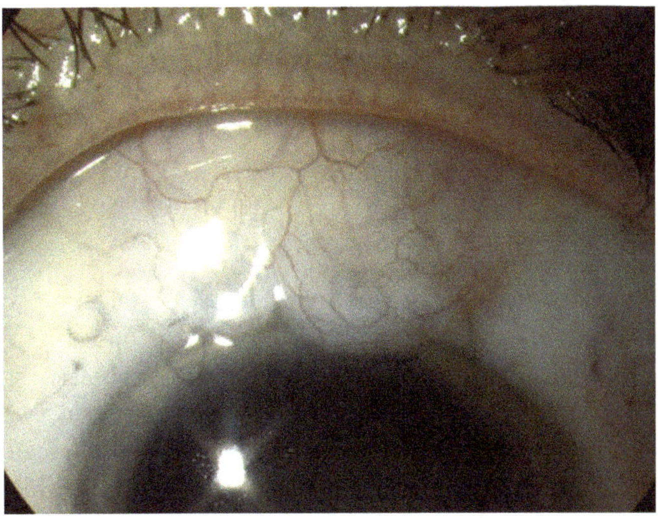

Figure 10.2. Trabeculectomy bleb in Behçet's uveitis.

Table 10.1. **Post-operative treatment regime.**

Drug	Dose
Oral prednisone	40 mg, 30 mg, 20 mg, 10 mg, 5 mg reducing every 5 days
Topical prednisolone acetate 1%	Hourly, tapering over 3–6 months
Topical antibiotic	Continue for 4 weeks
If signs of bleb fibrosis or inflammation: Subconjunctival 5-fluorouracil 5 mg AND/OR oral dexamethasone 20 mg OR oral triamcinolone 10 mg	

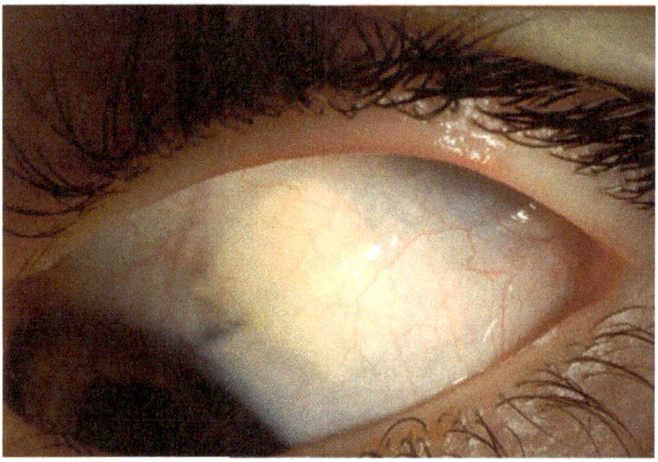

Figure 10.3. Molteno tube covered by scleral patch in uveitic glaucoma due to herpes zoster.

10.2.2 *Glaucoma Tube Surgery*

Tube surgery is indicated when trabeculectomy has failed, or would be unsuitable: adverse ocular surface, poor patient cooperation, difficult exposure, limited follow-up, or extensive peripheral anterior synechiae (PAS). A tube implant is recommended as the primary surgery in cases of Fuchs' uveitis syndrome and should be considered in pseudophakic patients. Tubes are routinely placed in the anterior chamber (which is possible even with some PAS present, Figures 10.3 and 10.4) or in the sulcus in

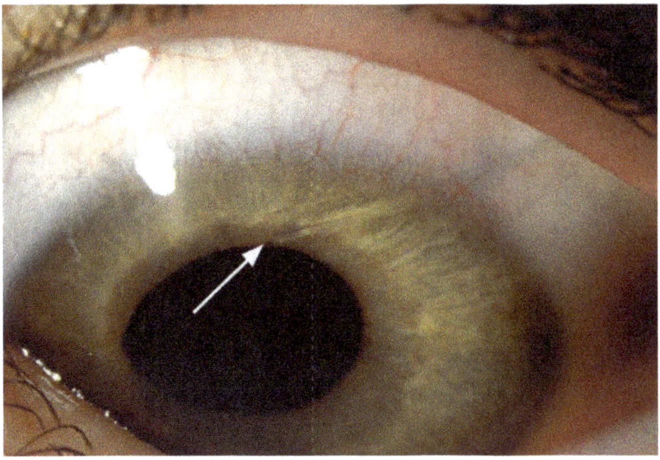

Figure 10.4. Molteno tube (arrow) in the anterior chamber of a patient with uveitic glaucoma due to herpes zoster.

pseudophakic patients, and even in the posterior segment if placed at the same time as a pars plana vitrectomy. There is long-term evidence for the use of Baerveldt,[8] Molteno[9] and Ahmed valve[10] glaucoma tubes in uveitic glaucoma. Recent innovations in tube design may prove to be of benefit in uveitis, including smaller plates, narrower lumens and adjustable valves, with the aim of reducing rates of hypotony.

10.2.3 *Laser in Uveitic Glaucoma*

Laser procedures are generally avoided in uveitis due to the propensity for inflammation. Selective laser trabeculoplasty has not been shown to be beneficial in uveitic glaucoma. Transscleral cyclodiode is pro-inflammatory, and increases the risk of phthisis. It is therefore not an ideal solution for uveitic glaucoma, but may be considered with reduced power in refractory cases, especially if there is a poor visual prognosis, and in those where other options are unsuitable.

10.2.4 *Closed Angle — Seclusio Pupillae and Peripheral Anterior Synechiae*

In the presence of pupil block, peripheral iridotomy (PI) is required to equalize the IOP between the anterior and posterior chamber. Surgical PI

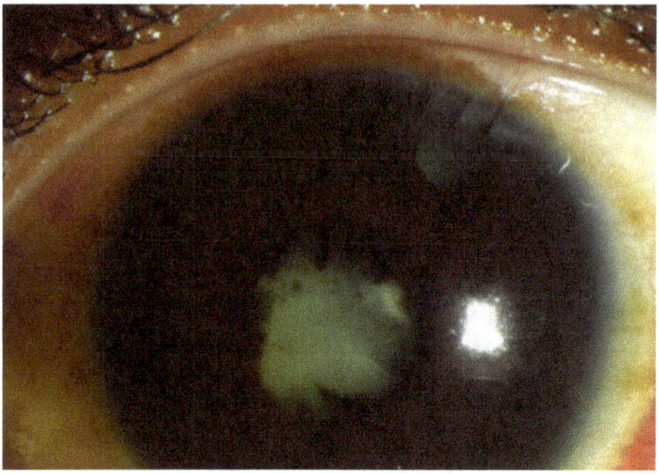

Figure 10.5. Surgical peripheral iridotomy in a patient with sarcoid uveitis.

is preferred (Figure 10.5) as it has greater longevity, lower rates of cataract, and less inflammation, than laser PI.[11] Multiple PIs are often required due to posterior synechiae forming septae and sectoral iris bombé. This can be achieved via microincision using an anterior vitrector. Goniosynechialysis might also be required to relieve recent PAS.

In the presence of extensive posterior synechiae, without pupil block, prophylactic PI can be considered to prevent, or temporarily treat, acute angle closure. Again, we recommend surgical PI in preference to YAG laser PI.

10.2.5 *Microincision Glaucoma Surgery (MIGS)*

There is an increasingly diverse range of new glaucoma surgical devices and techniques available to surgeons. Whilst there is a growing body of evidence for use in primary glaucomas, there is no clear evidence for a role in uveitic glaucoma. Currently we cannot recommend their use; however, conceptually some techniques have promise.

10.2.6 *Cataract Surgery with Uveitic Glaucoma*

Cataract is common in uveitis, and requires special consideration in the context of uveitic glaucoma (Figure 10.6). For a detailed discussion of

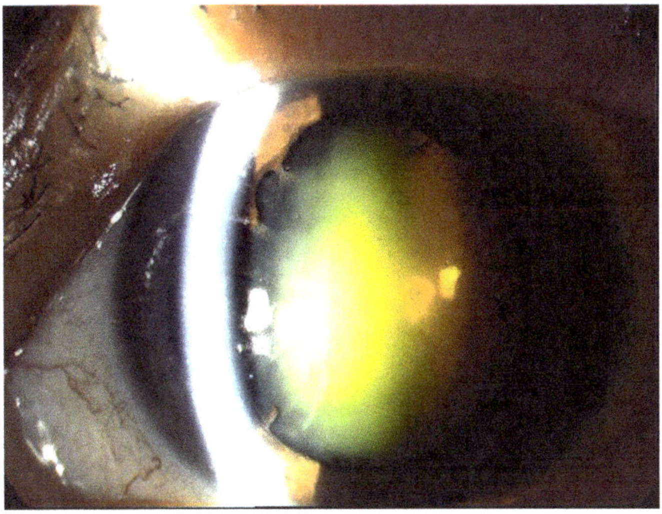

Figure 10.6. Cataract and posterior synechiae in a patient with uveitic glaucoma.

cataract surgery in uveitis, see Chapter 11. Cataract may be secondary to inflammation, steroid use, glaucoma drops or surgery. Both cataract and manifest GON reduce contrast sensitivity and can affect visual function.

The presence of cataract should be considered when planning glaucoma surgery. Best outcomes are achieved as separate procedures, but can be combined if necessary. Cataract surgery should not delay glaucoma surgery. However, after filtration surgery, cataract surgery is ideally delayed 6–12 months.

In patients who have had prior filtration surgery, there is a risk of failure in the post-operative period. Aggressive control of inflammation is required. We follow a regime similar to primary filtration surgery. Multifocal intraocular lenses are not a good choice in uveitic glaucoma because inflammatory deposits can build up on the lens and reduce its functionality.

10.2.7 Complications of Glaucoma Surgery

In eyes undergoing surgery with IOP over 30 mmHg, decompression retinopathy is a risk. This can be addressed with acetazolamide or a mannitol infusion 1 hour pre-operatively.

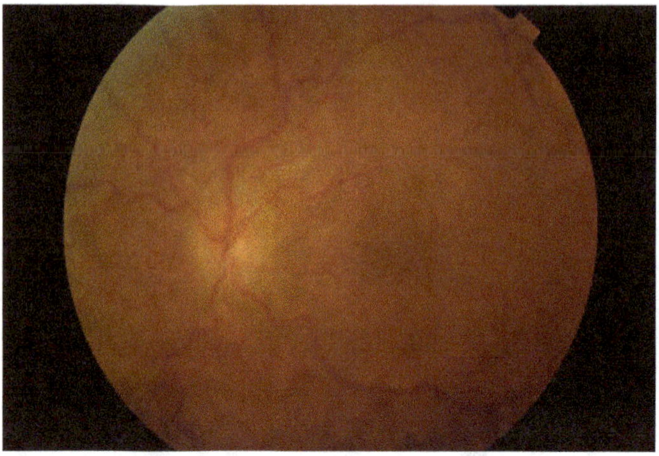

Figure 10.7. Hypotony following glaucoma surgery. Note the hypotony maculopathy including choroidal folds, vascular tortuosity, optic nerve edema and macular striae.

Early hypotony is a risk in any glaucoma filtration procedure, due to over-drainage or leak. However, in uveitis, post-operative inflammation can induce ciliary body shutdown. Hypotony is defined as an IOP $\leq$5 mmHg. It can affect visual acuity and ocular signs include corneal striae, edema, a shallow or flat anterior chamber, choroidal folds, vascular tortuosity, optic nerve edema and macular striae (Figure 10.7). Choroidal detachments are also a typical finding.

Other complications include post-operative inflammation and cataract formation. These are common complications and have already been discussed.

10.3 Vitreoretinal Surgery

Vitrectomy is used in eyes with uveitis for a number of reasons: firstly, to help provide a diagnosis of an infective pathogen or malignancy via vitreous, retinal or choroidal biopsy; secondly, to improve vision by removal of vitreous opacities and, in the case of endophthalmitis, to remove infective and inflammatory factors; and finally, to enable secondary maneuver like epiretinal peel or retinal detachment surgery. The key principle for any surgery on an eye with uveitis is to wait until there is minimal inflammation, usually after a 3-month period from when the eye is quiet. However, for diagnostic or retinal detachment vitrectomies then surgery may take place on a hot eye. In every case, the retinal surgeon needs to liaise closely with the consultant managing the uveitis, to ensure that maximal medical treatment is begun prior to surgery and inflammation is controlled as much as possible.

10.3.1 *Vitreous Biopsy*

Vitreous biopsy is performed for infectious uveitis, atypical inflammatory uveitis to rule out infectious agents and for suspected intraocular lymphoma.

For viral infections, an anterior chamber tap of aqueous fluid may be sufficient, particularly when PCR testing is available. In this setting, there are high rates of positive tests for HSV, VZV, EBV and CMV and a vitreous biopsy is often not required. For suspected bacterial or fungal infective endophthalmitis (Figure 10.8), a vitreous biopsy is more likely to yield a positive result (particularly if PCR testing is also used) and is recommended. Vitreous biopsies may be performed via needle aspiration, and in the case of endophthalmitis prior to injection with intravitreal antibiotics. Needle aspiration is performed with a sterile technique using speculum and 23 g or 25 g needle. Local anesthesia with either sub-tenon anesthetic

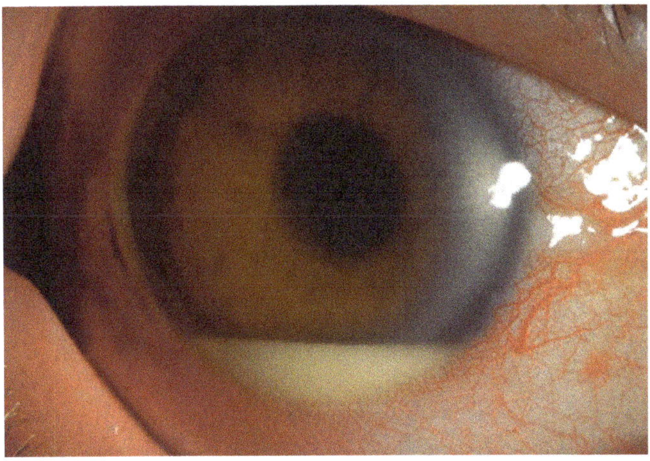

Figure 10.8. Coagulase negative staphylococcus endophthalmitis following intravitreal triamcinolone.

or subconjunctival anesthetic is required. Needle aspiration might be hampered when the vitreous is formed gel and the vitreous tap comes back dry, i.e., without any specimen. Even when a reasonable sample is collected via needle aspiration, the rate of positive identification of causative agents is not as high as a sample collected with a vitrector. We prefer to collect a vitreous sample under air using the vitrectomy machine, first described in 2003[12] and updated with small gauge vitrectomy probes by Tang *et al.* in 2020.[13] This enables at least a millilitre of pure vitreous to be collected under controlled conditions and gives a higher rate of positive results than needle aspiration samples.

Vitreous biopsy for ocular lymphoma is useful if lymphoma can be demonstrated but if the results are negative then lymphoma cannot always be excluded, leading to treatment dilemmas. It is important to have a close relationship with the pathologist when sending vitreous samples for testing for lymphoma, to ensure tests are expedited and appropriate handling of the sample occurs. Even in relatively large samples of vitreous the number of cells collected for testing may be small, causing difficulty in testing and thus reaching a diagnosis. In some patients, subretinal deposits can be aspirated to increase the number of cells available for testing, or retinal or choroidal biopsies of lesions can be obtained. In every case, it is important to inform the laboratory prior to the sample being taken and to ensure that the sample is handled in a way that enables the laboratory the best opportunity to use the sample. Retinal or choroidal samples are innately small and fragile, and careful handling is vital.

10.3.2 *Acute Infective Endophthalmitis*

While the Endophthalmitis Vitrectomy Study (EVS) was the gold standard for management of post-operative infectious endophthalmitis for many years,[14] more recently, there is increasing evidence that early vitrectomy (i.e., within 24 hours of presentation) improves visual outcome for most patients with endophthalmitis.[15,16] For this reason, some centers will consider vitreous biopsy combined with complete vitrectomy be performed as soon as practicable for these patients. It must be noted that injection of intravitreal antibiotics should occur as soon as possible after presentation and should not be delayed while waiting for a theatre slot (see Appendix A). Vitreous biopsy samples collected after intravitreal antibiotics given prior to surgery (for example, a tap and inject with a delayed same-day vitrectomy) may still manifest causative bacteria.[17] Broad spectrum intravitreal antibiotics should be injected into the vitreous cavity at the end of the vitrectomy, whether or not these have been given prior, to ensure a bactericidal concentration is maintained. Evidence for the role of intravitreal or oral steroid is still lacking and while some centers use these as adjuvant treatment, it is still not certain that they contribute to improved visual outcomes.

10.3.3 *Vitrectomy for Media Opacity*

Many patients with uveitis, either after an acute attack or from chronic inflammation, develop visually significant vitreous opacities which reduce vison and impede monitoring of retinal disease. For these reasons vitrectomy is indicated; however, unlike the situations described above, in most cases surgery should be delayed until the eye is quiet. The rule of thumb is to reduce inflammation to the lowest possible level and maintain this for at least 3 months before surgery is performed. Pre-operatively it is worth starting extra treatment to reduce inflammation, and post-operatively patients require close monitoring by their uveitis specialist to ensure their inflammation is well controlled. The patient's condition will determine if it is appropriate to perform a combined cataract extraction and IOL with the vitrectomy or not. In some situations, this may reduce the number of surgeries the patient undergoes and also reduce post-operative inflammation after the cataract surgery. Clinical experience suggests that cataract surgery is more likely to trigger inflammation than vitrectomy, presumably due to the release of lens proteins which have previously been isolated from the body's immune system. Adjuvants like intravitreal steroid can be delivered at the end of surgery to control inflammation but care must be taken to exclude infectious causes of uveitis prior to surgery, as intravitreal steroid can trigger uncontrollable progression of disease from infections. Toxoplasmosis prophylaxis should be utilized for patients with a history of previous toxoplasmosis retinochoroiditis, as they may experience recurrence following vitrectomy. Anecdotal evidence suggests that some patients have fewer or less severe episodes of uveitis after vitrectomy possibly due to the removal of inflammatory factors within the gel.

10.3.4 *Rhegmatogenous Retinal Detachment*

Rhegmatogenous retinal detachment (RRD) is more common in eyes with uveitis, particularly those of infectious etiology.[18] Entities like acute retinal necrosis (ARN) and progressive outer retinal necrosis (PORN) have high levels of detachment due to necrotic breaks in the retina. These detachments are challenging to treat as there is widespread necrosis and usual methods of retinopexy are often ineffective and can lead to further retinal breaks. Prophylactic barrier laser along the borders of necrotic areas has been advocated to prevent the progression to retinal detachment (Figure 10.9). Studies in ARN demonstrate mixed results and its effectiveness is unclear.[19,20] Laser burns should be placed along the border of the necrotic area, but only after good inflammatory control is achieved. Surgery for RRD tends to be technically difficult and in most cases oil tamponade is the best option, but failure and vision loss can occur in more than 50% of cases. For other forms of RRD associated with uveitis, the prognosis is not so dire. Treatment with vitrectomy and tamponade rather than scleral buckle is generally the preferred method as vitreous opacity may obscure retinal breaks. Proliferative vitreoretinopathy (PVR) is a common cause of failure or recurrent detachment in these eyes as the underlying inflammation is a significant risk factor for its development. For this

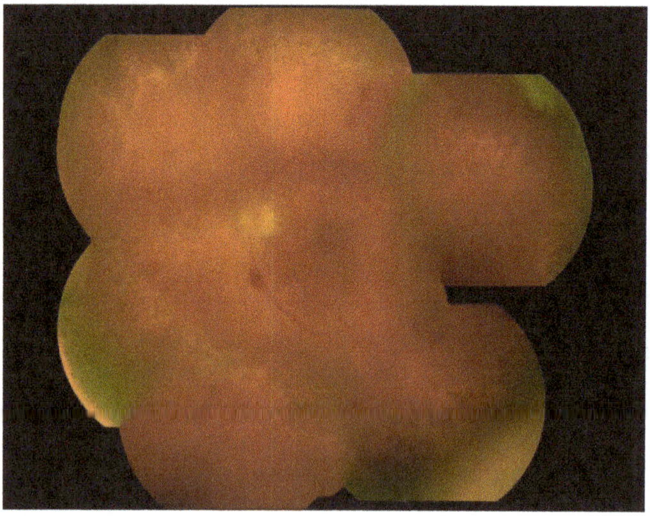

Figure 10.9. Barrier laser in acute retinal necrosis.

reason, it is important to aggressively control inflammation and treat any underlying infection.

10.3.5 *Epiretinal Membrane*

When operating for epiretinal membrane in the context of uveitis, most surgeons peel the inner limiting membrane as this reduces recurrences by removing a scaffold for the proliferation of the membrane.[21] The main concern both pre-operatively and post-operatively is control of associated cystoid macular edema. It is important that this is maximally controlled pre-operatively and the control continues after the surgery. In these cases, adjunctive therapy such as intravitreal steroid is very useful, although infective etiologies must be excluded before these are used. Plaque ERMs tend to have a poorer prognosis.

Teaching Points

- The most common technique for band keratopathy removal is chelation using Na_2 EDTA.
- If a uveitis patient has progressive GON and is on maximal therapy, regardless of their IOP they should be offered surgical intervention. These patients need optic nerve and visual field monitoring more often than in primary glaucoma as progression may be much faster.
- Surgical PIs are preferred to YAG laser in both pupil block and angle closure prophylaxis due to posterior synechiae, as they have greater longevity, lower rates of cataract, and cause less inflammation.
- Before any surgery in a uveitic eye it is advised to wait until there is a 3-month period of no inflammation. Exceptions to this rule may include when urgent diagnostic or retinal detachment vitrectomies are needed to decide whether the eye is quiet or not.
- Rhegmatogenous retinal detachments associated with uveitis tend to be treated with vitrectomy and tamponade, as vitreous opacities may block the view of retinal breaks rendering scleral buckles an inferior option. The necrotic breaks caused by ARN and PORN are very challenging to treat.

References

1. Jhanji V, Rapuano CJ, Vajpayee RB. Corneal calcific band keratopathy. *Curr Opin Ophthalmol* 2011;22(4):283–9.
2. Chan TC, Chow VW, Jhanji V, Wong VW. Different topographic response between mild to moderate and advanced keratoconus after accelerated collagen cross-linking. *Cornea* 2015;34(8):922–7.
3. Lee ME, Ouano DP, Shapiro B, Fong A, Coroneo MT. "Off-the-Shelf" K2-EDTA for calcific band keratopathy. *Cornea* 2018;37(7):916–918.
4. Ma T, Sims JL, Bennett S, Chew S, Niederer RL. High rate of conversion from ocular hypertension to glaucoma in subjects with uveitis. *Br J Ophthalmol* 2021;in press. doi:10.1136/bjophthalmol-2021-318809.
5. Daniel E, Pistilli M, Kothari S, *et al.* Risk of ocular hypertension in adults with noninfectious uveitis. *Ophthalmology* 2017;124(8):1196–1208.
6. Kanaya R, Kijima R, Shinmei Y, *et al.* Surgical outcomes of trabeculectomy in uveitic glaucoma: a long-term, single-center, retrospective case-control study. *J Ophthalmol* 2021;2021:5550776.
7. Wiese C, Heiligenhaus A, Heinz C. Changes in inflammatory activity after glaucoma filtration surgery in children with chronic anterior uveitis. *Ocul Immunol Inflamm* 2016;24(4):397–401.
8. Chhabra R, Tan SZ, Au L, Spencer AF, Fenerty CH, Jones NP. Long-term outcomes and complications of baerveldt glaucoma drainage implants in adults with glaucoma secondary to uveitis. *Ocul Immunol Inflamm* 2019;27(8):1322–9.
9. Molteno AC, Bevin TH, Herbison P, Houliston MJ. Otago glaucoma surgery outcome study: long-term follow-up of cases of primary glaucoma with additional risk factors drained by Molteno implants. *Ophthalmology* 2001;108(12):2193–200.
10. Bao N, Jiang ZX, Coh P, Tao LM. Long-term outcomes of uveitic glaucoma treated with Ahmed valve implant in a series of Chinese patients. *Int J Ophthalmol* 2018;11(4):629–34.
11. Betts TD, Sims JL, Bennett SL, Niederer RL. Outcome of peripheral iridotomy in subjects with uveitis. *Br J Ophthalmol* 2020;104(1):8–10.
12. Russell M, Polkinghorne PJ. Controlled aspiration pressure in methods for collecting pure vitreous samples during vitreous biopsy. *Retina* 2003;23(3):426.
13. Tang PH, Karkhur S, Nguyen QD. Obtaining undiluted vitreous sample using small gauge pars plana vitrectomy and air infusion. *Am J Ophthalmol Case Rep* 2020;19:100768.

14. Endophthalmitis Vitrectomy Study Group. Results of the Endophthalmitis Vitrectomy Study: A randomized trial of immediate vitrectomy and of intravenous antibiotics for the treatment of postoperative bacterial endophthalmitis. *Arch Ophthalmol* 1995;113(12):1479–96.
15. Dib B, Morris RE, Oltmanns MH, Sapp MR, Glover JP, Kuhn F. Complete and early vitrectomy for endophthalmitis after cataract surgery: an alternative treatment paradigm. *Clin Ophthalmol* 2020;14:1945–1954.
16. Welch S, Bhikoo R, Wang N, *et al.* Better visual outcome associated with early vitrectomy in the management of endophthalmitis. *Br J Ophthalmol* 2021; in press. doi:10.1136/bjophthalmol-2020-316846.
17. Bhikoo R, Wang N, Welch S, Polkinghorne P, Niederer RL. Factors associated with positive microbial culture in patients with endophthalmitis based on clinical presentation and multimodal intraocular sampling. *Asia Pac J Ophthalmol (Phila)* 2020;9(1):4–8.
18. Young-Zvandasara T, Brunner D, Welch S, *et al.* Rhegmatogenous retinal detachment presentation and surgery in uveitic eyes. *Br J Ophthalmol* 2021; in press. doi:10.1136/bjophthalmol-2021-319268.
19. Baltinas J, Lightman S, Tomkins-Netzer O. Comparing treatment of acute retinal necrosis with either oral Valacyclovir or intravenous Acyclovir. *Am J Ophthalmol* 2018;188:173–80.
20. Lau CH, Missotten T, Salzmann J, Lightman S. Acute retinal necrosis features, management, and outcomes. *Ophthalmology* 2007;114(4):756–62.
21. Rayess N, Vail D, Mruthyunjaya P. Rates of reoperation in 10 114 patients with epiretinal membranes treated by vitrectomy with or without inner limiting membrane peeling. *Ophthalmol Retina* 2021;5(7):664–9.

https://doi.org/10.1142/9789811251474_0011

Chapter 11

Cataract Surgery in Uveitis

Priya D Samalia, Joanne L Sims*†

11.1 Introduction

Uveitic cataracts develop because of chronic or recurrent intraocular inflammation and also due to ocular and systemic corticosteroid therapy that is used to treat inflammation.

Cataract surgery in the context of uveitis can be complex. Poor pupillary dilation due to posterior synechiae and pupillary membranes, floppy iris and zonular instability are just some of the challenges encountered during uveitic cataract surgery.

Each stage in cataract surgery — pre-operative, intra-operative, post-operative — needs to be well planned and executed to optimize the visual outcome.

11.2 Peri-operative Management

11.2.1 *Timing of Cataract Surgery*

It is important to carefully consider the timing and indications for surgery (Table 11.1).

11.2.2 *Pre-operative Approach*

11.2.2.1 *Control of Inflammation*

There is a general consensus to wait at least 3 months for uveitis to be quiescent prior to proceeding with cataract surgery. This reduces the risk

*The Royal Victorian Eye and Ear Hospital, Melbourne, Australia
†Greenlane Clinical Centre, Auckland District Health Board, Auckland, New Zealand

Table 11.1. Indications for cataract surgery.

Decreased vision with potential for improvement post-cataract removal
Cataract obscuring fundal view to enable adequate monitoring of posterior segment uveitis and uveitic complications
Lens-induced uveitis is an absolute indication as this is therapeutic
Urgent vitreoretinal surgery required and cannot be performed without cataract extraction
Child of amblyogenic age, where risk of amblyopia needs to be considered when cataract surgery is delayed
Contraindications
Poor control of uveitis
Active untreated cystoid macular edema
Active anterior segment inflammation other than that associated with lens-induced inflammation

of uveitic flares post-operatively.[2–6] In the case of Behçet's disease uveitis ideally should be quiescent for 6 months prior to cataract surgery. The risk of post-operative recurrence is linked to frequency of attacks 12 months before surgery.[7–8]

Prior to surgery consider a course of pre-operative steroids (topical ± systemic).[9–11] Steroids may be started up to 2 weeks prior to surgery (e.g., prednisolone acetate 1% and 0.5–1 mg/kg oral prednisone, intravitreal preservative-free triamcinolone or intravitreal dexamethasone implant, Table 11.2). In the presence of anterior uveitis without extensive posterior synechiae or posterior complications such as cystoid macular edema (CME), topical therapy alone may be adequate. In cases of anterior uveitis with extensive posterior synechiae, posterior/panuveitis uveitis, or previous cystoid macular edema, generally both topical and systemic/intravitreal corticosteroid/± systemic immunosuppression[12] should be used. Steroid pre-treatment is not essential for Fuchs' uveitis syndrome (FUS) or quiescent anterior uveitis off all treatment.

Steroid pre-treatment is essential for second eye cataract surgery if there was a poor outcome with the first eye, a history of cystoid macular edema, posterior segment uveitis, if iris manipulation will be required during surgery, and in an only eye. If there is suboptimal control of uveitis and there is an urgent need to operate (i.e., unable to wait at least 3 months once quiescent), consider pre-operative intravenous methylprednisolone.[9]

Table 11.2. Suggested pre-operative steroid regimen for uveitic cataract surgery.

Clinical scenario	Pre-operative steroid regimen
Anterior uveitis, no extensive posterior synechiae	Topical steroid 1 week prior
Anterior uveitis with extensive posterior synechiae, intermediate or posterior uveitis, or a history of previous CME	Topical steroid 1 week prior Oral prednisone 1 mg/kg starting 3–7 days prior Consider intravitreal triamcinolone or dexamethasone implant at time of surgery
CME pre-operatively	Ideally postpone surgery until controlled If surgery required despite CME, add intra-operative triamcinolone or dexamethasone implant
Suboptimal control of uveitis	Consider pre-operative intravenous methylprednisolone +/– intravitreal steroid

CME = cystoid macular edema

If the patient is already on immunomodulatory therapy (biologic and non-biologic) for their uveitis, this should continue peri-operatively.

11.2.2.2 *Consider Prophylaxis for Infectious Etiologies*[9]

1. Herpetic Uveitis: Up to 40% recurrence of disease can be observed post-operatively. Consider starting acyclovir or valacyclovir the day of surgery and continue for 3–6 months post-op (see Chapter 6).[13]
2. Ocular Toxoplasmosis: There is an increased risk of reactivation of ocular toxoplasmosis up to 36% within 4 months after surgery (Figure 11.1). Antibiotic prophylaxis should be considered (see Chapter 6, Table 6.9).[9]

11.2.2.3 *Pre-operative Assessment of Visual Potential*[9,14,15]

Before surgery it is important to assess for signs that may indicate worse visual prognosis, such as the presence of a relative afferent pupillary defect, hypotony, CME (ideally postpone until resolved), optic disc edema, optic atrophy, macular scar, or subretinal neovascularization. A B-scan ultrasonography should be performed if there is no fundal view through a dense cataract.

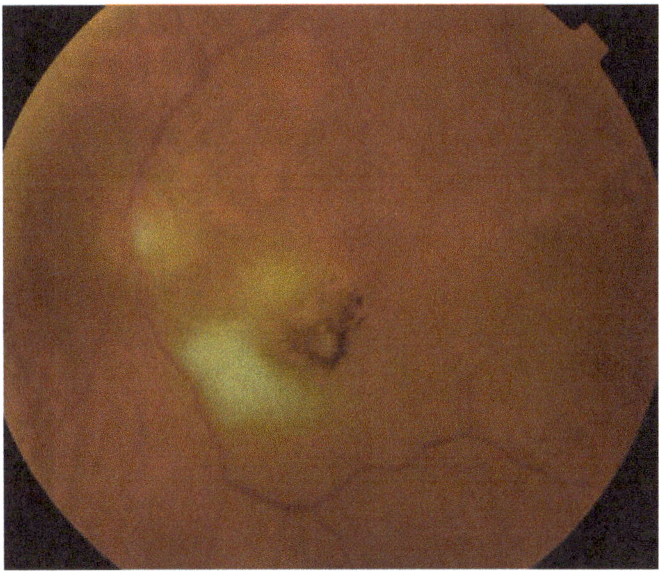

Figure 11.1. Reactivation of ocular toxoplasmosis.

11.2.2.4 *Pre-operative Assessment of Risk of Hypotony*[16]

Before surgery the patient must be assessed for signs of risk of hypotony, including low intraocular pressure (IOP) (≤6 mmHg even when quiet), phacodonesis without evident zonulysis, seclusio pupillae with normal IOP, diffusely thickened choroid or effusions on B-scan ultrasonography.[16] Ultrasonography of ciliary body may demonstrate ciliary body atrophy or cyclitic membrane.[17]

11.2.2.5 *Careful Pre-operative Counselling*

Patient expectations should be managed, including a discussion around increased risk of surgical complications, prolonged visual recovery, visual potential, need for compliance with therapy, and induced presbyopia. Also consider visual needs, state of other eye, refraction of other eye, and need for surgery in the other eye.

11.2.3 Intra-operative Approach

11.2.3.1 *Anesthesia*

Regional anesthesia is preferred over topical anesthesia due to the need for iris manipulations, as this can cause unnecessary patient discomfort and movement.

11.2.3.2 *Wounds*

A temporal clear corneal incision approach has the advantage of preserving the superior conjunctiva.

- Ocular hypertension and uveitic glaucoma occur in up to 41.8% of patients with uveitis.[18]
- Preserving the superior conjunctiva will provide healthy tissue for trabeculectomy surgery if required in the future.

There is an increased risk of bleeding and hyphema during incisions, known as Amsler Sign and is seen in FUS.

11.2.3.3 *Pupil Management*

Uveitic eyes often have poor dilation due to posterior synechiae and pupillary membranes (Figure 11.2). Intra-operative pharmacologic methods to assist dilation include:

- Topical mydriatic
- Intracameral mydriatics
- Anterior chamber infusion with balanced salt solution with 1:1000 adrenaline

Intra-operative surgical approaches for pupil dilation include:

- Specialized viscoelastic device to viscodilate the pupil and perform synechiolysis with viscodissection (e.g., cohesive healon, healon GV, viscoadaptive healon 5)

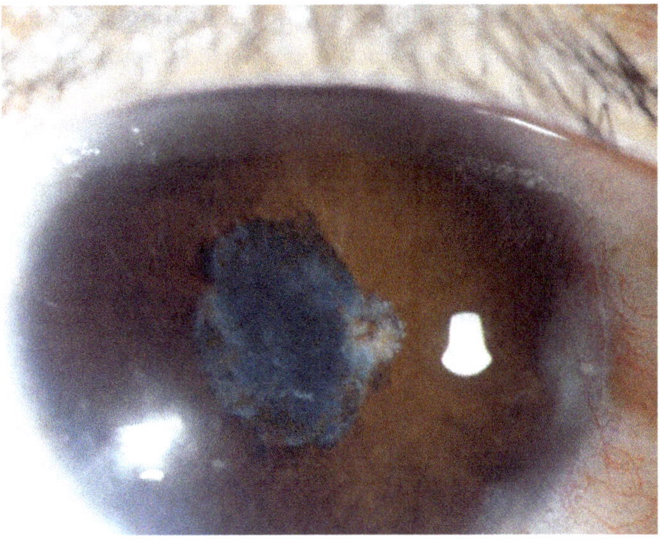

Figure 11.2. Pupillary membrane.

- Avoiding instrument pupil stretch as this tends to make the iris more floppy
- A pupillary membrane can be nicked with a needle then peeled off with micrograsping forceps[9]
- Surgical pupil expanders can be used (e.g., iris hooks, Malyugin ring)[9]
- If pupil expanders are insufficient to dilate the pupil then sphincterotomies can be performed

11.2.3.4 *Lens Capsule Management*

Trypan blue dye can improve visibility, particularly for dense cataracts, to assist in performing the capsulorhexis. In cases of very small pupils the capsular stain can be more effective if applied after the pupil has been expanded and viscoelastic removed from the anterior chamber. Alternatively, the capsular dye can be 'painted' onto the anterior capsule beneath the viscoelastic. Aim for the capsulorhexis to be central and of adequate size, just smaller than the diameter of the intraocular lens (IOL) optic (5.5–6 mm) to prevent post-operative adhesion formation.[19] An adequately sized capsulorrhexis also decreases the risk of post-operative anterior capsule phimosis.

There may be an increased risk of posterior capsular rupture due to weakened zonules. If zonular weakness is detected, capsule hooks can stabilize the capsule while working followed by a capsular tension ring.

11.2.3.5 *Cataract Extraction*

Phacoemulsification is the preferred technique. Extracapsular cataract extraction is more inflammatory.[20] It is important to minimize phaco power. Soft lens techniques such as bowling out lens may be needed. Completing cortical clean-up is essential, as residual cortex will incite more post-operative inflammation. Polishing the posterior capsule will reduce post-operative inflammation and the risk of posterior capsule opacification.

11.2.3.6 *Intraocular Lens Implant (IOL)*

Risk of IOLs in uveitis patients include:

- Dense IOL precipitates
- Cyclitic membranes
- Cocooned IOL

In general, hydrophobic acrylic square-edged IOL in the bag are preferred as they demonstrate lower risk of post-operative inflammation, lower rates of posterior capsule opacification, low rates of CME and superior visual outcomes.[21–23] Surface modifications such as heparin coating may provide a more hydrophilic surface that may reduce adhesion of fibrin and white blood cells.[23] Most avoid silicone IOLs[23] and prolene haptics as these tend to be more pro-inflammatory.[9,19]

Anterior chamber IOLs (ACIOLs) and iris-supported posterior chamber IOLs should be avoided where possible due to risk of provoking anterior uveitis. Scleral fixation of three-piece IOL is safer if there is a posterior capsule tear and no capsular support. There is also a general preference is to avoid multifocal IOLs due to poorer quality vision and risk of decentration.

IOL implants remain contentious in pediatric uveitic cataracts but can be considered in well-controlled cases. Older studies demonstrated high rates of hypotony and cyclitic membranes in JIA uveitis[24–27] but more recently there have been good outcomes with IOL implantation at the time of cataract surgery with meticulous control of uveitis for at least 6 months prior to surgery.[12,28] Generally superior visual outcomes have been demonstrated with IOL placement,[23] but one could consider leaving aphakic patients with any of the following:

- Significant flare
- Hypotony
- Non-compliance
- Patients who have failed IOL in contralateral eye, or in pediatric patients

11.2.3.7 *Wound Closure*

The need for frequent topical corticosteroid use post-operatively may theoretically inhibit wound healing and therefore sutured wound closure should be considered, particularly in pediatric cases.[9]

11.2.3.8 *Intra-operative Medications*

Intracameral or subconjunctival antibiotics are recommended as part of standard care. An intravitreal, sub-tenon or periocular steroid injection at end of surgery could reduce the risk of post-operative relapse. Intracameral dexamethasone may help control early post-operative inflammation and prevent fibrin formation, especially if the iris has been manipulated.[29]

11.2.4 *Post-operative Approach*

Uveitis patients are at a higher risk of post-operative complications, including[9,30]:

- Corneal edema
- Recurrence or exacerbation of uveitis
- Glaucoma or hypotony

- Cystoid macular edema
- Posterior capsule opacification
- IOL inflammatory deposits
- Anterior capsule phimosis
- IOL fibrous encapsulation
- IOL dislocation

The post-operative plan is aimed at reducing inflammation and monitoring closely, to minimize risk of complications and optimize management if they do occur. If post-operative inflammation occurs, more frequent topical steroids are required to control the inflammation and a longer treatment duration, for example initial intensive topical steroid (i.e., prednisolone acetate 1% drops every hour during waking hours), followed by slow taper and treating for at least 2 months. Patients may need topical steroid post-operatively for a prolonged period to prevent IOL deposits. Post-operative cycloplegics are needed to prevent recurrent posterior synechiae and should be continued until anterior chamber cells are +0.5 or less.

If high-dose oral steroids were started pre-operatively, they should be continued for 1 week post-operatively then tapered by 5 mg per week to maintenance. Subjects require more regular follow-up. Typically patients are reviewed on day one post-operatively, then 1–2 weeks post-operatively, with further follow-up based on degree of post-operative inflammation. CME may occur even up to 6 months post-operatively, so ongoing checks are necessary.

11.3 Managing Post-operative Complications

11.3.1 *Cystoid Macular Edema*

Post-operative CME occurs between 12%[31] and 44% of subjects with uveitis undergoing cataract surgery (Table 11.3),[32] compared to 0.1%[33] to 4%[31] in non-uveitic eyes following uncomplicated cataract surgery (Figure 11.3). Although many cases resolve without affecting vision, untreated chronic cases can eventually lead to atrophic macular changes and permanent vision loss. Patients will present with blurring of vision or metamorphopsia.

Table 11.3. Risk factors for the development of post-operative cystoid macular edema in uveitis.

Patient factors	Operative factors
Uveitis i. Longer duration ii. Intermediate and panuveitis iii. Age >50 years	Complicated cataract surgery (posterior capsule rupture, vitreous incarceration into incision site)
Pre-existing epiretinal membrane	Retained lens fragment
Previous vein occlusions	ACIOL
Prior topical prostaglandin treatment	Secondary IOL
History of CME in other eye	
Other eye diseases, e.g., retinitis pigmentosa	
Diabetes	
Smoker	

CME = cystoid macular edema, ACIOL = anterior chamber intraocular lens, IOL = intraocular lens

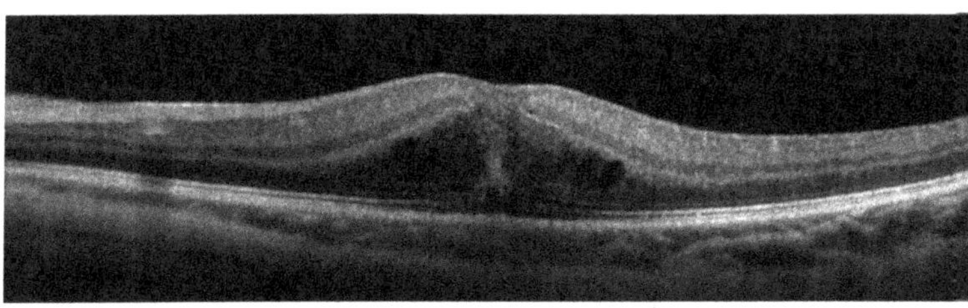

Figure 11.3. Cystoid macular edema on optical coherence tomography.

11.3.1.1 *Prevention of CME*

Post-operative CME can be prevented with strict pre-operative control of uveitis and initiation of pre-operative steroids. Uveitic eyes treated with peri-operative oral corticosteroids had a 7-fold reduction in post-operative CME (relative risk 0.14, P = 0.05).[4] Uveitic eyes with active inflammation within 3 months before surgery had increased risk of CME (relative risk 6.19, P = 0.04).[4] Other commonly used protocols include periocular/intraocular steroids or extensive post-operative topical NSAIDs.[19]

11.3.1.2 *Management of CME*

CME is managed early, even if visual acuity is good, using a stepwise approach. Mechanical factors should be corrected, for example, anterior

Table 11.4. Specific treatments targeted to CME.

Pharmacological treatment	Topical steroid and topical NSAID are less effective when used in isolation for uveitic CME, but are useful as adjunctive treatment
	Periocular steroid
	Intraocular steroid
	Anti-VEGF[34] or methotrexate intravitreal injection[35]
Surgical treatment	Vitrectomy can be considered if no response to medical treatment, particularly if apparent vitreomacular disturbance[36]
	Role when there is no mechanical component is not established, and the elimination half-life of triamcinolone in vitrectomized eyes is 3.2 days versus 18.6 days in non-vitrectomized eyes[37]

vitrectomy or YAG laser vitrectomy to vitreous incarceration if present, or removal of any retained lens fragments. Any active inflammation must be controlled aggressively, as this can contribute to resolution of CME. Additionally, specific treatment can be used to resolve the CME (Table 11.4). It is important to review patients following discontinuation of eye drops as CME can rebound.

11.3.1.3 *POINT Trial*[38]

Purpose: periocular triamcinolone (PTA) vs intravitreal triamcinolone (ITA) vs intravitreal dexamethasone implant (IDI)

Main Outcomes: ITA and IDI were superior to PTA for treating uveitic CME with modest increase in risk of IOP elevation

- Improvement in best corrected visual acuity (BCVA) at 8 weeks
- Both IVTA and IDI treatments demonstrated visual improvements of 5 letters greater than PTA group at 8 weeks ($P < 0.004$):
  - PTA 4.37 letters
  - ITA 9.70 letters
  - IDI 9.53 letters
- All treatments demonstrated improvement in central subfoveal thickness (CST). IVTA and IDI had larger reductions in CST than PTA at 8 weeks ($P < 0.0001$)
- Reduction in CST at 8 weeks:
  - PTA 23%
  - ITA 39%
  - IDI 46%

Table 11.5. General risk factors for posterior capsule opacification.

Patient factors	Operative factors
Young patient	Retained lens matter during surgery
Diabetes	IOL design (controversial)
Uveitis	1. Square-edged designs reduce PCO risk
Retinitis	2. PMMA IOL demonstrate highest rates of PCO[32]
pigmentosa	3. Lowest rates with acrylic IOL compared to PMMA and silicone[40]
	Inadequate cortical clearance

- The risk of IOP ≥ 24 mmHg was higher in ITA (HR 1.83, CI 0.91–3.65) and IDI (HR 2.52, 95% CI 1.29–4.91) than PTA group at 8 weeks. There was no significant difference between the two intravitreal treatment groups.

11.3.2 *Posterior Capsule Opacification*

Posterior capsule opacification (PCO) is common after uveitic cataract surgery and develops up to 58% of cases.[39] Risk is reduced with strict pre-operative uveitis control, good cortical clean-up and intra-operative capsule polish (Table 11.5).

Management of PCO is typically with Nd:YAG posterior capsulotomy. Treatment should be postponed for a post-operative period of at least 3–6 months and patients covered with topical steroid for 1 week post-procedure with careful follow-up. There is an increased risk of complications including rise in IOP, CME and possibly retinal detachment after YAG capsulotomy.[41]

11.3.3 *IOP Problems and Glaucoma*

Uveitic eyes are prone to IOP fluctuations and glaucoma can be exacerbated post-operatively. Meticulous control of uveitis as well as the IOP are important in management (Table 11.6). The increased need for topical steroid peri-operatively may exacerbate IOP, and systemic steroid may allow reduction of local steroid in these cases. IOP is managed medically where possible, as further surgery soon after cataract surgery will increase inflammation and have higher risk of failure.

Table 11.6. Overview of management of uveitic glaucoma post-operatively.

Look for contributing factors for high IOP

1. Shallow anterior chamber: exclude aqueous misdirection, pupil block, suprachoroidal hemorrhage
2. Deep anterior chamber: consider retained viscoelastic, retained soft lens matter, inflammation, hyphema, steroid-response

Corticosteroid to control inflammation

1. Topical steroid titrated to degree of inflammation
2. Systemic steroid in severe inflammation, or consider in steroid responders as may allow reduction in topical steroid requirements

Medical/laser IOP management

1. Aqueous suppressant
2. Pilocarpine should be avoided
3. Selective laser trabeculoplasty generally avoided in uveitis (limited data) and post-operatively as may exacerbate inflammation and lead to peripheral anterior synechiae
4. Cycloablation, avoided if possible as potential for severe flare of inflammation and complications including phthisis

Surgical IOP management

1. Pupil block can arise post-operatively if anterior uveitis is uncontrolled and leads to reformation of posterior synechiae
   i. Surgical peripheral iridectomy preferred and combine with synechiolysis, high failure rate with laser peripheral iridotomy
   ii. Intense topical corticosteroid post-procedure
2. Trabeculectomy is rarely indicated in the acute post-operative period
   i. Use antimetabolite to reduce failure
   ii. Risk of hypotony
   iii. Following cataract surgery, ideally wait at least 6 months before trabeculectomy, else increased risk of failure
3. Glaucoma Drainage Device
   i. If hypotony risk use smaller plate, no adjuvant antimetabolite, supramid intraluminal suture, ligature sutures around tube
4. MIGS
   i. Exact role in uveitis still to be determined, e.g., Xen implant

11.3.4 *Hypotony*

Hypotony can develop even following uncomplicated cataract surgery in a uveitic eye and can lead to poor visual outcomes. Risk factors for hypotony include poor inflammatory control, patients with juvenile idiopathic arthritis,[32] presence of cyclitic membranes (Figure 11.4)

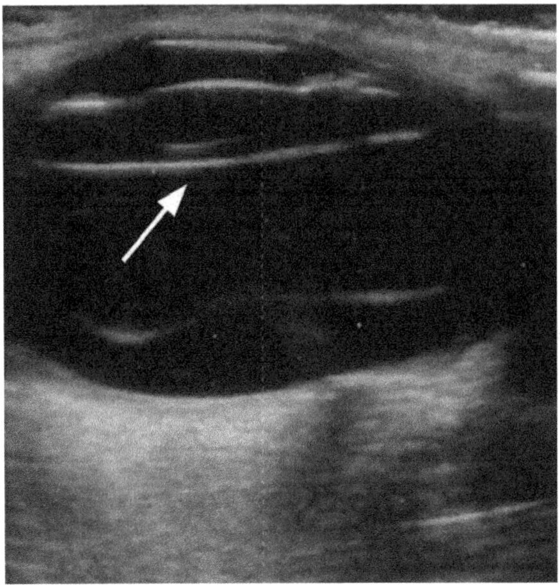

Figure 11.4. Ultrasound demonstrating a cyclitic membrane (arrow).

or following cyclodiode laser. Prevention of hypotony includes strict pre-operative uveitis control and intensive topical/systemic steroid peri-operatively.

11.3.4.1 *Management of Hypotony*

1. Assessment for contributing factors:
   - Low IOP and **shallow** anterior chamber: wound leak (must be sutured if identified), choroidal effusions
   - Low IOP and **deep** anterior chamber: suggest ciliary body shut down, retinal detachment
2. Increase topical steroid (may get IOP rise response)
3. Atropine to deepen anterior chamber and reduce risk of aqueous misdirection
4. Reform anterior chamber if needed
5. Consider intraocular sodium hyaluronate[42]
6. Consider intravenous methylprednisolone[43]
7. Drain choroidal effusion if kissing

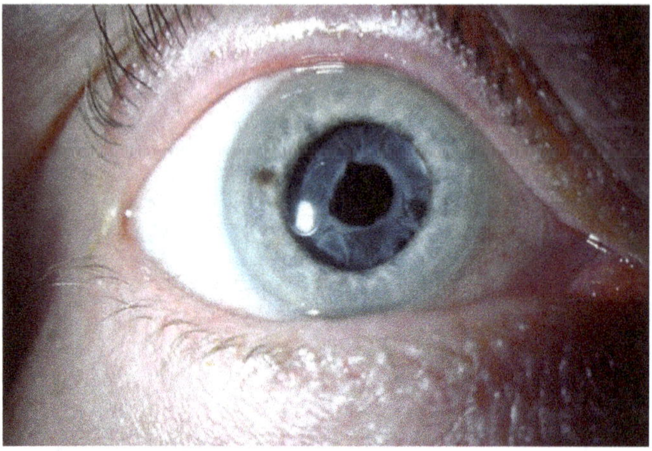

Figure 11.5. Anterior capsule phimosis.

Hypotony management can be challenging if there are no easily reversible factors, and if longstanding can lead to permanent structural damage in the retina or even phthisis.

11.3.5 *Anterior Capsule Phimosis*

Capsular phimosis (Figure 11.5) can develop at any stage but risk is increased in uveitis particularly if there are any intra-operative difficulties such as zonular weakness or a small capsulorrhexis. Complications of anterior capsule phimosis include IOL decentration/dislocation, pseudophakodonysis, and hyperopic shift due to IOL posterior vaulting as the capsular bag contracts.

Risk can be reduced by utilizing a large capsulorrhexis, meticulous cortical removal as presence of lens epithelial cells on the anterior capsule increases risk, and Nd:YAG relaxing incisions in high-risk patients.

11.3.5.1 *Management Options of Capsule Phimosis*

In patients able to cooperate Nd:YAG anterior capsulotomy can be attempted, though it may be unsuccessful in thick phimosis. An alternative surgical approach can be tried using vitreous cutter or capsule scissors/forceps. If capsule contraction is severe and zonules are weak, IOL exchange may need to be performed. Capsulotomy enlargement with a femtosecond laser has also been achieved.

11.3.6 *Recurrence or Exacerbation of Uveitis*

Varied rates of uveitis recurrences or worsening have been reported, depending on the follow-up duration, type of uveitis and type of cataract surgery, but can occur in as many as 50%.[32] Risk factors include the type of surgery as extracapsular cataract extraction or small incision cataract surgery has higher risk than phacoemulsification.[20,44] Presence of pre-operative anterior segment inflammation is also a risk factor, as is the type of uveitis. Lower recurrence occurs with good pre-operative uveitic control, meticulous cortical clearance, and using hydrophobic acrylic IOL or heparin-coated IOL.

If recurrence occurs then escalation of corticosteroid therapy and occasionally other immune suppressive treatment such as immunomodulatory drugs will be needed.

11.3.7 *Other Complications*

11.3.7.1 *IOL Deposits*

Risk factors include active uveitis and also plate-haptic silicone IOLs.[32]

To prevent IOL deposits from occurring, strict pre-operative control of inflammation is needed, with intensive topical steroid whilst inflamed, and implanting either an acrylic IOL or a heparin surface-modified IOL (Figure 11.6).[23]

Management includes intensive topical steroid to reduce inflammation. Nd:YAG laser may be used to clear large deposits and, rarely, IOL exchange is required.

11.3.7.2 *Malpositioned IOL*

IOL subluxation or dislocation can occur in 0.2–0.3%[32] and can occur early or late (Figure 11.7). Early dislocation is due to loss of capsular support and zonular integrity, while late dislocation occurs because of progressive zonular dehiscence. If subluxation impairs vision or leads to worsened control of uveitis, then surgical intervention is required to remove or re-position the IOL.

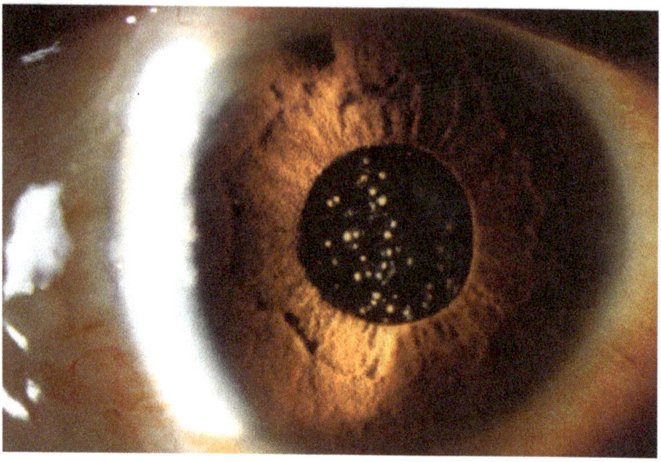

Figure 11.6. IOL deposits.

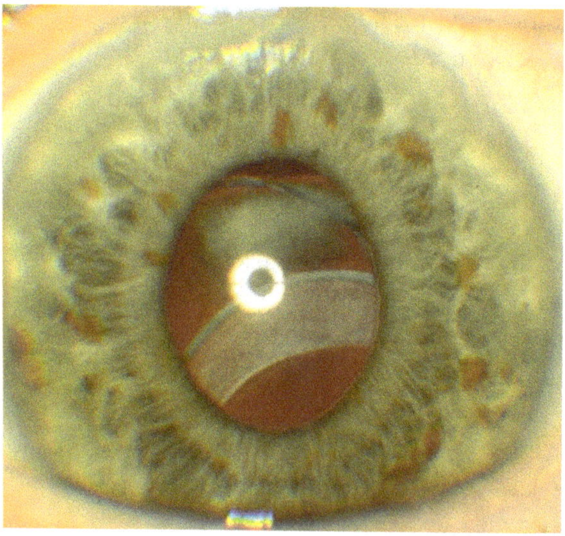

Figure 11.7. Inferior subluxation of three-piece intraocular lens.

11.3.7.3 *Retinal Detachment*

Retinal detachment is common in patients with uveitis, occurring in 1.6% of eyes, with higher rates in infectious uveitis and chronic disease. The risk may increase following cataract surgery. All patients should be counselled to present to ophthalmology if there is an increase in floaters, flashes or a black curtain over the vision, and particular care should be taken in performing examination of the peripheral retina for breaks at each post-operative visit.

11.3.7.4 *Floaters*

Floaters are a common symptom in patients with uveitis. Following cataract surgery, the improved media clarity may result in increased visibility of floaters. All patients with previous intermediate uveitis and/or vitreous opacities should be counselled that floaters may be more visible following surgery, and consideration should be given to performing combined phacovitrectomy in patients with significant floaters.

11.4 Special Notes on Pediatric Uveitic Cataracts

Cataract is a common complication of uveitis in the pediatric population, occurring in up to two-thirds of patients,[28] and is of even more significance in the pediatric population due to the risk of amblyopia. The management of pediatric uveitic cataracts is complex and involves a multidisciplinary team approach with combined management with parents/caregivers, uveitis specialists, pediatric ophthalmologists, pediatricians and optometrists.

11.4.1 *Additional Considerations for Pediatric Uveitic Cataracts*

1. Indications of cataract extraction: risk of amblyopia needs to be considered when cataract surgery is delayed
2. Aggressive pre-, intra- and post-operative control of inflammation is imperative to optimize visual outcomes[28,45,46]
3. Timing of surgery: ideally aim for quiescent uveitis for ≥3 months[28] and if possible ≥6 months[44]
4. If band keratopathy is managed with EDTA chelation, allow at least 3 months before performing cataract surgery to allow refraction to stabilize.

11.4.2 Choice of Surgical Technique: Phacoaspiration Versus Pars Plana Approach

Cataract surgery in children can be performed using phacoaspiration with an anterior approach, or through the pars plana. Pars plana vitrectomy with pars plana lensectomy is preferred over phacoaspiration particularly in cases with presence of cyclitic membranes, atrophic ciliary body on ultrasound biomicroscopy, the presence of vitreous membrane or dense opacities or in the case of pre-operative hypotony.[45]

11.4.3 Aphakic Correction Versus IOL Implantation

IOL implantation is contentious in the pediatric population but can be considered if uveitis control has been good for a long time.[28] When considering IOL implantation a hydrophobic, acrylic IOL is preferred. In general, multifocal IOLs should be avoided as retinal damage (secondary to uveitis) affecting vision may make them intolerable. It is also difficult to perform retinoscopy through them for disease monitoring. Leaving an eye aphakic requires the availability of aphakic correction and that the child can tolerate aphakic contact lenses (especially if unilateral surgery needed). The risk of topical steroid use in the presence of contact lenses also needs consideration.

11.4.4 Management of Posterior Capsule

Primary posterior capsulotomy with limited anterior vitrectomy is generally considered for those under 5–8 years of age due to high rates of posterior capsule opacification. Primary posterior capsulotomy should be approximately 1.0–1.5 mm smaller than anterior capsulotomy (~4–4.5 mm).

11.4.5 Start Amblyopia Treatment As Soon As Able Post-operatively

Delay of resolution of post-operative inflammation can delay treatment of ambloyopia.[46]

11.5 Outcomes

Overall 59.3–82% achieve post-operative best corrected visual acuity of 6/12 or better, compared to 96% in non-uveitic eyes.[9]

Proportion of those achieving a visual outcome of 6/12 or better is also dependant on the underlying uveitic entity[9]:

- Anterior uveitis 91.1–94.5%
- Fuchs' uveitis syndrome 92%
- Posterior/panuveitis 57.4%
- Vogt-Koyanagi-Harada disease 67.1–68%
- Behçet's disease 12.2–16.7%[5]
- Sympathetic ophthalmia 33.3%[1]

Good peri-operative management, in particular meticulous control of uveitis leading up to surgery, and careful monitoring and treatment post-operatively can enhance visual outcomes and reduce need for further intervention.

Teaching Points

- Pre-operative, intra-operative and post-operative planning are required to optimize the visual outcome in uveitic eyes.
- For most uveitis patients there should be a 3-month quiescent period before cataract surgery. However, in Behçet's disease it needs to be 6 months. Topical, oral, intravitreal or even intravenous steroids should be considered pre-operatively to control the uveitis.
- Due to the high recurrence of herpetic uveitis and ocular toxoplasmosis after cataract surgery, prophylaxis should be considered.
- A temporal incision is preferable in cataract surgery to leave healthy conjunctiva if trabeculectomy surgery is ever needed in the future.
- Hydrophobic acrylic square-edged IOL in the bag are the most suitable for uveitis patients as they have a lower rate of post-operative inflammation, posterior capsule opacification and CME, as well as superior visual outcomes.

- Intravitreal, sub-tenon or periocular steroid delivery at the end of cataract surgery reduces the risk of post-operative uveitis relapses.
- PCO occurs in up to 58% of uveitic cataract surgery. Treatment with YAG laser should occur at least 3–6 months after surgery.

References

1. Rojas B, Foster CS. Cataract surgery in patients with uveitis. *Curr Opin Ophthalmol* 1996;7:11–6.
2. Rojas B, Zafirakis P, Foster CS. Cataract surgery in patients with uveitis. *Curr Opin Ophthalmol* 1997;8:6–12.
3. Elgohary MA, McCluskey PJ, Towler HM, Okhravi N, Singh RP, Obikpo R, *et al.* Outcome of phacoemulsification in patients with uveitis. *Br J Ophthalmol* 2007;91:916–21.
4. Bélair ML, Kim SJ, Thorne JE, Dunn JP, Kedhar SR, Brown DM, *et al.* Incidence of cystoid macular edema after cataract surgery in patients with and without uveitis using optical coherence tomography. *Am J Ophthalmol* 2009;148:128–35.e2.
5. Kadayifçilar S, Gedik S, Eldem B, Irkeç M. Cataract surgery in patients with Behçet's disease. *J Cataract Refract Surg* 2002;28:316–20.
6. Foster CS, Fong LP, Singh G. Cataract surgery and intraocular lens implantation in patients with uveitis. *Ophthalmology* 1989;96:281–8.
7. Matsuo T, Takahashi M, Inoue Y, Egi K, Kuwata Y, Yamaoka A, *et al.* Ocular attacks after phacoemulsification and intraocular lens implantation in patients with Behçet disease. *Ophthalmologica* 2001;215:179–82.
8. Akova YA, Küçükerdönmez C, Gedik S. Clinical results of phacoemulsification in patients with uveitis. *Ophthalmic Surg Lasers Imaging* 2006;37:204–11.
9. Chan NSW, Ti SE, Chee SP. Decision-making and management of uveitic cataract. *Indian J Ophthalmol* 2017;65:1329–39.
10. Herbort CP, Jauch A, Othenin-Girard P, Tritten JJ, Fsadni M. Diclofenac drops to treat inflammation after cataract surgery. *Acta Ophthalmol Scand* 2000;78:421–4.
11. Dada T, Dhawan M, Garg S, Nair S, Mandal S. Safety and efficacy of intraoperative intravitreal injection of triamcinolone acetonide injection after phacoemulsification in cases of uveitic cataract. *J Cataract Refract Surg* 2007;33:1613–8.
12. Smith JR, Matthews JM, Conrad D, Hall AJ, Niederer RL, Singh-Grewal D, Tay-Kearney ML, Wells JM, Zagora SL, Australian and New Zealand Juvenile

Idiopathic Arthritis-Uveitis Working Group, McCluskey PJ. Recommendations for the management of childhood juvenile idiopathic arthritis-type chronic anterior uveitis. *Clin Exp Ophthalmol* 2021;49(1):38–45.

13. Herpetic Eye Disease Study Group. Acyclovir for the prevention of recurrent herpes simplex virus eye disease. *N Engl J Med* 1998;339:300–6.
14. Murthy SI, Pappuru RR, Latha KM, Kamat S, Sangwan VS. Surgical management in patient with uveitis. *Indian J Ophthalmol* 2013;61:284–90.
15. Ram J, Gupta A, Kumar S, Kaushik S, Gupta N, Severia S, *et al.* Phacoemulsification with intraocular lens implantation in patients with uveitis. *J Cataract Refract Surg* 2010;36:1283–8.
16. Agrawal R, Murthy S, Ganesh SK, Phaik CS, Sangwan V, Biswas J, *et al.* Cataract surgery in uveitis. *Int J Inflam* 2012;2012:548453.
17. Tran VT, LeHoang P, Herbort CP. Value of high-frequency ultrasound biomicroscopy in uveitis. *Eye (Lond)* 2001;15:23–30.
18. Ma T, Sims JL, Bennett S, Chew S, Niederer RL. High rate of conversion from ocular hypertension to glaucoma in subjects with uveitis. *Br J Ophthalmol* 2021; in press. doi: 10.1136/bjophthalmol-2021–318809.
19. Moshirfar M, Somani AN, Motlagh MN, Ronquillo YC. Management of cataract in the setting of uveitis: a review of the current literature. *Curr Opin Ophthalmol* 2020; 31(1):3–9.
20. Hazari A, Sangwan V. Cataract surgery in uveitis. *Indian J Ophthalmol* 2002;50(2):103–7.
21. Leung TG, Lindsley K, Kuo IC. Types of intraocular lenses for cataract surgery in eyes with uveitis. *Cochrane Database Syst Rev* 2014;3:CD007284.
22. Van Gelder RN, Leveque TK. Cataract surgery in the setting of uveitis. *Curr Opin Ophthalmol* 2009;20:42–5.
23. Mehta S, Linton MM, Kempen JH. Outcomes of cataract surgery in patients with uveitis: a systematic review and meta-analysis. *Am J Ophthalmol* 2014;158(4):676–92.e7.
24. Foster CS, Barrett F. Cataract development and cataract surgery in patients with juvenile rheumatoid arthritis-associated iridocyclitis. *Ophthalmology* 1993;100:809–17.
25. Fox GM, Flynn HW, Jr, Davis JL, Culbertson W. Causes of reduced visual acuity on long-term follow-up after cataract extraction in patients with uveitis and juvenile rheumatoid arthritis. *Am J Ophthalmol* 1992;114:708–14.
26. BenEzra D, Cohen E. Cataract surgery in children with chronic uveitis. *Ophthalmology* 2000;107:1255–60.
27. Quiñones K, Cervantes-Castañeda RA, Hynes AY, Daoud YJ, Foster CS. Outcomes of cataract surgery in children with chronic uveitis. *J Cataract Refract Surg* 2009;35:725–31.

28. Schmidt DC, Al-Bakri M, Rasul A, Bangsgaard R, Subhi Y, Bach-Holm D, Kessel L. Cataract surgery with or without intraocular lens implantation in pediatric uveitis: a systematic review with meta-analyses. *J Ophthalmol* 2021;2021:5481609.
29. Gungor SG, Bulam B, Akman A, Colak M. Comparison of intracameral dexamethasone and intracameral triamcinolone acetonide injection at the end of phacoemulsification surgery. *Indian J Ophthalmol* 2014;62:861–4.
30. Foster RE, Lowder CY, Meisler DM, Zakov ZN. Extracapsular cataract extraction and posterior chamber intraocular lens implantation in uveitis patients. *Ophthalmology* 1992;99:1234–41.
31. Bélair ML, Kim SJ, Thorne JE, Dunn JP, Kedhar SR, Brown DM, Jabs DA. Incidence of cystoid macular edema after cataract surgery in patients with and without uveitis using optical coherence tomography. *Am J Ophthalmol* 2009;148(1):128–35.e2.
32. Llop SM, Papaliodis GN. Cataract surgery complications in uveitis patients: a review article. *Semin Ophthalmol* 2018;33(1):64–9.
33. Han JV, Patel DV, Squirrell D, McGhee CN. Cystoid macular edema following cataract surgery: A review. *Clin Exp Ophthalmol* 2019;47(3):346–56.
34. Ghasemi Falavarjani K, Parvaresh MM, Modarres M, Hashemi M, Samiy N. Intravitreal bevacizumab for pseudophakic cystoid macular edema; a systematic review. *J Ophthalmic Vis Res* 2012;7(3):235–9.
35. Taylor SR, Habot-Wilner Z, Pacheco P, Lightman S. Intraocular methotrexate in the treatment of uveitis and uveitic cystoid macular edema. *Ophthalmology* 2009;116(4):797–801.
36. Tranos P, Scott R, Zambarakji H, Ayliffe W, Pavesio C, Charteris DG. The effect of pars plana vitrectomy on cystoid macular edema associated with chronic uveitis: a randomised, controlled pilot study. *Br J Ophthalmol* 2006;90(9):1107–10.
37. Beer PM, Bakri SJ, Singh RJ, Liu W, Peters GB III, Miller M. Intraocular concentration and pharmacokinetics of triamcinolone acetonide after a single intravitreal injection. *Ophthalmology* 2003;110(4):681–6.
38. Thorne JE, Sugar EA, Holbrook JT, Burke AE, Altaweel MM, Vitale AT, Acharya NR, Kempen JH, Jabs DA, Multicenter Uveitis Steroid Treatment Trial Research Group. Periocular Triamcinolone vs. intravitreal Triamcinolone vs. intravitreal dexamethasone implant for the treatment of uveitic macular edema: the PeriOcular vs. INTravitreal corticosteroids for uveitic macular edema (POINT) trial. *Ophthalmology* 2019;126(2):283–95.
39. Krishna R, Meisler DM, Lowder CY, Estafanous M, Foster RE. Long-term follow-up of extracapsular cataract extraction and posterior chamber

intraocular lens implantation in patients with uveitis. *Ophthalmology* 1998;105(9):1765–9.

40. Kawaguchi T, Mochizuki M, Miyata K, Miyata N. Phacoemulsification cataract extraction and intraocular lens implantation in patients with uveitis. *J Cataract Refract Surg* 2007;33(2):305–9.
41. Steinert RF, Puliafito CA, Kumar SR, Dudak SD, Patel S. Cystoid macular edema, retinal detachment, and glaucoma after Nd:YAG laser posterior capsulotomy. *Am J Ophthalmol* 1991;112(4):373–80.
42. Küçükerdönmez C, Beutel J, Bartz-Schmidt KU, Gelisken F. Treatment of chronic ocular hypotony with intraocular application of sodium hyaluronate. *Br J Ophthalmol* 2009;93(2):235–9.
43. Edmunds MR, Madge SN. Profound hypotony maculopathy in a first episode of bilateral idiopathic acute anterior uveitis. *BMC Ophthalmol* 2015;15:116.
44. Bhargava R, Kumar P, Sharma SK, Kumar M, Kaur A. Phacoemulsification versus small incision cataract surgery in patients with uveitis. *Int J Ophthalmol* 2015;8(5):965–70.
45. Yangzes S, Seth NG, Singh R, Gupta PC, Jinagal J, Pandav SS, Gupta V, Gupta A, Ram J. Long-term outcomes of cataract surgery in children with uveitis. *Indian J Ophthalmol* 2019;67(4):490–5.
46. O'Rourke M, McCreery K, Kilmartin D, Brosnahan D. Pediatric cataract in the uveitis setting. *Eur J Ophthalmol* 2021;31(5):2651–8.

https://doi.org/10.1142/9789811251474_0012

Chapter 12 Practical Approach to Managing the Uveitis Patient

Rachael Niederer,[*,†] Sue Lightman,[‡,§] Oren Tomkins-Netzer[¶,||]*

12.1 Case 1 — Acute Anterior Uveitis (AAU)

A 35-year-old woman complains of a red and painful right eye. She reports blurred vision and sensitivity to light. No known previous medical or ocular history.

12.1.1 *History and Symptoms*

Patients with AAU typically complain of new onset ocular pain that developed over several days, followed by blurred vision. The pain is of a deep boring type and not sharp or irritating, as is seen with cases of conjunctivitis or conjunctival foreign bodies. Other symptoms include a red eye, photophobia and new floaters.

Patients will occasionally confuse the symptoms with ocular surface inflammation including viral conjunctivitis, which could delay seeking

* Department of Ophthalmology, Auckland District Health Board, Auckland, New Zealand
† University of Auckland, Auckland, New Zealand
‡ UCL Institute of Ophthalmology, University College London, London, UK
§ University of the Highlands and Islands, Inverness, UK
¶ Uveitis Service, Ophthalmology Department, Lady Davis Carmel Medical Center, Haifa, Israel
|| Ruth and Bruch Rappaport Faculty of Medicine, Technion — Israel Institute of Technology, Haifa, Israel

medical treatment. AAU typically does not have ocular discharge and is painful instead of irritating.

It is important to ascertain if this is a first event and whether the patient can recall any prodrome, such as beginning treatment with new medication, recent viral infection or underlying systemic condition (see Table 12.1 for related conditions).

Table 12.1. Etiologies related to AAU.

Condition	Clinical findings	Investigations
HLA-B27-associated uveitis (see Chapter 5)	*Hx*: known seronegative spondyloarthropathy or inflammatory bowel disease *Symptoms*: arthralgia; previous gastrointestinal complaints; previous urinary complaints; skin lesions or rashes *Signs*: hypopyon	HLA-B27 Sacroiliac and lumbar spine X-ray Refer to a rheumatologist
Tubulointerstitial nephritis and uveitis (TINU, see Chapter 5)	*Hx*: recent systemic flu-like illness *Signs*: bilateral disease	β-2-microglobulin levels ESR Urine analysis for casts Refer to a nephrologist
Phacolytic uveitis	*Signs*: a mature or hypermature cataract	
Infectious endophthalmitis (see Chapter 6)	*Hx*: recent intraocular surgery or trauma, intravenous drug user, indwelling vascular catheter, diabetes mellites *Signs*: painful, injected eye; hypopyon; vitritis; retinal hemorrhage, vasculitis, retinitis	Vitreous biopsy and intravitreal injection of antibiotics
Viral uveitis (see Chapter 6)	*Signs*: raised intraocular pressure	Consider anterior chamber biopsy and PCR for CMV, HSV, VZV
Drug-induced uveitis (see Chapter 7, Table 7.1)	*Hx*: related drugs Rifabutin Systemic fluoroquinolone Bisphosphonates Sulfonamides	

(*Continued*)

Table 12.1. (*Continued*)

Condition	Clinical findings	Investigations
	Diethylcarbamazine Anticancer immunotherapies Etanercept	
Vaccine-related uveitis	*Hx*: recent vaccination Influenza BCG Hepatitis A Hepatitis B MMR Varicella Human papillomavirus (HPV) COVID-19	

BCG = Bacilli Calmette-Guerin; CMV = cytomegalovirus; COVID = coronavirus disease; ESR = erythrocyte sedimentation rate; HLA = human leukocyte antigen; HPV = human papillomavirus; HSV = herpes simplex virus; MMR = measles-mumps-rubella; PCR = polymerase chain reaction; VZV = varicella zoster virus

Systems review: Patients should be asked about arthralgia, lower back pain, gastrointestinal complaints and skin rashes.

12.1.2 *Examination and Signs*

Visual acuity ranges from normal to moderately reduced.

The **conjunctiva** is typically mildly to moderately injected and ciliary flush can be seen. The **cornea** is clear, unless the intraocular pressure (IOP) is elevated or the endothelium is covered with extensive keratic precipitates (KPs, Figure 12.1). These are commonly located in the lower third of the cornea (Arlt's triangle) but can also be diffusely spread over the entire cornea. KPs can be small and discrete (stellate, see Chapter 5, Figure 5.7) or large (mutton fat or granulomatous). Granulomatous KPs are considered related to granulomatous systemic diseases (tuberculosis, sarcoidosis), but are a non-specific sign.

The **anterior chamber** is the main site of inflammation with cells and flare the prominent findings. The extent of inflammation can vary from a few occasional cells (+0.5) to a hypopyon, and fibrin strands across the pupil (Tables 12.2 and 12.3). Consider Behçet's disease if hypopyon occurs in a white eye. Examining for posterior synechia is important and

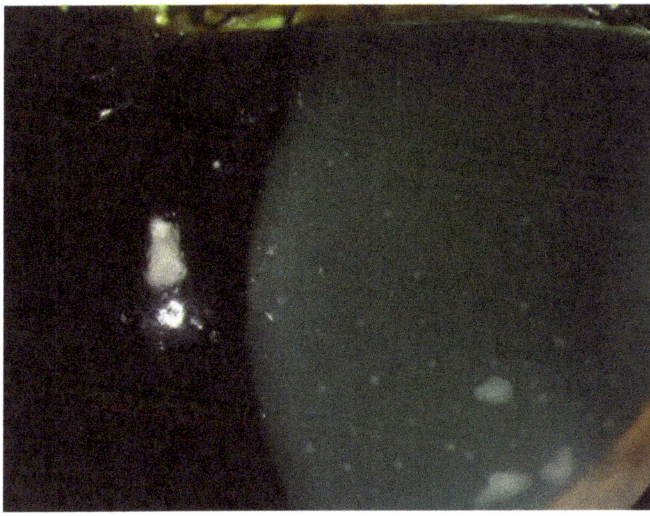

Figure 12.1. Granulomatous keratic precipitates in a patient with acute anterior uveitis.

Table 12.2. SUN Working Group grading for anterior chamber cells.[1]

Grade	Cell number
0	<1
0.5+	1–5
1+	6–15
2+	16–25
3+	25–50
4+	>50

Table 12.3. SUN Working Group grading for anterior chamber flare.[1]

Grade	Flare description
0	None
1+	Faint
2+	Moderate (iris and lens details clear)
3+	Marked (iris and lens details hazy)
4+	Intense (fibrin or plastic aqueous)

pupils should always be dilated. The **lens** tends to be clear on first events but repeat relapses can result in development of a cataract. **IOP** can range from elevated to low and requires repeat monitoring during treatment and follow-up. The **retina** should always be examined and a hyperemic optic nerve or macula edema can be found, particularly in children or young adults.

12.1.3 *Investigations*

Need for systemic investigations depends on findings during the history, review of systems and ocular examination. In most cases patients should undergo a complete blood count, liver function test, urine analysis, erythrocyte sedimentation rate, C-reactive protein and test for syphilis (see Chapter 4). Other investigations should focus on common etiologies related to AAU and depend on combinations of ocular and systemic findings (Table 12.1). In cases of AAU with raised IOP, consider performing an anterior chamber tap and polymerase chain reaction test (PCR) for a viral cause.

In a case of first event of unilateral AAU in a young patient, with no findings on review of systems or relevant history, one can consider not performing systemic investigations.

12.1.4 *Early Management*

Control of the intraocular inflammation using topical corticosteroids is the cornerstone of treatment. The goal of treatment is to rapidly achieve a state of no inflammation. Frequency of treatment depends on the extent of inflammation seen on examination, but hourly treatment is a common starting dose. Treatment is reduced weekly with repeat follow-ups to ascertain inflammatory control and IOP control (see Chapter 9).

Short- to medium-acting topical mydriatics are used to keep the pupil mobile and prevent the development of posterior synechia while inflammation is active. Depending on the half-life of the drug, repeat daily installations may be needed to maintain pupil mobility (Table 12.4).

Antihypertensive medications are used in cases with ocular hypertension and continued until IOP returns to normal values.

Table 12.4. Commonly used mydriatics.

Agent	Onset of action	Duration of action
Phenylephrine HCl	30–60 min	3–5 hrs
Tropicamide	20–40 min	4–6 hrs
Cyclopentolate HCl	30–60 min	1–2 d
Atropine sulfate	45–120 min	7–14 d

12.1.5 *Managing Complications*

If **posterior synechia** are found on examination an attempt should made to break them to prevent future development of pupillary block. Posterior synechia can be broken pharmacologically or mechanically. Pharmacological synechiolysis is performed using mydriatic agents. These can be given topically by repeat instillation of combinations of drugs or subconjunctival injection. Long-acting mydriatics should not be used during active inflammation so that new posterior synechia with a fully dilated pupil do not develop.

Posterior synechia that remain for longer than 72 hours are less likely to break pharmacologically and mechanical synechiolysis should be considered. This is usually performed during elective cataract surgery. In case of pupillary block with increased IOP, penetrating iridectomy should be performed immediately.

If **cystoid macular edema** (CME) is suspected an optical coherence tomography (OCT) scan should be performed. In case of CME consider adding systemic corticosteroids at a dose of 1 mg/kg/day on a tapering regime or local corticosteroid injections (see Chapter 9). Repeat OCT scans are done during follow-up to demonstrate response to treatment.

12.2 Case 2 — Recurrent Anterior Uveitis (RAU)

A 32-year-old man has repeat episodes of a red painful eye. On examination there are signs of anterior uveitis and according to his previous ocular history this is his third relapse over the last 2 years. He reports lower back pain for the past several months.

Some patients with anterior uveitis have repeat relapses, requiring re-initiation of topical and/or systemic immunosuppression. Recurrent anterior uveitis (RAU) is defined as relapsing inflammation separated by >3 months without treatment.[1]

12.2.1 *History and Symptoms*

Relapses typically occur in a single eye, though they can alternate between sides. Symptoms include pain or photophobia, circumlimbal redness and anterior chamber cells and flare. Patients with anterior uveitis usually complain of pain, redness, blurred vision, and photophobia.[2]

Systems review: Patients should be questioned about systemic signs like unexplained fever, pain in the joints or back, recent trips to endemic regions, gastrointestinal complaints, rashes, and any family medical history of rheumatologic or neurologic diseases.

Although RAU can be associated with systemic findings, in over 50% of cases there is no evidence of systemic disease (Table 12.5). The most common non-infectious systemic association is with ankylosing spondylitis (HLA-B27 positive), which affects predominantly young males and is characterized by acute unilateral recurrent anterior uveitis. Ankylosing

Table 12.5. Etiologies related to recurrent anterior uveitis (RAU).

Condition	Clinical findings	Investigations
HLA-B27-associated uveitis (see Chapter 5)	*Hx*: known seronegative spondyloarthropathy or inflammatory bowel disease *Symptoms*: arthralgia; previous gastrointestinal complaints; previous urinary complaints; skin lesions or rashes *Signs*: hypopyon; recurrent alternating disease	HLA-B27 Sacroiliac and lumbar back X-ray Refer to a rheumatologist
Viral uveitis (see Chapter 6)	Signs: raised intraocular pressure	Consider anterior chamber biopsy and PCR for CMV, HSV, VZV
Posner-Schlossman syndrome (see Chapter 5)	*Signs*: mild inflammation, non-granulomatous KPs, raised intraocular pressure	

CMV = cytomegalovirus; HLA = human leukocyte antigen; HSV = herpes simplex virus; KP = keratic precipitates; PCR = polymerase chain reaction; VZV = varicella zoster virus; HLA = human leukocyte antigen

spondylitis is most commonly associated with RAU, up to a third of which develop uveitis.[3] Sacroiliitis with morning stiffness that improves with exercise is the most common systemic symptom (see Chapter 5).[4]

12.2.2 *Examination and Signs*

Visual acuity ranges from normal to severely reduced.

The **cornea** may show granulomatous or non-granulomatous KPs. The degree of **anterior chamber** inflammation varies from few cells to a fibrinous hypopyon (see Chapter 5, Figure 5.1). **IOP** is usually normal but may be elevated following recurrent relapses. Subsequently, recurrent episodes of intraocular inflammation can lead to intraocular complications including posterior synechia, cataract, glaucoma and CME.

12.2.3 *Investigations*

Systemic investigations should be completed for all patients with RAU, focusing on general inflammatory indices (complete blood count, erythrocyte sedimentation rate, C-reactive protein) and HLA-B27. Additional tests include syphilis serology, serum angiotensin-converting enzyme (ACE) and tests for tuberculosis (see Chapter 4). Following a complete review of systems, more directed tests for possible gastrointestinal, axial or dermatologic involvement should be considered. If indicated, refer patients to a rheumatologist or gastroenterologist for further evaluation. A chest and sacroiliac X-ray should be considered in all patients, particularly those complaining of morning stiffness or low back pain. In cases of RAU with raised IOP and signs suggestive of CMV or herpetic uveitis (see Chapter 6), consider performing an anterior chamber tap and PCR for a viral cause.

12.2.4 *Early Management*

Topical corticosteroids are effective in managing episodes of active anterior uveitis in patients. In most cases, a rapid tapering of treatment maintains inflammatory control.

In cases with frequent relapses (>2 per year), long-term treatment at ≤2 times/day should be considered to prevent further relapses. Treatment at this dose can be maintained for months before an attempt is made to discontinue. Studies in children with juvenile idiopathic arthritis (JIA)-associated uveitis demonstrated that if the inflammation is controlled at this dose, the incidence of cataract formation was 0.0/eye year (see Chapter 9).[5,6]

If prevention of relapses cannot be maintained with topical treatment, systemic corticosteroids then 2nd-line immunosuppression agents can be added (see Chapter 10).

12.3 Case 3 — Chronic Anterior Uveitis (CAU)

A 23-year-old woman with known anterior uveitis in her left eye returns with complaints of pain and blurred vision. She has had previous similar episodes that responded to topical corticosteroids but relapsed several weeks after stopping treatment. Her last relapse was 2 months ago and she is now still taking corticosteroids drops at a frequency of 3 times a day.

Chronic anterior uveitis (CAU) is defined as persisting inflammation of the anterior chamber with relapses in under 3 months after discontinuing treatment. This includes cases that relapse after treatment was stopped and those when inflammation relapses during tapering.

12.3.1 *History and Symptoms*

Patients with CAU will return to the ophthalmologist with renewed symptoms as the treatment is tapered or discontinued. Typically, symptoms recur within 4 weeks of stopping treatment, but relapses can occur even after months. Symptoms tend to be similar to those of acute anterior uveitis, but in patients still receiving corticosteroids active inflammation may be asymptomatic. Therefore, patients with CAU need to continue follow-up, even if quiescent.

Past medical history: ask about constitutional symptoms (malaise, fever, weight loss), pulmonary complaints, arthralgia, rashes and contact with known tuberculosis patients.

Systems review: Causes of CAU include both infectious and non-infectious diseases, and patients should complete an extensive medical history and review of systems (see Table 12.6 for related conditions).

Table 12.6. Etiologies related to chronic anterior uveitis (CAU).

Condition	Clinical findings	Investigations
Fuchs' uveitis syndrome (see Chapter 5)	*Signs*: unilateral, low-grade inflammation, diffuse non-granulomatous, stellate KPs, heterochromia	
Sarcoidosis (see Chapter 5)	*Hx*: pulmonary complaints *Signs*: bilateral, granulomatous KPs, iris nodules, peripheral anterior synechia	ACE, CBC (for lymphopenia) CXR
Juvenile idiopathic arthritis-associated uveitis (see Chapter 5)	Young children *Hx*: often pre-existing JIA *Symptoms*: no history of an injected eye or painful eye, arthralgia *Signs*: ocular complications found at presentation (cataract, posterior synechia, band keratopathy)	ANA, referral to a rheumatologist
Tubulointerstitial nephritis and uveitis (TINU, see Chapter 5)	*Hx*: recent systemic flu-like illness *Signs*: bilateral disease	β-2-microglobulin levels ESR Urine analysis for casts Refer to a nephrologist
Herpetic keratouveitis (see Chapter 6)	*Signs*: unilateral, corneal opacifications, sectoral iris atrophy, raised intraocular pressure	Serology for HSV, VZV
Tubercular uveitis (see Chapter 6)	*Hx*: pulmonary disease *Signs*: granulomatous KPs	PPD, IGRA (see Chapter 4) CXR
Syphilitic uveitis (see Chapter 6)	*Signs*: granulomatous KPs, rash over palms or soles	Syphilis serology (see Chapter 4)

ACE = angiotensin-converting enzyme; ANA = anti-nuclear antibody; CXR = chest X-ray; HSV = herpes simplex virus; Hx = history; IGRA = interferon-gamma release assay; PPD = purified protein derivative (a type of tuberculin skin test); VZV = varicella zoster virus

12.3.2 *Examination and Signs*

Ocular findings are similar to those seen in acute anterior uveitis. The presence of complications is more likely as the inflammation persists.

Visual acuity ranges from normal to severely reduced.

The **cornea** may have KPs, which could be granulomatous or non-granulomatous. Unilateral inflammation with diffuse stellate KPs suggests Fuchs' uveitis syndrome (FUS, see Chapter 5, Figure 5.7). Presence of band keratopathy at presentation, with no history of previous uveitis, suggests ongoing, low-grade inflammation and is typical in children with juvenile idiopathic arthritis (JIA)-associated uveitis (see Chapter 5, Figure 5.11).

With repeat relapses the **iris** may develop atrophy, which can be diffuse or sectoral. Sectoral iris atrophy is suggestive of herpetic uveitis (see Chapter 6, Figure 6.3). With repeat relapses heterochromia may develop, suggesting FUS (see Chapter 5, Figure 5.8). Anterior or posterior synechia can develop during active inflammation, and if not resolved within 72 hours may persist for years (see Chapter 5, Figure 5.10). Tent-shaped peripheral anterior synechia covering the irido-corneal angle suggests a diagnosis of sarcoidosis (see Chapter 2, Figure 2.13). **IOP** can be elevated or low, but is commonly high in herpetic uveitis. In cases with extensive inflammation, particularly children, posterior involvement can be found. The **optic disc** can become swollen and hyperemic, and macular edema can develop. These posterior findings improve with control of the anterior inflammation, though specific treatment is needed in persistent cases.

12.3.3 *Investigations*

Systemic investigation should be completed for all patients with CAU (Table 12.6). Commonly performed tests include ACE, serology for syphilis, tests for tuberculosis and serology for Lyme disease in endemic regions. Consider performing an anterior chamber tap and PCR for herpes simplex virus, varicella zoster virus and cytomegalovirus. A chest X-ray should also be ordered in most patients and a urine analysis completed if not previously done. Other blood tests and imaging should be directed based on clinical findings, medical history and review of systems.

In children with no history of previous uveitis consider testing ANA and referring to a rheumatologist to rule out JIA (see Chapter 4).

12.3.4 *Early Management*

Treatment of active CAU is similar to that for acute anterior uveitis; control of the inflammation with corticosteroids is the cornerstone to treatment. Mydriatics and antihypertensive drugs should be used as indicated.

Tapering of treatment should be gradual. Once inflammation control is achieved with topical corticosteroids given at ≤2 times/day, maintain treatment for an extended time to prevent relapse. Treatment at this dose can be maintained for months before an attempt is made to discontinue (see Chapter 9).

If inflammation is not controlled with topical corticosteroids at a dose of ≤2 times/day, systemic corticosteroids should be introduced. An acceptable dose of systemic prednisone for controlling anterior uveitis is 0.5 mg/kg on a tapering regimen. In children with JIA-associated uveitis, methotrexate is used as a first-line systemic drug.

12.3.5 *Managing Complications*

Ocular complications in CAU are similar to those that develop in AAU or recurrent anterior uveitis and are related to uncontrolled inflammation.

Careful consideration should be given to adverse effects of extensive treatment with corticosteroids. IOP should be measured at every follow-up and signs of cataract progression noted. Extensive use of corticosteroids typically results in development of a posterior subcapsular cataract (Figure 12.2), which may require surgery if affecting visual acuity or visualization of the retina.

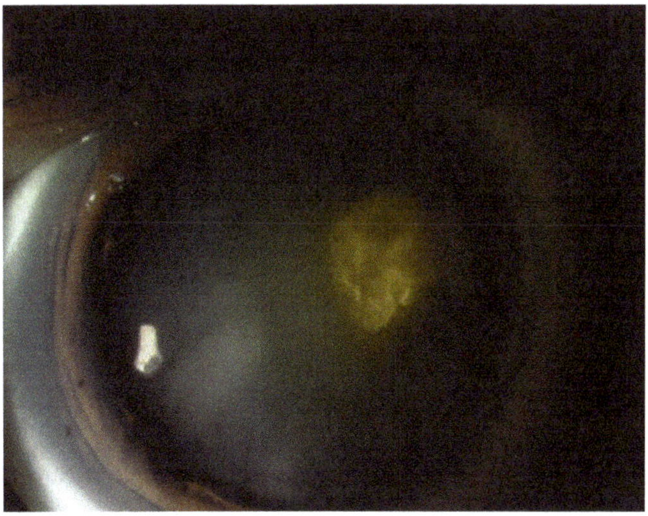

Figure 12.2. Posterior subcapsular cataract in a patient with sarcoidosis.

12.4 Case 4 — Intermediate Uveitis (IU)

An 18-year-old woman complains of blurred vision and new floaters in her right eye. She is systemically healthy with no previous ocular complaints.

In intermediate uveitis (IU) the main site of inflammation is in the vitreous cavity, and vitreous cells and haze are needed to make a diagnosis of vitritis. However, because of the proximity of the vitreous to the anterior chamber and retina, the inflammation can manifest as symptoms related to these structures.

12.4.1 *History and Symptoms*

Patients with IU complain of blurred, hazy, painless reduced vision, accompanied by new floaters. If there is spillover of cells into the anterior chamber, symptoms of anterior uveitis are also reported including a red, painful eye or photophobia. Vitritis can result in the development of CME, an epiretinal membrane, a swollen optic disc and cataract.

Past medical history: Patient history should concentrate on the duration of symptoms, frequency of recurrences or any complaints that may suggest a systemic disease. Fatigue, night sweats or pulmonary complaints are suggestive of sarcoidosis or tuberculosis. Arthritis can be related to Lyme disease or sarcoidosis, and rashes to Lyme disease, syphilis or sarcoidosis. Special focus should be on neurologic complaints due to an association with multiple sclerosis in up to 10% of patients with IU.

Systems review: Causes of IU include both infectious and non-infectious diseases and patients should complete an extensive medical history and review of systems (see Table 12.7 for related conditions). In up to two-thirds of cases the investigations are negative and a diagnosis of idiopathic IU is reached.

12.4.2 *Examination and Signs*

Visual acuity is usually reduced and patients complain of floaters.

In the **anterior chamber** cells and flare can be seen with an increase in **IOP**. The **vitreous** will have cells and haze (scored based on the SUN classification, see Chapter 2, Table 2.11). Finding snowballs is indicative

Table 12.7. Etiologies related to intermediate uveitis (IU).

Condition	Clinical findings	Investigations
Multiple sclerosis-associated uveitis (see Chapter 5)	*Symptoms*: systemic neurological complaints or deficits, history of previous optic neuritis	Complete neurological examination, brain MRI
Sarcoidosis (see Chapter 5)	*Hx*: pulmonary complaints *Signs*: bilateral	CBC, ACE, CXR
Lyme disease (see Chapter 6)	*Hx*: residence in an endemic region	Serology for *Borrelia burgdorferi*
Tubercular uveitis (see Chapter 6)	*Hx*: exposure to patients with active TB or from endemic region, pulmonary complaints	PPD, IGRA (see Chapter 4) CXR
Syphilitic uveitis (see Chapter 6)	*Signs*: rash over palms or soles	Syphilis serology (see Chapter 4)
Primary vitreoretinal lymphoma/primary central nervous system lymphoma (see Chapter 7)	*Hx*: age at presentation 5th–6th decade *Signs*: dense vitreous cells in veil pattern, subretinal infiltrates	Vitreous biopsy for cytology, IgH gene rearrangement and IL-10:IL-6 ratio

ACE = angiotensin-converting enzyme; bMRI = brain magnetic resonance imaging; CXR = chest X-ray; IGRA = interferon-gamma release assay; IL = interleukin; PPD = purified protein derivative (a type of tuberculin skin test)

of vitritis (see Chapter 2, Figure 2.21), though they may persist even years after the inflammation is quiet. Their presence is used to determine IU but do not reflect active inflammation. In disease relapses more snowballs can appear and patients typically complain of new floaters. Careful examination of the inferior retina and vitreous is needed to detect snowbanks and they must be followed for developing neovascularization, retinal traction and rarely retinal detachment (see Chapter 2, Figure 2.22).

Examination of the **retina** can reveal a hyperemic, swollen **optic disc**, foveal thickening and peripheral vascular sheathing (Figure 12.3). Presence of subtle subretinal lesions may suggest birdshot chorioretinitis (see Chapter 5, Figure 5.23).

Ocular investigations should include a fluorescein angiography to determine optic nerve involvement, CME or vascular leakage (Figure 12.4). Consider ICG looking for granulomatous disease in the choroid or birdshot chorioretinitis, and consider autofluorescence to look for subtle changes in vitreoretinal lymphoma. OCT is used to document CME and response to treatment (Figure 12.5) and to assess epiretinal membrane.

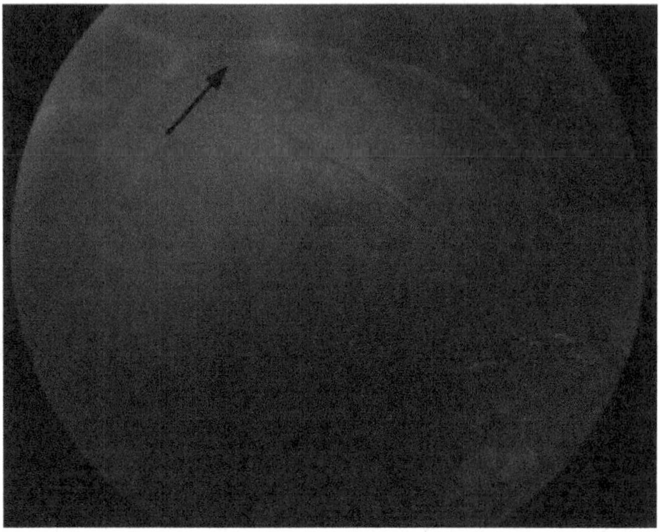

Figure 12.3. Vascular sheathing in a patient with intermediate uveitis.

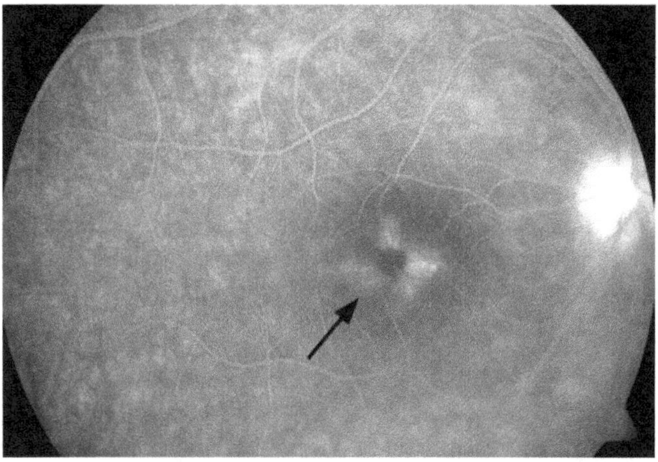

Figure 12.4. Fluorescein angiography showing cystoid macular edema appearing as a petaloid pattern (arrow) and a hot disc, in a patient with intermediate uveitis.

12.4.3 *Investigations*

Systemic investigations should be completed for all patients with IU (Table 12.7). Patients should undergo tests for ACE, serology for syphilis and tests for tuberculosis (see Chapter 4). Serology for Lyme disease

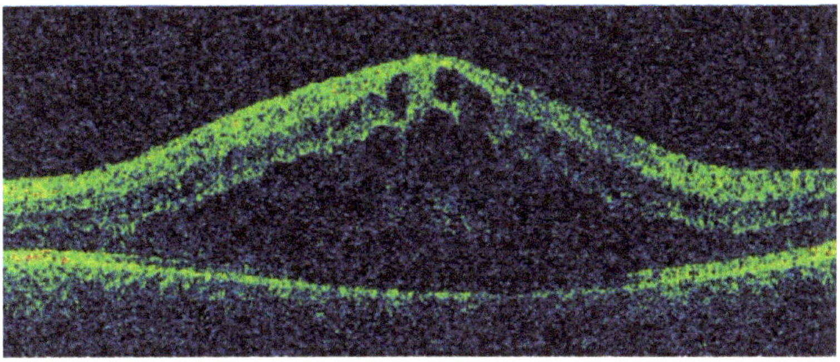

Figure 12.5. Optical coherence tomography of cystoid macular edema in a patient with multiple sclerosis-associated intermediate uveitis.

should be performed if patient is from an endemic region. Consider investigations for TINU if aged <40 years or if creatinine is abnormal. A chest X-ray should also be ordered. Other blood tests and imaging should be directed based on clinical findings, medical history and review of systems.

Following the introduction of modern treatment options for multiple sclerosis, a neurologic exam should be conducted, and consider referring patients to a neurologist for complete evaluation, including a brain magnetic resonance imaging, and initiate early systemic treatment if needed.

12.4.4 *Early Management*

Treatment of active IU depends on the extent of visual deterioration, presence of complications like CME or raised IOP and patient complaints of floaters. In patients with mild inflammation, no complications and no visual complaints, treatment may not be required, and patients can just be followed.

When the decision to treat is made, choice of treatment is based on whether the disease is bilateral and if there is a systemic disease. If an infective cause is identified, specific treatment is needed to address the underlying illness.

In non-infectious IU, treatment focuses on the ocular complications. In general, if only one eye is active, local periocular or intravitreal injections can be used (see Chapter 9). However, in bilateral disease, or if a systemic disease is associated with the IU, systemic immunosuppression is required. Because IU is a chronic disease and relapses are common, treatment is given for long periods of time. Corticosteroids should be tapered to a safe dose (≤7.5 mg/day) and if quiescent disease cannot be maintained, 2nd-line immunosuppression and biologics agents should be used.

Local injections can be used as adjunctive treatment to systemic medication in cases of persistent or asymmetric disease. For vitritis, periocular corticosteroid injections may be adequate, but CME usually requires intravitreal injections (see Chapter 9 – results of the POINT study).[7]

Long-term studies demonstrate that with good inflammatory control, visual acuity can be maintained and the majority of patients retain good vision.[8]

12.5 Case 5 — Panuveitis

A 40-year-old woman presents with photophobia, floaters and blurring of vision. On examination she has panuveitis.

Panuveitis is a common clinical presentation. The differential diagnosis can be found in Chapter 2, Table 2.15 and includes inflammatory disease such as sarcoidosis, Vogt-Koyanagi-Harada syndrome (VKH), sympathetic ophthalmia and Behçet's disease, infectious causes such as toxoplasmosis, syphilis, endophthalmitis, tuberculosis and acute retinal necrosis, and also masquerade syndromes such as lymphoma or trauma.

12.5.1 *History and Symptoms*

Patients with panuveitis will often present with floaters and visual blur. Pain, photophobia and redness are features in more acute presentations if the anterior chamber is involved, but some chronic cases may have anterior chamber inflammation without symptoms. Attention should be paid to the speed of onset of symptoms, whether symptoms are bilateral or unilateral, and whether they have had a fluctuating or recurrent course.

Past ocular history, in particular previous ocular surgery or trauma, should be sought. Past medical history is important, including any pre-existing diagnosis of sarcoidosis, tuberculosis, human immunodeficiency virus (HIV), and other immune compromise.

Systems review should include constitutional symptoms (fevers, malaise), shortness of breath or cough (for sarcoidosis or tuberculosis), mouth or genital ulcers, arthritis, skin rashes or shortness of breath (for Behçet's disease), central nervous system symptoms (for lymphoma and VKH). Patients should be asked for any history of rash, in particular rash over tattoos (sarcoidosis) or rash over palms of hands (syphilis). Risk factors for syphilis and HIV should be asked, and patients should also be asked about possible intravenous drug use as this can increase risk for endogenous endophthalmitis. See Table 12.8 for symptoms and investigations of possible etiologies.

Table 12.8. Etiologies related to panuveitis.

Condition	Clinical findings	Investigations
Sarcoidosis (see Chapter 5)	*Symptoms*: cough, shortness of breath *Signs*: granulomatous uveitis, multifocal choroiditis, vasculitis	Serum ACE, CBC (for lymphopenia) CXR
Vogt-Koyanagi-Harada syndrome (see Chapter 5)	*Symptoms*: headache, neck stiffness, tinnitus *Signs*: bilateral disease, optic nerve swelling, multifocal retinal detachments	Lumbar puncture Audiometry
Sympathetic ophthalmia (see Chapter 5)	*Hx*: previous surgery or trauma *Signs*: Dalen Fuchs' nodules	
Behçet's disease (see Chapter 5)	*Hx*: mouth and genital ulcers, DVT/PE *Symptoms*: explosive onset *Signs*: hypopyon in a white eye, retinitis, hemorrhage	HLA-B51 Refer to rheumatologist
Toxoplasmosis (see Chapter 6)	*Hx*: may have previous episodes *Signs*: retinochoroiditis adjacent to retinal scar, or retinitis with no scar in primary toxoplasmosis; may have elevated intraocular pressure	Toxoplasmosis serology Toxoplasmosis PCR from anterior chamber or vitreous if atypical

(*Continued*)

Table 12.8. (*Continued*)

Condition	Clinical findings	Investigations
Syphilitic uveitis (see Chapter 6)	*Hx*: may have risk factors for sexually transmitted infection *Symptoms*: rash over palms of hands *Signs*: placoid retinitis, optic nerve swelling	Syphilis serology (see Chapter 4)
Tubercular uveitis (see Chapter 6)	*Hx*: may have TB exposure *Symptoms*: cough, shortness of breath *Signs*: granulomatous uveitis, multifocal choroiditis	PPD, IGRA (see Chapter 4) CXR
Acute retinal necrosis (see Chapter 6)	*Hx*: may have history of neonatal encephalitis/meningitis *Signs*: peripheral retinitis and hemorrhage	Anterior chamber or vitreous tap for viral PCR
Infectious endophthalmitis (see Chapter 6)	*Hx*: recent surgery or bacteremia/candidemia	Anterior chamber or vitreous tap for microscopy Blood cultures and systemic workup if suspected endogenous

ACE = angiotensin-converting enzyme; CBC = complete blood count; CXR = chest X-ray; DVT = deep vein thrombosis; IGRA = interferon-gamma release assay; IL = interleukin; PE = pulmonary embolism; PCR = polymerase chain reaction; PPD = purified protein derivative (a type of tuberculin skin test)

12.5.2 *Examination and Signs*

Visual acuity ranges from normal to severely reduced.

The **conjunctiva** may be injected or white. The **cornea** may show granulomatous (Figure 12.6) or non-granulomatous KPs (see Chapter 5, Figure 5.7). **Anterior chamber** inflammation can be graded using the SUN grading system (Table 12.2). Posterior synechiae may be present and **iris** nodules should be specifically looked for within the body of the iris (Bussacca) and along the pupillary margin (Koeppe) (Figure 12.7).

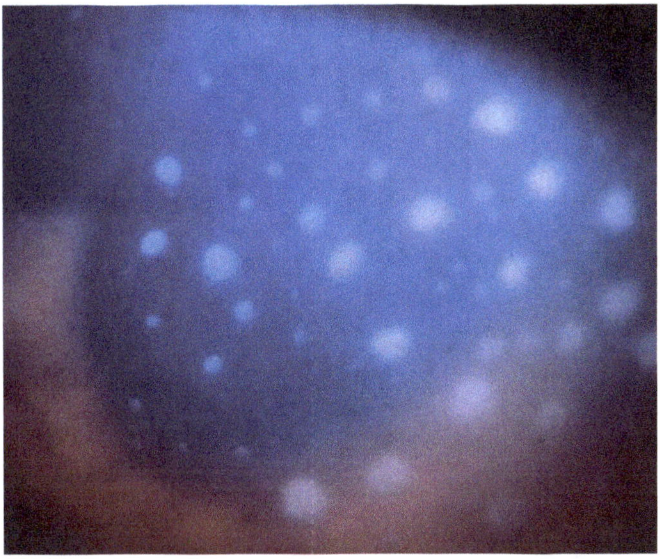

Figure 12.6. Mutton fat keratic precipitates in a patient with tuberculosis.

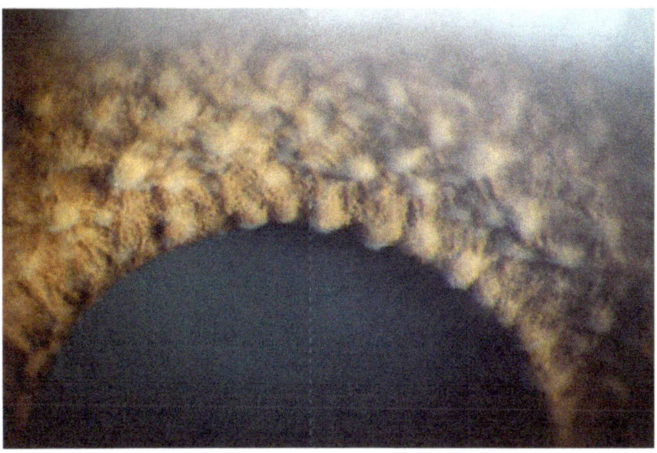

Figure 12.7. Koeppe nodule.

Gonioscopy may reveal peripheral anterior synechiae (in particular tent-shaped peripheral anterior synechiae in sarcoidosis, see Chapter 2, Figure 2.13) and possibly angle nodules (Berlin nodules). **IOP** is usually normal, but may be elevated in infectious etiologies, particularly varicella zoster virus (VZV), herpes simplex virus (HSV) or toxoplasmosis, or in

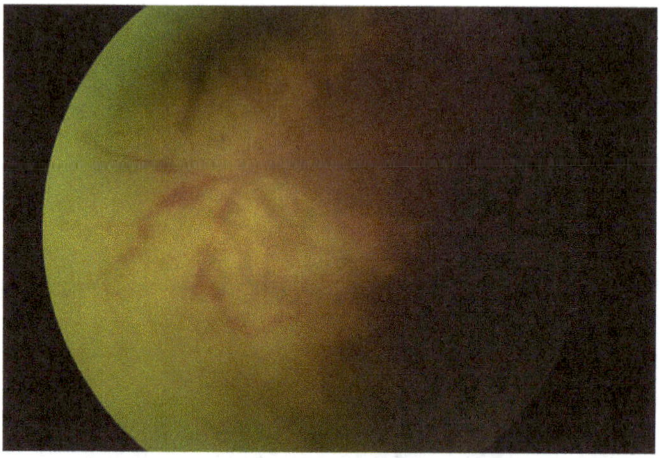

Figure 12.8. Retinitis in acute retinal necrosis.

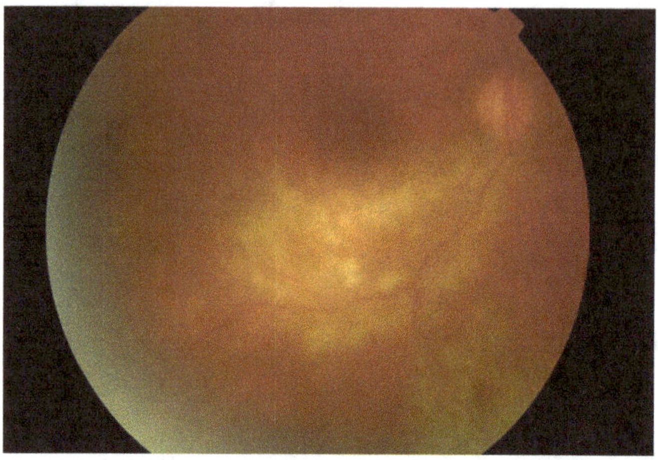

Figure 12.9. Retinitis in cytomegalovirus.

delayed presentations with chronic disease (see Chapter 2, Table 2.13). Cataract may give evidence of chronic inflammation.

Anterior **vitreous** inflammation and vitreous haze may be graded by SUN grading (see Chapter 2, Tables 2.7 and 2.9). Dilated fundal examination may reveal clues to the etiology. **Retinitis** is suggestive of infectious etiology (Figures 12.8 and 12.9) or Behçet's disease (Figure 12.10) (see Chapter 2, Table 2.10). A scar adjacent to an area of retinitis may strongly suggest a diagnosis of toxoplasmosis (Figure 12.11). Peripheral retini-

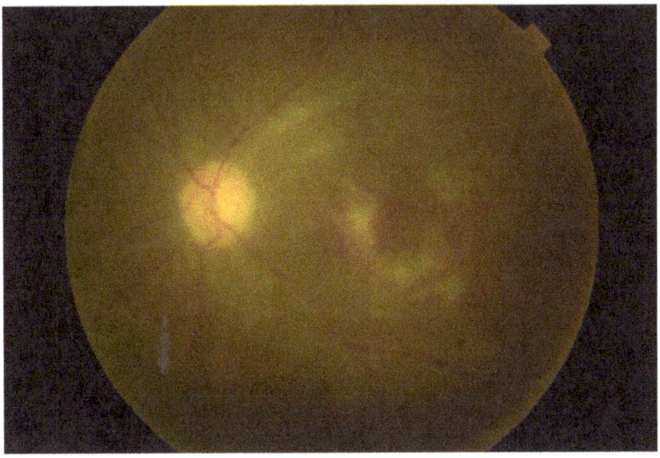

Figure 12.10. Retinitis in Behçet's disease.

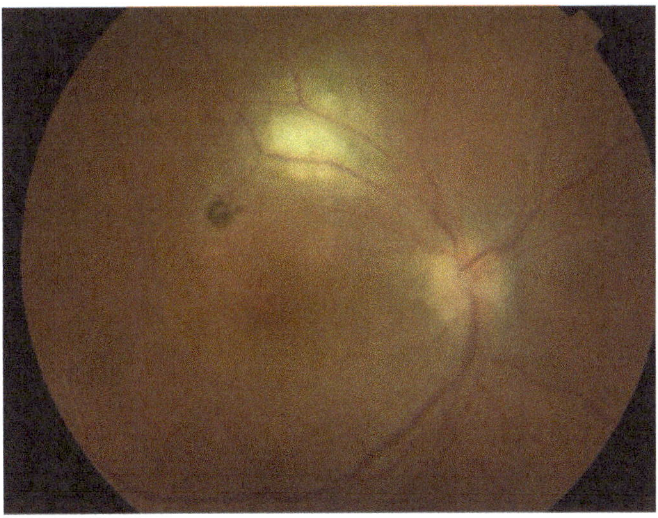

Figure 12.11. Toxoplasmosis retinochoroiditis.

tis associated with retinal hemorrhages and vascular occlusion ("ghost vessels") suggests a diagnosis of acute retinal necrosis (Figure 12.12). Serous retinal detachments are found in patients with VKH or sympathetic ophthalmia (Figure 12.13). **Vasculitis** may be graded as occlusive or non-occlusive and with arterial, venous or both (see Chapter 2, Table 2.11). **Choroidal** involvement may be suggestive of sarcoidosis,

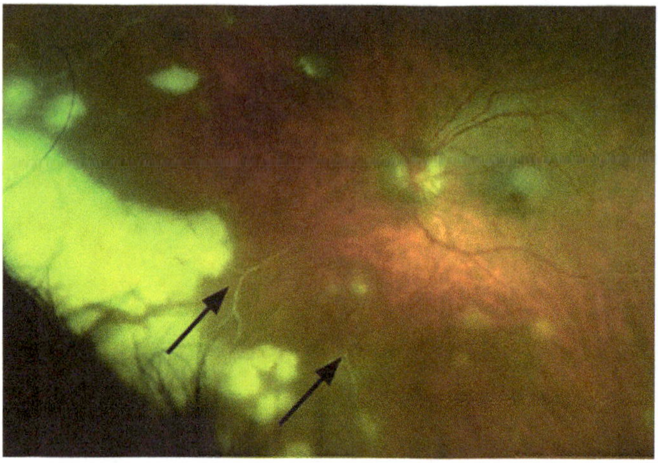

Figure 12.12. Acute retinal necrosis. Note the occluded vessels ('ghost vessels', arrows).

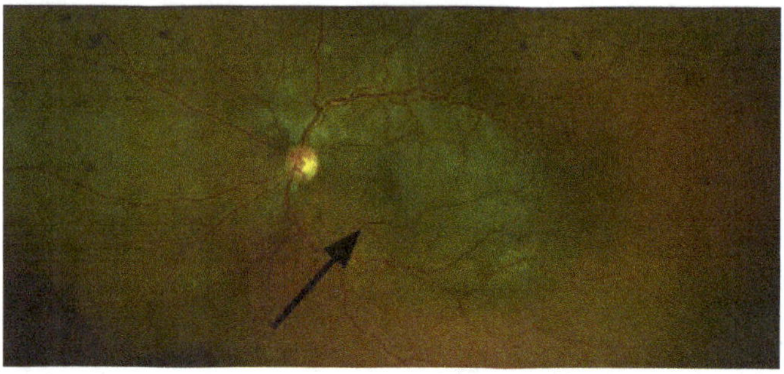

Figure 12.13. Serous retinal detachment in post-vaccine VKH-like uveitis (arrow).

tuberculosis or other infectious etiology (Figures 12.14 and 12.15) (see Chapter 2, Table 2.12). **Optic nerve** swelling is a non-specific sign but occurs frequently in VKH (Figure 12.16) and may be more common in subjects with sarcoidosis.

12.5.3 *Investigations*

Investigations should be targeted towards the suspected etiology and include workup for possible need of immunomodulatory therapy. Some diagnoses will be able to be made clinically, such as classic toxoplasmosis or acute retinal necrosis (see Chapter 6), but most will require further tests.

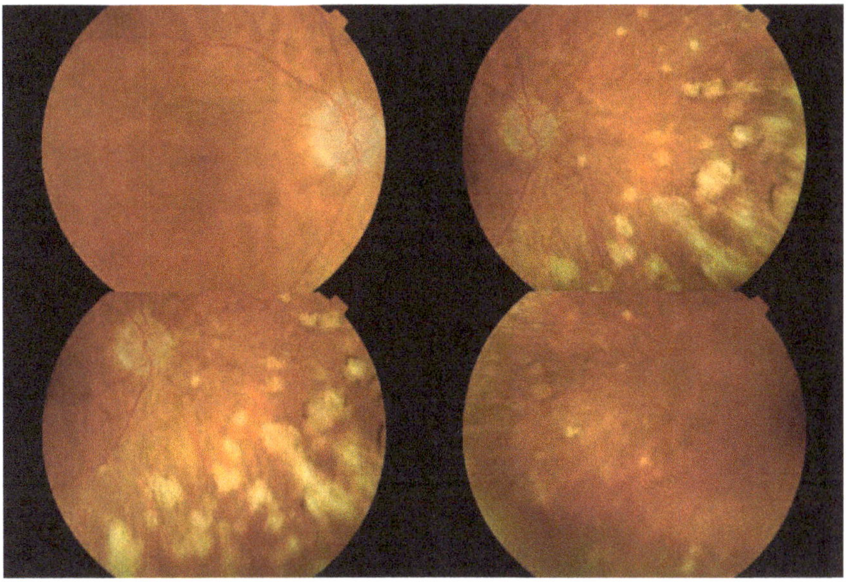

Figure 12.14. Panuveitis due to sarcoidosis with choroidal involvement.

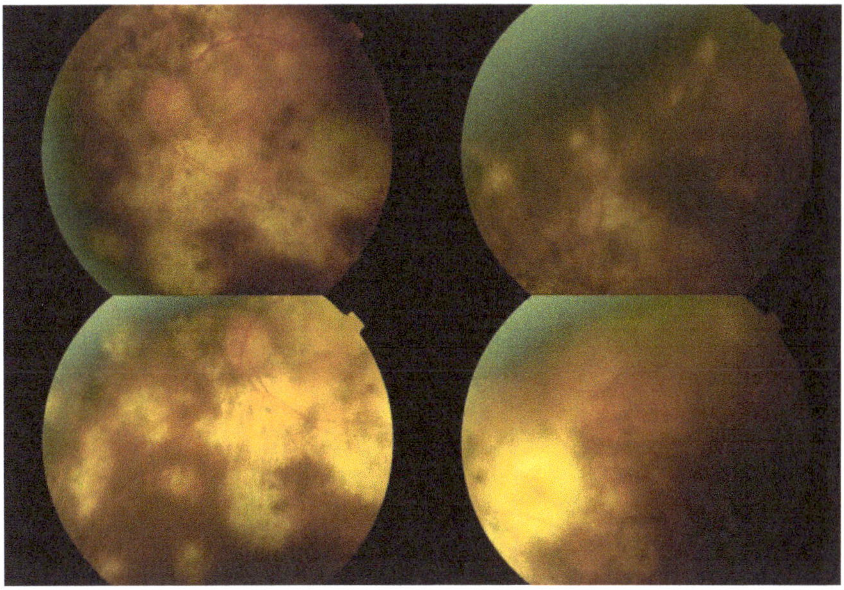

Figure 12.15. Panuveitis due to tuberculosis with choroidal involvement.

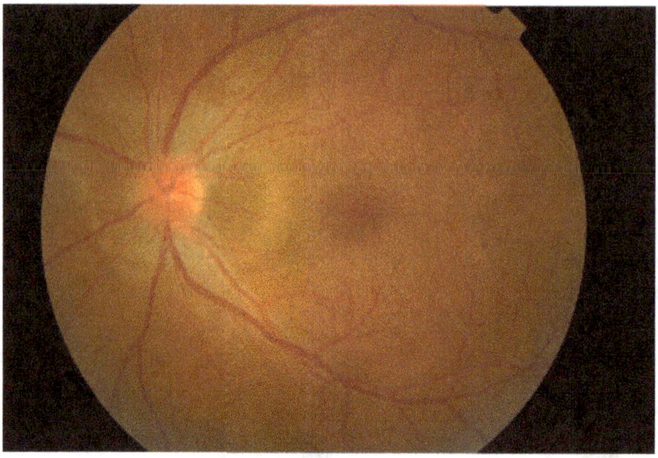

Figure 12.16. Optic nerve swelling in Vogt-Koyanagi-Harada syndrome.

If retinitis is present then vitreous (and/or anterior chamber) tap for PCR for HZV, HSV, toxoplasmosis and cytomegalovirus (CMV) is indicated. Depending on the degree of suspicion, empiric treatment should be commenced prior to confirmation via PCR. Toxoplasmosis serology and syphilis serology should be included in the blood workup.

In the absence of retinitis, routine investigations for panuveitis would generally include full blood count, erythrocyte sedimentation rate and/or C-reactive protein, assessment of liver function and kidney function (may be impaired in systemic disease, but also important for immunomodulatory therapy workup), ACE (for sarcoidosis), tests for tuberculosis, syphilis serology and chest X-ray. Other targeted tests for sarcoidosis may include CT chest and/or punch biopsy of any skin (or tattoo) lesions.

12.5.4 *Early Management*

If the presentation is classic for infectious etiology, then the appropriate treatment regimen should be started (see Chapter 6). If retinitis is present but the diagnosis is unclear, then an appropriate empiric treatment regimen whilst awaiting PCR results and serology could include valacyclovir 2 g po tds, trimethoprim/sulfamethoxazole 960 mg po bd +/– oral prednisone (0.5–1 mg/kg po od). The treatment could then be tailored as results came back.

If non-infectious uveitis is believed to be the most likely diagnosis, then initial treatment may include either oral prednisone (typically 0.5–1 mg/kg po od with a tapering course) or with local therapy, usually orbital floor steroid, intravitreal triamcinolone or a slow-release dexamethasone implant. Care should be taken to exclude infectious etiology as steroid may worsen infectious uveitis.

Anterior segment inflammation should be treated with topical steroid and IOP-lowering agents, and cycloplegics used as needed.

12.6 Case 6 — Panuveitis with Dense Vitritis

A 50-year-old man presents with unilateral uveitis. He has 2+ anterior chamber cells and a dense vitritis, with no view to the fundus.

When there is dense vitritis (Figure 12.17), the diagnosis may be severe intermediate uveitis or there may also be posterior involvement that is unable to be seen due to the uveitis. The most important diseases to rule out include infections such as acute retinal necrosis, endophthalmitis (including endogenous endophthalmitis), toxoplasmosis and syphilis that can worsen in the absence of adequate targeted treatment. Non-infectious etiologies such as sarcoidosis, Behçet's disease and idiopathic disease

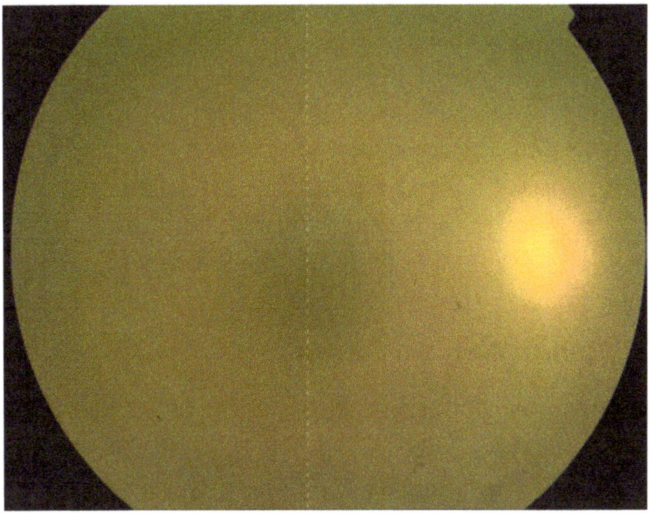

Figure 12.17. Dense vitritis with limited fundal view.

should also be considered. Lymphoma will rarely cause a dense vitritis precluding fundal view.

12.6.1 *History and Symptoms*

Onset of disease is important: infectious causes and also Behçet's disease will typically have a rapid onset over days to one week. Sarcoidosis and idiopathic disease are frequently of slower onset and sarcoidosis may demonstrate a grumbling course.

Past ocular history: ask specifically for history of previous uveitis, and in particular previous toxoplasmosis retinochoroiditis. Subjects with acute retinal necrosis may give history of previous involvement of the other eye. Ask about recent ocular surgery, previous glaucoma surgery or trauma as they may be associated with endophthalmitis.

Past medical history: ask about known systemic disease, in particular sarcoidosis or Behçet's disease, and for immune suppression (associated with increased risk of infection etiology). History of previous sexually transmitted disease or HIV infection increases the likelihood of syphilis co-infection. Intravenous drug use, recent surgery or central venous lines may be associated with endogenous endophthalmitis. Childhood history of neonatal encephalitis or meningitis should prompt consideration of subsequent HSV-2 acute retinal necrosis.

Systems review should include recent fever or malaise which may suggest endogenous endophthalmitis or active systemic inflammation (such as sarcoidosis or Behçet's disease). Ask patients about inflammatory joint pain, shortness of breath, cough and any neurological symptoms. See Table 12.9 to review clinical findings and investigations.

12.6.2 *Examination and Signs*

Visual acuity is usually severely reduced, commonly 6/60 or worse.

The **conjunctiva** is usually injected. If the conjunctiva is white, consider Behçet's disease or sometimes chronic disease with late presentation such as sarcoidosis panuveitis (see Chapter 5). The **cornea** may show KPs which may be granulomatous or non-granulomatous. The **anterior chamber** reaction can be graded using the SUN grading system (Tables 12.2 and 12.3). As with panuveitis, there may be posterior synechiae, and **iris** nodules should be looked for.

Vitritis is dense in subjects with no fundal view. Sometimes a fundal view may be obtained in these cases by using indirect with a small bright beam, or widefield imaging may sometimes yield a better view than obtained at the slit lamp.

12.6.3 *Investigations*

Vitreous sampling is the most important investigation in subjects with dense vitritis to look for an infectious etiology. A sample should be sent for microscopy and culture, and also for PCR looking for HSV, VZV and toxoplasmosis. If endophthalmitis is suspected then consideration should be given to vitrectomy rather than vitreous tap.

Blood tests should be sent for full blood count, erythrocyte sedimentation rate and/or C-reactive protein, assessment of liver function and kidney function, serum ACE (for sarcoidosis), QuantiFERON-gold (for tuberculosis), syphilis serology and toxoplasmosis serology. If there is suspicion of granulomatous disease, then chest X-ray should be ordered.

12.6.4 *Early Management*

Emperic therapy is important in cases where there is no fundal view, as it is impossible to exclude serious infection such as acute retinal necrosis until PCR results return. If there is a suspicion of endophthalmitis then intravitreal antibiotics can be given at the time of the vitreous tap, typically vancomycin 1 mg in 0.1 mL and ceftazidime 2.25 mg in 0.1 mL (see Appendix A). Emperic treatment with valacyclovir 2 g po tds, trimethoprim/sulfamethoxazole 960 mg po bd +/– oral prednisone (0.5–1 mg/kg po od). This will provide cover for acute retinal necrosis and toxoplasmosis while awaiting results. Medication can then be stopped once the PCR results return.

12.7 Case 7 — Retinitis

A 30-year-old man presents with blurring of vision. A patch of retinitis is noted on his fundal examination with some associated hemorrhage.

Table 12.9. Etiologies related to retinitis.

Condition	Clinical findings	Investigations
Acute retinal necrosis (see Chapter 6)	*Hx*: may have neonatal encephalitis/meningitis *Signs*: peripheral retinitis and hemorrhage	Anterior chamber or vitreous tap for viral PCR
CMV retinitis (see Chapter 6)	*Hx*: immunosuppression, HIV/AIDS *Symptoms*: scotoma or blur, no inflammatory symptoms *Signs*: central burnt-out retinitis with peripheral active disease and hemorrhage	Clinical diagnosis Anterior chamber or vitreous tap for viral PCR to confirm or for atypical cases
Toxoplasmosis retinochoroiditis (see Chapter 6)	*Hx*: may have previous episodes *Signs*: retinochoroiditis adjacent to retinal scar, may have elevated intraocular pressure	Clinical diagnosis Toxoplasmosis serology Anterior chamber or vitreous tap for PCR in atypical cases PCR is less useful in primary infection
Syphilis retinitis (see Chapter 6)	*Hx*: may have risk factors for sexually transmitted infection *Symptoms*: rash over palms of hands *Signs*: placoid retinitis, optic nerve swelling	Syphilis serology (see Chapter 4) Always consider HIV co-infection
Behçet's disease (see Chapter 5)	*Hx*: mouth and genital ulcers, DVT/PE *Symptoms*: explosive onset *Signs*: hypopyon in a white eye, retinitis, hemorrhage	HLA-B51 Refer to rheumatologist

AIDS = acquired immunodeficiency syndrome; DVT = deep vein thrombosis; HIV = human immunodeficiency virus; PCR = polymerase chain reaction

Retinitis is a serious vision-threatening presentation in uveitis. The most common causes include acute retinal necrosis (due to HSV or VZV), CMV retinitis, syphilis and Behçet's disease (see Chapter 2, Table 2.10). Toxoplasmosis retinochoroiditis may also include areas of retinitis (Figure 12.18). Many cases may be diagnosed by typical clinical presentation and constellation of clinical history and signs, but systemic investigations and vitreous sampling are extremely useful in a typical cases.

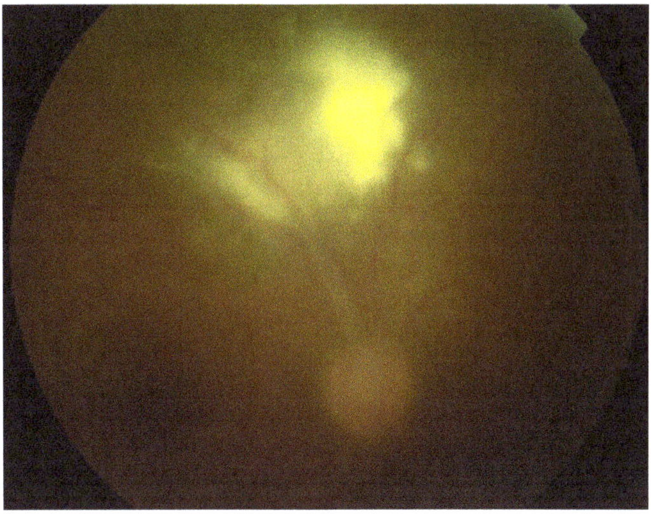

Figure 12.18. Dense retinochoroiditis in toxoplasmosis reactivation.

12.7.1 *History and Symptoms*

Patients typically present with floaters, photophobia and visual blur. Asymptomatic presentations or presenting only with scotoma is important as it may point to CMV with an absence of inflammatory signs (see Chapter 6). Ethnicity is important as people from the Silk Road regions are more likely to develop Behçet's disease (see Chapter 5).

Past ocular history may include previous episodes of toxoplasmosis. In subjects with Behçet's there is sometimes a history of previous vein occlusion.

Past medical history should be asked, in particular history of immune suppression such as chemotherapy, hematological malignancy, immune suppressant medication or a history of HIV/AIDS. Patients with Behçet's disease may report a known diagnosis, mouth or genital ulcers, or previous deep vein thrombosis or pulmonary embolism.

Systems review should include history of mouth or genital ulcers, arthritis, skin rashes or shortness of breath (seen in Behçet's disease). History of risk behavior for HIV or syphilis should be sought. See Table 12.9 for history, examination and investigations for different etiologies with retinitis.

12.7.2 Examination and Signs

Visual acuity may be normal to severely reduced, depending on location of retinitis and amount of vitritis.

The **conjunctiva** may be injected. **Cornea** is usually clear but may show KPs. In herpetic disease these are often pigmented and mid-sized. **Anterior chamber** cells can be graded with the SUN grading (Table 12.2). The **iris** may show posterior synechiae. **IOP** may be elevated, particularly in HSV, VZV or toxoplasmosis.

Anterior **vitreous** cell and haze are variable and dependent on immune function. Subjects with CMV tend to have little or no vitreous cell. Progressive outer retinal necrosis in AIDS will also have no vitreous inflammation.

Retinal examination will show retinitis which may be dense (particularly in toxoplasmosis, Figure 12.18) or granular in appearance (especially viral etiology or toxoplasmosis when immunosuppressed, Figure 12.19). CMV will show burnt-out areas of scar with active retinitis at the borders (Figure 12.20). Toxoplasmosis may show retinal scars from previous episodes. Syphilis retinitis is usually placoid, poorly defined and may have yellow-white discrete spots of retinitis (Figure 12.21). There may be associated hemorrhage, subretinal fluid and/or vasculitis.

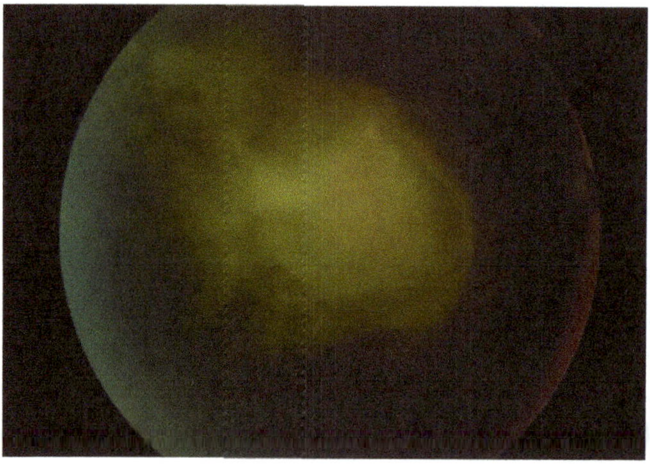

Figure 12.19. Granular appearance of toxoplasmosis retinochoroiditis in patient with HIV.

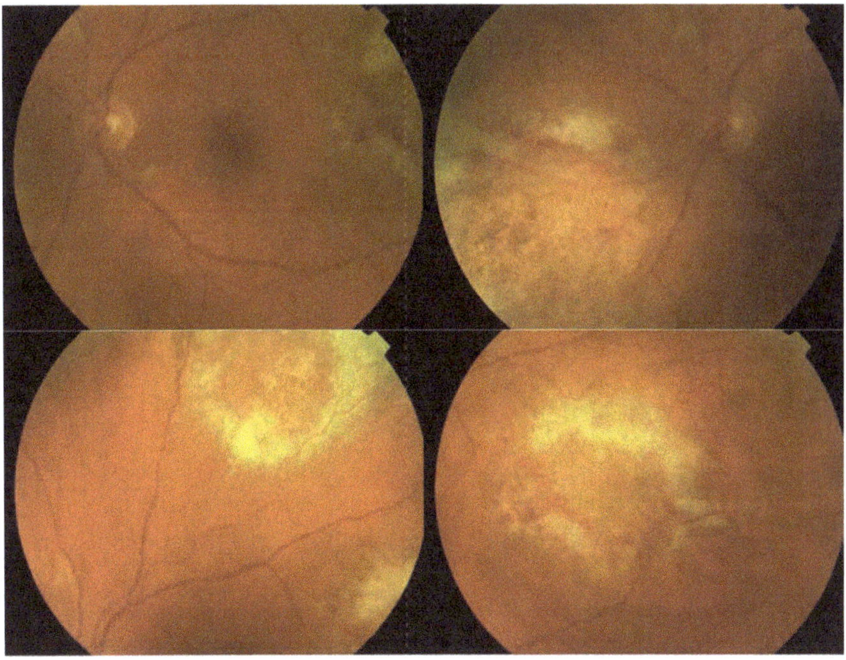

Figure 12.20. CMV retinitis in HIV-positive patient.

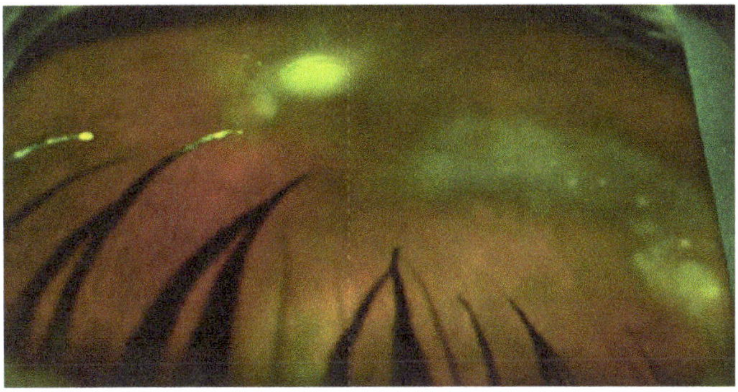

Figure 12.21. Syphilis retinitis.

12.7.3 *Investigations*

Investigations need to be carefully targeted to the clinical presentation. Standard tests include full blood count, liver and renal function (to inform treatment decisions), HIV and syphilis serology. If syphilis serology is positive, HIV must be ruled out. Toxoplasmosis serology may be of value, but 20–70% of the population will be IgG positive for toxoplasmosis (depending on local seroprevalence), so a positive IgG does not make a definitive diagnosis. Positive IgM for toxoplasmosis is of value as it indicates recent infection (see Chapter 4). Serology for HSV, VZV or CMV is not usually helpful as it will be positive in 90% of the normal population. Consider testing HLA-B51 if a diagnosis of Behçet's is suspected.

Where the diagnosis is unclear, vitreous or anterior chamber tap for PCR for HSV, VZV, CMV and toxoplasmosis is useful. In primary toxoplasmosis PCR may be less useful.

12.7.4 *Early Management*

When the diagnosis may be made clinically, appropriate targeted therapy can be initiated. See Chapter 6 for detailed discussion of treatment of infectious retinitis. For typical cases the following regimens may be considered.

Toxoplasmosis: trimethoprim/sulfamethoxazole 960 mg po bd for 6 weeks with tapering oral prednisone course, starting dose 0.5–1 mg/kg/day, commencing 24 hours after antibiotics started. Consider triple therapy (pyrimethamine, sulfadiazine, folinic acid — see Chapter 6, Table 6.9) if macular disease or if immunosuppressed. Consider intravitreal clindamycin if macular disease or if unable to tolerate systemic antibiotics.

Acute retinal necrosis: take anterior chamber or vitreous tap to determine etiology, consider intravitreal foscarnet, start valacyclovir 2 g po tds, can consider dropping to 1 g po tds if HSV.

CMV: start oral valgancyclovir 900 mg po bd for induction, liaise with medical or infectious disease team to treat underlying immunosuppression, can reduce to 900 mg po od for maintenance.

Behçet's disease: will require either high dose oral prednisone (0.5–1 mg/kg od) or IV methylprednisolone 1 g po od for 3 days then tapering course of oral prednisone. High risk of vision loss so consider early initiation of anti-TNF therapy.

Where the diagnosis is in doubt then empiric therapy is recommended with valacyclovir 2 g po tds, trimethoprim/sulfamethoxazole 960 mg po bd +/– oral prednisone (0.5–1 mg/kg po od). This will provide cover for acute retinal necrosis and toxoplasmosis while awaiting results of screening investigations and PCR from vitreous tap.

12.8 Case 8 — Multifocal Choroiditis

A 30-year-old woman presents with photopsias. A multifocal choroiditis is observed on dilated fundal examination.

Multifocal choroiditis may be the presenting sign for systemic diseases such as sarcoidosis or tuberculosis (Table 12.10). It may also occur in white dot syndromes, such as punctate inner choroiditis, multifocal choroiditis, presumed ocular histoplasmosis or birdshot chorioretinitis, or in idiopathic disease. Rarely, other infections may present with multifocal choroiditis, such as cryptococcus or pneumocystis carnii, but usually only in the presence of significant immunosuppression (see Chapter 2, Table 2.12).

Table 12.10. Etiologies related to multifocal choroiditis.

Condition	Clinical findings	Investigations
Sarcoidosis (see Chapter 5)	*Symptoms*: cough, shortness of breath *Signs*: granulomatous uveitis, multifocal choroiditis, vasculitis	Serum ACE, CBC (for lymphopenia) CXR
Tubercular uveitis (see Chapter 6)	*Hx*: may have TB exposure *Symptoms*: cough, shortness of breath *Signs*: granulomatous uveitis, multifocal choroiditis	PPD, IGRA (see Chapter 4) CXR
Punctate inner choroiditis (see Chapter 5)	*Hx*: myopia in young females *Symptoms*: often present with blur from CNVM *Signs*: small punched-out scars in posterior pole, if CNVM may have hemorrhage and/or subretinal fluid	
Multifocal choroiditis (see Chapter 5)	*Hx*: may be myopic *Symptoms*: floaters and blur *Signs*: vitritis, multifocal scars both within and outside of arcades, if CNVM may have hemorrhage and/or subretinal fluid	

(Continued)

Table 12.10. (*Continued*)

Condition	Clinical findings	Investigations
Presumed ocular histoplasmosis syndrome (see Chapter 6)	*Hx*: lived in endemic regions *Signs*: small 'histo' spots, may have linear lesions	
Birdshot chorioretinitis (see Chapter 5)	*Symptoms*: floaters and blur *Signs*: vitritis, poorly defined 'birdshot' lesions, more prominent nasal retina	HLA-A29

ACE = angiotensin-converting enzyme; CBC = complete blood count; CNVM = choroidal neovascularization membrane; CXR = chest X-ray; DVT = deep vein thrombosis; IGRA = interferon-gamma release assay; PPD = purified protein derivative (a type of tuberculin skin test); TB = tuberculosis

12.8.1 *History and Symptoms*

Ethnicity and country of origin are important in the history. Subjects from areas where tuberculosis is endemic may be more likely to present with multifocal choroiditis due to tuberculosis. White dot syndromes may be more common in Caucasian patients. Consider presumed ocular histoplasmosis in subjects from USA particularly living near Ohio and Mississippi river valleys.

Multifocal choroiditis may be an incidental finding in an uninflamed eye (particularly punctate inner choroiditis and sarcoidosis), or may be associated with significant intraocular inflammation, presenting with floaters, visual blur and photophobia (for example multifocal choroiditis with panuveitis, tuberculosis, sarcoidosis). Sometimes multifocal choroiditis will present with complications of the disease, particularly choroidal neovascular membrane, presenting with blur and distortion of vision.

Some patients may report a viral prodrome prior to onset of white dot syndromes (such as punctate inner choroiditis or multifocal choroiditis).

Past ocular history of myopia is important as punctate inner choroiditis is more common in high myopes.

Past medical history of tuberculosis or sarcoidosis is important. Consider also history suggestive of undiagnosed sarcoidosis, such as previous Bell's palsy, cardiac conduction defects or 'adult-onset asthma'. History of immunosuppression should be looked for, as this may suggest increased risk of more atypical infections.

Systems review should include history of weight loss or malaise (sarcoidosis and tuberculosis), fevers (tuberculosis), shortness of breath or cough (sarcoidosis and tuberculosis), skin rash (sarcoidosis) and inflammatory joint pain (sarcoidosis).

12.8.2 *Examination and Signs*

Visual acuity is usually normal, unless there is associated inflammation, macular lesions, or complications such as choroidal neovascular membrane.

The **conjunctiva** is frequently white. **Cornea** may show granulomatous or non-granulomatous KPs. **Anterior chamber** cells can be graded with the SUN grading (Table 12.2). Subjects with punctate inner choroiditis will have no inflammation. There may be posterior synechiae and **iris** nodules (particularly tuberculosis or sarcoidosis, Figure 12.22). **IOP** is usually normal, but may be elevated if there is chronic inflammation.

Vitreous may be uninflamed or may show anterior vitreous cells and/or vitreous haze and snowballs. **Retina** may show signs of

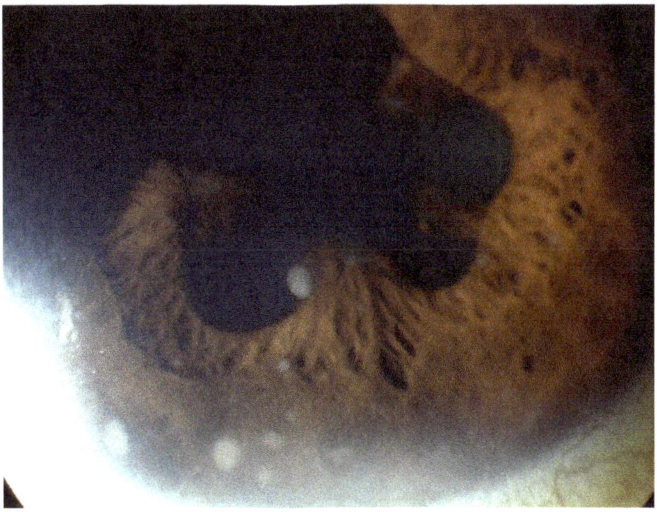

Figure 12.22. Granulomatous keratic precipitates and posterior synechiae in a patient with tuberculosis.

punched-out chorioretinal scars which may involve the macula or be peripheral (Figures 12.23 and 12.24). Patients with punctate inner choroiditis are more likely to have lesions within the macula (Figure 12.25), while patients with multifocal choroiditis are more likely to have lesions outside of the arcades (Figure 12.26). In patients with presumed ocular histoplasmosis, there may be linear or curvilinear near-confluent atrophic scars throughout

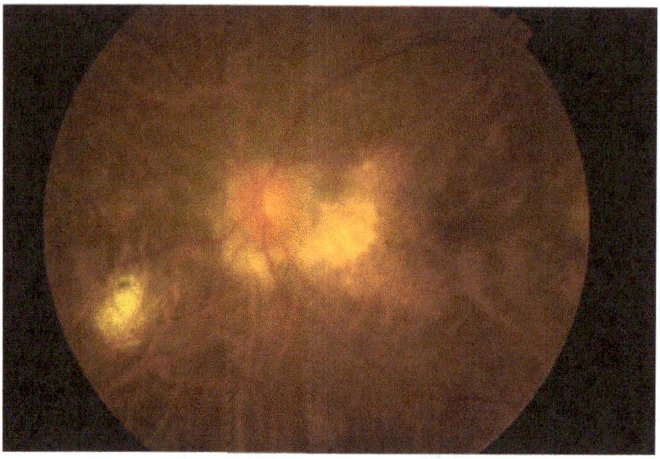

Figure 12.23. Multifocal choroidal granulomas in tuberculosis.

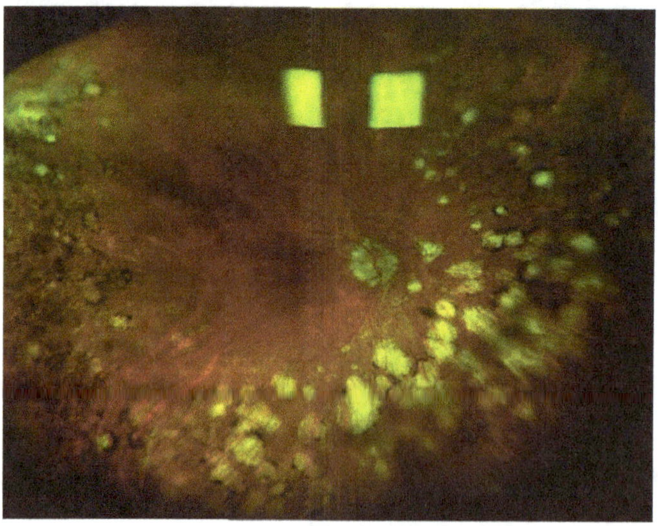

Figure 12.24. Peripheral multifocal choroiditis in sarcoidosis.

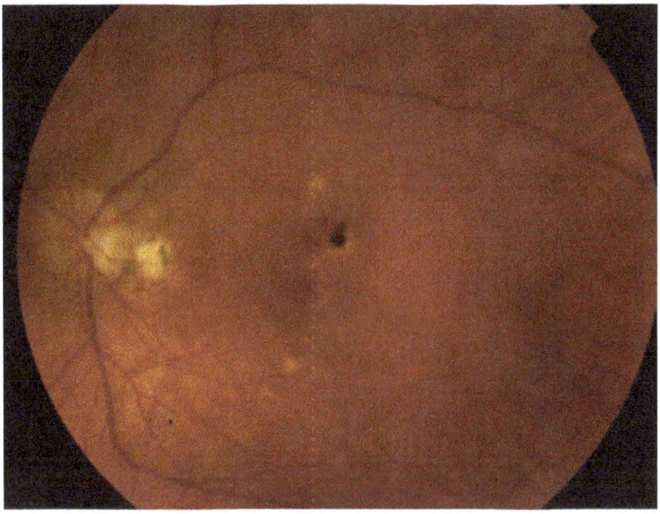

Figure 12.25. Punched out chorioretinal scars in a patient with punctate inner choroiditis.

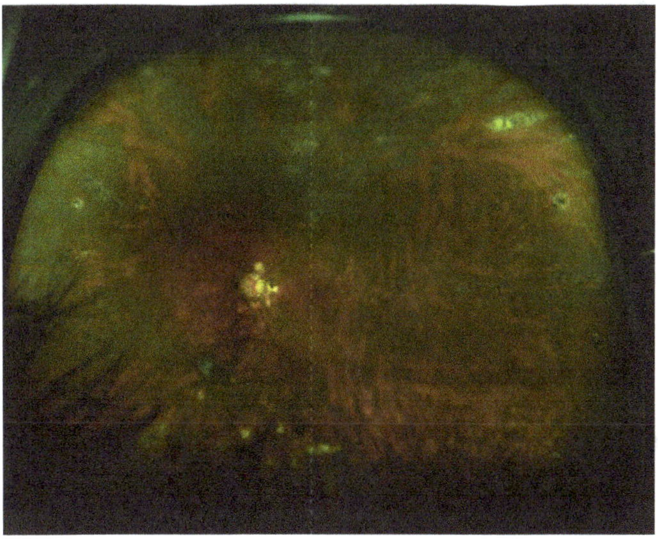

Figure 12.26. Multifocal choroiditis with panuveitis.

the retinal periphery (Figure 12.27). Lesions in birdshot chorioretinitis are subtle and are more numerous in the nasal retina (Figure 12.28). There may be signs of active inflammation, including fuzzy borders and overlying vitreous cell. Choroidal neovascular membrane may be present, associated with retinal hemorrhage and subretinal fluid.

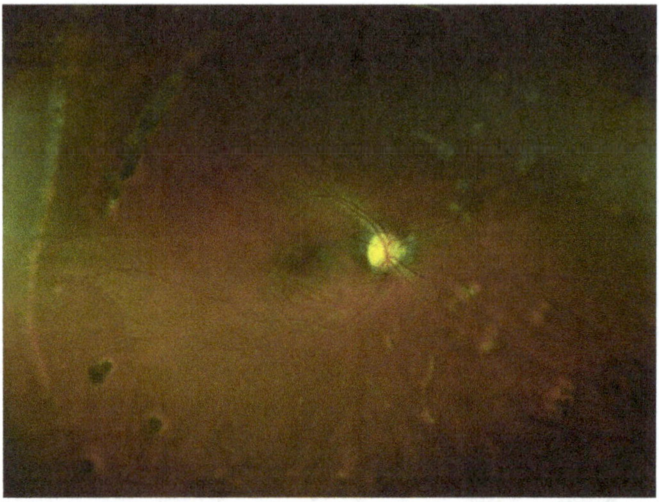

Figure 12.27. Presumed ocular histoplasmosis syndrome.

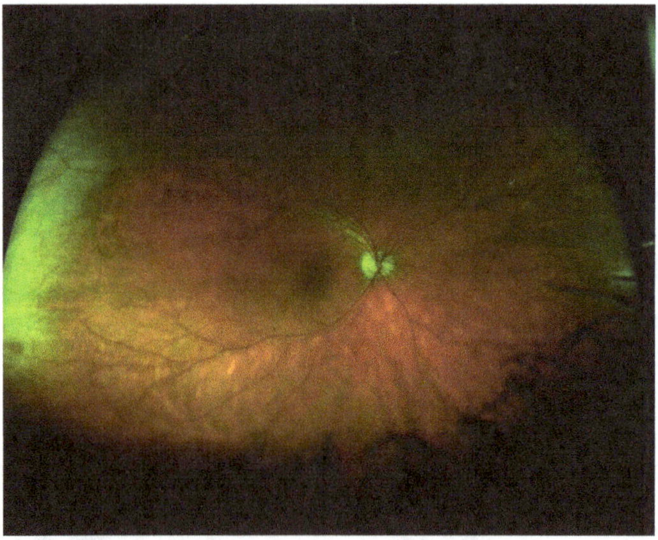

Figure 12.28. Birdshot chorioretinitis.

12.8.3 *Investigations*

Initial investigations are aimed at looking for underlying systemic disease, in particular sarcoidosis and tuberculosis (see Chapter 4). Blood tests should include full blood count (lymphopenia is common in sarcoidosis), serum ACE, QuantiFERON gold, as well as liver function tests (abnormal liver function is common in sarcoidosis). Syphilis serology is always requested as it can be a masquerade. HLA-A29 should be checked if there is suspicion of birdshot chorioretinitis. Chest X-ray should be performed looking for sarcoidosis and tuberculosis. Other tests should be performed as indicated by the clinical history and examination (may include blood cultures and further systemic workup if immunosuppressed).

12.8.4 *Early Management*

Anterior chamber or vitreous inflammation should be treated with topical, periocular or systemic steroid as required for the degree of inflammation. As long as there are no signs of active pulmonary tuberculosis, it is acceptable to start steroids whilst awaiting the other tuberculosis investigations.

If choroidal neovascular membrane is present, this will require treatment with intravitreal anti-VEGF agents +/– oral steroid.

If multifocal choroidal lesions are inactive and there is no vision-threatening disease, then observation may be appropriate. Consider initiating immune suppression therapy if new active vision-threatening lesions were to develop or in all subjects with birdshot chorioretinitis.

References

1. Jabs DA, Nussenblatt RB, Rosenbaum JT. Standardization of uveitis nomenclature for reporting clinical data. Results of the First International Workshop. *Am J Ophthalmol* 2005;140(3):509–16.
2. Hogan MJ, Kimura SJ, Thygeson P. Signs and symptoms of uveitis. I. Anterior uveitis. *Am J Ophthalmol* 1959;47(5 Pt 2):155–70.
3. Wakefield D, Clarke D, McCluskey P. Recent developments in HLA B27 anterior uveitis. *Front Immunol* 2020;11:608134.
4. Chang JH, McCluskey PJ, Wakefield D. Acute anterior uveitis and HLA-B27. *Surv Ophthalmol* 2005;50(4):364–88.
5. Thorne JE, Woreta FA, Dunn JP, Jabs DA. Risk of cataract development among children with juvenile idiopathic arthritis-related uveitis treated with topical corticosteroids. *Ophthalmology* 2010;117(7):1436–41.
6. Kramer M, Tomkins-Netzer O. Cataract risk and topical corticosteroids among children with juvenile idiopathic arthritis-related uveitis. *Ophthalmology* 2020;127(4S):S19–S20.

7. Thorne JE, Sugar EA, Holbrook JT, *et al.* Periocular Triamcinolone vs. intravitreal Triamcinolone vs. intravitreal dexamethasone implant for the treatment of uveitic macular edema: the PeriOcular vs. INTravitreal corticosteroids for uveitic macular edema (POINT) trial. *Ophthalmology* 2019;126(2):283–95.
8. Niederer RL, Sharief L, Bar A, *et al.* Predictors of long-term visual outcome in intermediate uveitis. *Ophthalmology* 2017;124(3):393–8.

https://doi.org/10.1142/9789811251474_bmatter

Appendix A Administration of Frequently Used Drugs in Uveitis

Antibiotics

Intravitreal antibiotics

IVT Vancomycin	1 mg in 0.1 mL
IVT Ceftazadime	2.25 mg in 0.1 mL
IVT Amikacin	0.25 mg in 0.1 mL
IVT Clindamycin	1 mg in 0.1 mL

Systemic antibiotics

IV Penicillin G	12–24 MU od 10–15 days (tertiary syphilis)
PO Doxycycline	100 mg bd (for *Bartonella henselae* neuroretinitis)

Treatment for ocular toxoplasmosis

Classic triple therapy protocol

PO Pyrimethamine	200 mg load then 25 mg od
PO Sulfadiazine	2 g load then 1 g qid use for 4–6 weeks
PO Folinic acid	10 mg every other day

Alternative treatment options

PO Clindamycin	300 mg qid
PO Trimethoprim/ sulfamethoxazole	960 mg bd

Antifungals

Intravitreal antifungals

IVT Amphotericin B	5–10 μg in 0.1 mL
IVT Voriconazole	100 μg in 0.1 mL

Systemic antifungals	
PO Fluconazole	200 mg bd
PO Voriconazole	200 mg bd
IV Amphotericin B	1–1.5 mg/kg/day

Antivirals

Intravitreal antivirals	
IVT Foscarnet	2.4 mg in 0.1 mL twice weekly
IVT Gancyclovir	2 mg in 0.1 mL
Systemic antivirals	
IV Acyclovir	10 mg/kg q8h 10–14 days then oral
IV Foscarnet	60 mg/kg q8h 2–3 weeks then 90–120 mg/kg q24h
IV Gancyclovir	5 mg/kg q12h for 2–3 weeks then 5 mg/kg q24h
PO Valacyclovir	1000–2000 mg q8h
PO Valgancyclovir	900 mg bd induction then 900 mg od maintenance

Intravitreal immunosuppression

IVT Triamcinolone	4 mg in 0.1 mL or 2 mg in 0.05 mL
IVT Methotrexate	400 μg in 0.1mL
IVT Dexamethasone	0.4 mg in 0.1 mL (for endophthalmitis)

IV = intravenous; IVT = intravitreal; PO = oral; od = once daily; bd = twice a day; tid = three times a day; qid = four times a day; q8h = every 8 hours; q12h = every 12 hours

https://doi.org/10.1142/9789811251474_bmatter

Appendix B Frequently Asked Questions in Uveitis Clinic

1. **What is the chance of relapse following a first episode of acute anterior uveitis?**
   Relapses of uveitis are uncommon. For most people there is only a single event. However, relapses can occur even after months or years of quiet disease. The first month after stopping treatment is the most at risk of a relapse. For most types of uveitis the cause of relapses is unknown.
2. **How long does the inflammation last?**
   According to the SUN definition active uveitis lasts up to 3 months in acute cases. In chronic cases active disease can last longer, requiring long-term treatment. Disease may relapse even months or years after becoming quiescent.
3. **How long do I need to continue taking treatment? Is the treatment forever?**
   Treatment is usually not required forever. In acute cases treatment is needed until the inflammation is under control, typically under 3 months. In chronic disease, treatment may be needed for longer, depending on disease activity. Once inflammation control is achieved, treatment is tapered down gradually to a low, safe dose. At that dose treatment is typically maintained for at least 2–5 years, before an attempt is made to stop treatment.
4. **Does uveitis cause blindness?**
   The risk of blindness in uveitis depends on the type of uveitis and risk of ocular complications. In anterior uveitis the risk of blindness is low, but in posterior uveitis with posterior pole involvement, vision loss may develop due to optic nerve or macular pathology. With adequate inflammation control, follow-up and treatment adjustment, further vision deterioration can be avoided in most cases.

5. **Is uveitis a genetic disease? Are my children at risk?**
Uveitis is not a genetic disease, though some causes of non-infectious uveitis may be related to susceptible genetic variants (e.g., HLA-A29 in birdshot chorioretinitis; HLA-B27 in spondyloarthropathies; HLA-B51 in Behçet's disease). Genetic counselling is not warranted for uveitis.
6. **If everything is quiet how often should I have a follow-up appointment?**
Depending on the type of uveitis and frequency of relapses, follow-ups are scheduled to monitor disease activity, response to treatment and risk of relapse. The frequency may range from every few months to follow-up visits only during relapses (recurrent anterior uveitis),
7. **Can I self-medicate when I feel a relapse?**
Because signs and symptoms of active disease may not always be clear, self-medication is not encouraged. However, in cases where patients are clear when they have active disease and have no issues with elevated intraocular pressure, self-medication is possible to prevent delay in treatment.
8. **Are uveitis relapses induced by stress?**
Non-infectious uveitis is an autoimmune condition. Whilst stress can impact on your immune function, there is no clear evidence currently that stress will increase the chance of a uveitis flare. Whilst general lifestyle measures to reduce stress may help patients in other ways, patients should not be encouraged to make major life changes such as changing their occupation or stop working.
9. **Is uveitis contagious? Is herpetic uveitis contagious?**
Most uveitis is non-infectious and is not contagious. Important exceptions are syphilis and also HIV-related diseases. Herpetic disease (HSV, HZV) is only infectious if there are vesicles that have not scabbed over. You cannot catch shingles, but people who are not immune to HZV can catch chickenpox from contact with HZO vesicles. Toxoplasmosis is not infectious, but in acute infection (IgM positive) it can be passed to the fetus in pregnant women.
10. **If I have a relapse, how soon do I need to see an ophthalmologist?**
The speed at which you should see an ophthalmologist depends on the severity of symptoms, risk of vision loss, and whether it is your only eye. Generally within 24–48 hours is advised, but some patients (such as those with Behçet's disease) should usually be seen the same day.

11. **Should I change my diet to reduce inflammation?**
Over the last 10 years there has been increased interest in the role of the microbiome (and diet) in inflammation. Research into this is still developing, however, and at present there is no clear evidence that altering your diet will help with uveitis symptoms or disease recurrence.
12. **What does undifferentiated uveitis mean? Why have you not been able to find a cause?**
Most uveitis is non-infectious uveitis, which occurs due to autoimmune disease. This may occur in association with a systemic autoimmune disease, such as ankylosing spondylitis or sarcoidosis, or it may occur in isolation, affecting only your eye. When we use the term undifferentiated or idiopathic uveitis, we mean that screening for associated systemic disease has been negative, and the inflammation appears to be isolated to your eyes. In the setting of recurrent or chronic uveitis, screening may be repeated every couple of years, or if new symptoms arise.
13. **Is my cataract due to the steroid drops you have been giving me?**
Cataract may occur due to uncontrolled inflammation in your eye, or it may occur as a response to the steroid used to treat the inflammation. Studies in patients with juvenile idiopathic arthritis-associated uveitis have shown that topical steroid up to twice a day is not associated with an increased risk of cataract and may be used long-term.
14. **How long will I need to be on immunosuppression?**
When we commence immunosuppressive treatment for uveitis, we will normally treat for a minimum of 2 years. Some patients may require much longer immunosuppression. Studies in children have shown an approximately 50% rate of recurrence on cessation of immunosuppression, and a higher rate of recurrence if there is less than 2 years of disease quiescence, or less than 3 years total treatment.

https://doi.org/10.1142/9789811251474_bmatter

Index

www.ingramcontent.com/pod-product-compliance
Lightning Source LLC
LaVergne TN
LVHW010331220926
848484LV00004BB/876
* 9 7 8 9 8 1 1 2 5 1 4 6 7 *